Current Diagnostic Pediatrics

Series Editor: Alan R. Chrispin

A.R. Chrispin I. Gordon
C. Hall C. Metreweli

Diagnostic Imaging of the Kidney and Urinary Tract in Children

With 271 Figures in 418 Separate Illustrations

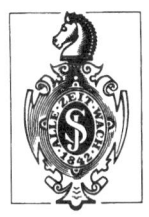 Springer International 1980

Series Editor

Dr. Alan R. Chrispin
The Hospital for Sick Children, Great Ormond Street
London WC1N 3JH, England

Dr. Isky Gordon
Dr. Christine Hall
Dr. Constantine Metreweli

The Hospital for Sick Children,
Great Ormond Street, London WC1N 3JH, England

ISBN-13:978-1-4471-3099-4   e-ISBN-13:978-1-4471-3097-0
DOI: 10.1007/978-1-4471-3097-0

Library of Congress Cataloging in Publication Data. Main entry under title: Diagnostic imaging of the kidney and urinary tract in children. (Current diagnostic pediatrics) Bibliography: p. Includes index. 1. Pediatric urology – Diagnosis. 2. Urinary organs – Radiography. 3. Pediatric radiography. 4. Diagnosis, Ultrasonic. 5. Radioisotopes in urology. 6. Radioisotopes in pediatrics. I. Chrispin, A. R., 1930– . II. Series. [DNLM: 1. Kidney – Radiography. 2. Kidney – Radionuclide imaging. 3. Urography – In infancy and childhood. 4. Urinary tract – Radionuclide imaging. 5. Kidney diseases – In infancy and childhood. 6. Urinary tract infections – In infancy and childhood. 7. Ultrasonics – Diagnostic use. 8. Tomography, Coputerized axial – In infancy and childhood. WICU788DP WS320 D536] RJ469.R33D52   618.92'607572   79-29646.

2128/3140-543210

To Marilyn and Gill

Preface

All unsuccessful revolutions are the same, but each successful one is different in its own distinctive way. The reason why revolutions occur is that new forces attain increasing significance and classic institutions are incapable of accomodating these forces. Such has been the pattern of events in the English, American and French revolutions. These successful revolutions produced a new dynamic and new perspectives. One English revolutionary put this succinctly: "Let us be doing, but let us be united in doing".

This book sets out what is a revolution in the perspectives of diagnostic imaging of the kidney and urinary tract. Forces which have brought about this revolution are the advent of reliable techniques in radioisotope studies, ultrasonics and computerized tomographic (CT) scanning. This last modality carries with it specific problems for routine paediatric work and its role in the study of kidney and urinary tract problems is discrete and circumscribed. However, in conjunction with classic radiology, each of these techniques yields information of a different type and so a synthesis of data accrues.

To achieve a successful synthesis of data it is essential that departments concerned with diagnostic imaging are self-contained and have within their orbit, and most preferably in one location, a range of diagnostic equipment appropriate for the task. At The Hospital for Sick Children for routine fluoroscopic work the Department has a Siemens Infantoskop with an over-table X-ray tube and an under-table high-performance image intensifier and TV chain with a videotape recorder. For routine radiographic work, including tomography, high performance falling load generators are used in conjunction with rare earth screen/film combinations to reduce radiation dose. Philips ultrasound equipment is located in a room adjacent to the fluoroscopy unit and a few metres from the rooms containing the standard radiographic equipment. Also nearby radioisotope work is carried out on a Nuclear Enterprises gamma camera with its associated data-processing and display facility. CT scanning facilities have proved to be of limited help in further diagnosis but are close at hand. The immediacy of information provided by ultrasonics study is important in its own right. The integration of ultrasonics study into the radiographic, fluoroscopic and radioisotope investigations can prove decisive in their conduct and make for a more meaningful result than would otherwise be the case.

The objective of this book is to help to indicate those techniques which may be most appropriately used, in an integrated way, to give that information which is essential to the rational management of the individual child's problem. There is only very limited detail given about the incidence, in statistical terms, of particular lesions and age and sex. And the reason is simple and logical. In the case of each individual child such data may suggest what is probable, but it does not indicate what is certain.

There are distinctions to be made between a Department of Diagnostic Imaging and a racecourse, because the favourite horse does not always win, children with problems are not racehorses and doctors should not be professional gamblers. For the individual child there must be that essential element of confidence and certainty if the next steps in management are to be rational and beneficial.

When considering an individual child's problem the clinician ascertains a range of facts which, by a process of induction, lead to the formulation of certain questions to which answers must be sought. The questions are then put to the department responsible for the investigatory work, and, a close liason is maintained between the clinical team and the department. The investigatory path which is then followed is that deemed most likely to give the answers to the questions. This approach makes for incisive thinking before surgical incisions. It provides that element of confidence and certainty essential for management of the clinical problem. It avoids risks and gambles inherent in the notion that, for example, the intravenous urogram will alone provide the answers in children who appear to have renal mass lesions. Finally, it obviates unnecessary, time-consuming, expensive and possibly hazardous investigation.

The structure of this book is, therefore, orientated to solving problems and its structure is based on this concept. The first chapter is devoted to a brief outline of those clinical circumstances which lead to investigation. Then follow two issues of central importance in the majority of patients in the paediatric age range; these are the problems of obstruction and reflux in the urinary tract. In considering these subjects the concept of preserving kidney function and the potential for growth lie to the fore and determine prognosis. It is the same in the many variants of cystic disease of the kidney, acutely acquired kidney lesions and the multiplicity of congenital anomalies which affect performance and development of the kidney and urinary tract. Malignant disease has its own specific features, but malignant disease in infants and children can (in for example Wilms' tumour) carry a vastly better prognosis than neoplasms in later life. No consideration of these subjects would be complete without a discussion of adrenal gland lesions. Traumatic injury is dealt with only in so far as it carries long-term implications for the future of the individual child. Finally, kidney and adrenal lesions are the principal causes of systemic hypertension in children and careful analysis and investigation can lead to dramatic steps in management which carry a good prognosis.

It has to be acknowledged that, as in all branches of medicine, failures in management do occur and these must be analyzed. Sometimes it is impossible to avoid failure because the potential for development and a good prognosis is simply not there. Nevertheless new techniques must be used to diminish the numbers of children in whom failure occurs. Techniques must be appropriate, but they must always be used as kindly as possible and as safely as possible. One imperative is to reduce potential radiation hazard and in this respect radioisotope and ultrasonic studies have clear-cut advantages. As the revolution in imaging proceeds the newer techniques will be fully validated. Specific points where this is necessary and how this can be achieved are indicated.

As authors we believe this book will be stimulating. It has been designed to be of importance to all concerned with the care of infants and children suffering from renal and urological disorders, in particular those radiologists concerned with diagnosis, paediatricians and paediatric surgeons, nephrologists and urologists. This book describes the current position and gives pointers for the future. The future is there to be created and this means a better future for children – this is the objective of this endeavour.

September, 1979

ALAN R. CHRISPIN
ISKY GORDON
CHRISTINE HALL
CONSTANTINE METREWELI

Contents

Acknowledgements

The authors are deeply indebted to Miss M. Sugarhood and Mrs. G. Porter who have typed and produced the manuscript. They have also kept the meticulous records of patients' studies without which this book could not have been written.

Miss Margaret Riocreux, Superintendent Radiographer, and the Radiographers in the Department of Paediatric Radiology at The Hospital for Sick Children have, through their skills and kindness, made it possible for so many children to be helped at the outset of their lives. This volume is a reflection of that help.

1 The Clinical Context

1.1 Introduction

Incisive thinking about an individual infant or child's problem demands clinical acumen. And this is an amalgam of clinical knowledge, experience and the capacity for experience. Astute clinical assessment provides the pointers for likely diagnoses. The objective of using imaging techniques is to confirm or refute diagnostic possibilities. As the investigatory process develops interactions between the findings from imaging and clinical assessments provide the synthesis of hard data on which rational management is based.

Very often the analysis of the clinical context defines, in a fairly direct way, that circle in which the diagnostic possibilities lie. Sometimes, however, imaging techniques will extend the circumference of the diagnostic circle which then encompasses additional diagnostic possibilities.

The consideration of diagnostic possibilities has to begin somewhere and so this chapter is devoted to defining those primary circles which contain certain clinical diagnostic possibilities. The starting point in drawing each of these circles is the symptom or symptom complex as it affects the individual child. Some clinical features, such as mass lesions palpable in the abdomen or systemic hypertension have such obvious connotations for imaging procedures that they are dealt with directly and separately in succeeding pages. The scope of the survey of symptoms and symptom complexes presented here is annotated at the head of this chapter; the detail now follows.

1.2 Renal Failure

1.2.1 Renal Failure in the Very Young

In the very young neonate overt clinical and biochemical evidence of renal failure may not be present because insufficient time has elapsed since the moment of the infant's delivery. Clinical features, such as anuria, oliguria, polyuria, or findings suggesting obstructive uropathy, may be present and indicate renal failure is impending. A major perinatal catastrophe associated with hypoxia or exsanguination may precipitate acute kidney damage with cortical, medullary or tubular necrosis being the consequence.

Once renal failure has become manifest uraemia is present. Commonly this is described in terms of its prerenal, renal and post-renal components, but this is a rather simplistic approach in the paediatric context. In the acute phase of renal failure in the infant vomiting, diarrhoea and abdominal distension with ileus, may produce both major elements of prerenal uraemia and also renal parenchymal damage because of the inevitable change in blood flow and supply to the kidney. Nevertheless prompt medical measures can alleviate the prerenal components of the uraemic state and in this way reveal the underlying extent of uraemia due to lesions of the kidney and urinary tract.

Renal failure in infancy has certain life-threatening connotations of immediate significance. It may be associated with hyponatraemia and circulatory collapse or hyperkalaemia and circulatory arrest.

Convulsions may result from either hyper – or hyponatraemia or hypocalcaemia. There is a susceptibility to infection and sepsis. Acute kidney and urinary infection may precipitate a clinical crisis in those with obstructive uropathy or primary reflux. In the very young infant urinary infection in an essentially normal urinary tract may be associated with septicaemia, jaundice and renal failure. Indeed these grave clinical features may constitute the cardinal presentation.

*Causes of Renal Failure
in the Neonate and Young Infant*

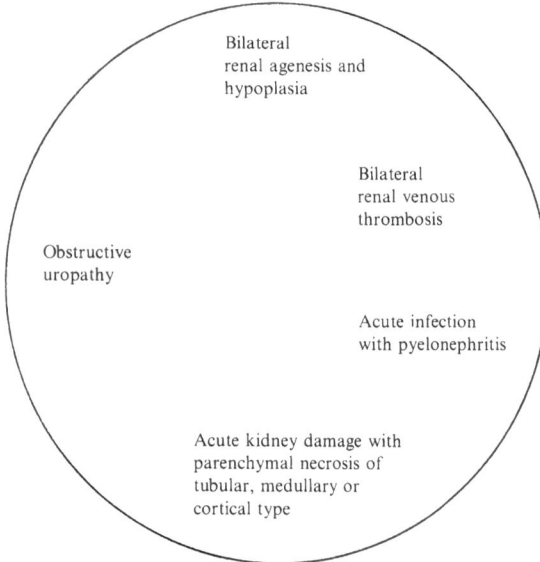

1.2.2 Protracted Renal Failure

Failure to thrive and grow normally is a common manifestation of chronic renal insufficiency in older infants and young children. In such circumstances there is often anorexia and a low calorie intake. Retardation of skeletal maturation may be observed on skeletal radiographs and rachitic changes may occur either with or without clinically evident bowing deformities of the limbs.

When the kidney's ability to conserve water is impaired polyuria develops because of the obligatory diuresis and then the urine has a fixed low specific gravity. These are features common to a very wide range of disorders in which the renal parenchyma is damaged or has failed to develop as the child has grown. And very often an element of somatic growth failure parallels the development of renal failure.

Be this as it may, the relationship between failure to thrive and grow and the onset of renal failure is neither clear cut nor direct. A number of children present quite suddenly with end-stage renal failure and yet they have grown well up to what must represent some critical moment in their life.

Systemic hypertension (with oedema, heart failure and pulmonary oedema, or hypertensive encephalopathy) may be one way in which renal failure is suspected and then investigated. The causes of hypertension declaring in this way are numerous. But not all patients who have hypertension necessarily have renal failure and in such children there is always good development of at least a proportion of the renal parenchyma.

In summary, infants and children who have protracted kidney failure may have
(i)   clinical evidence of an illness, often with growth failure, extending back over a considerable period of time, or
(ii) clinical evidence of a more acute illness which represents an end-point of a previously cryptic problem.

Protracted renal failure always implies a kidney parenchymal problem. This problem may be intrinsic to the kidney itself, as with hypoplasia. Alternatively it may be a feature (and a dominant feature) of a more generalized disease process, such as disseminated lupus erythematosis, which is but one of many examples of nephritis. And yet again, the parenchymal problem may be a consequence of a lesion in

Causes of Protracted Renal Failure

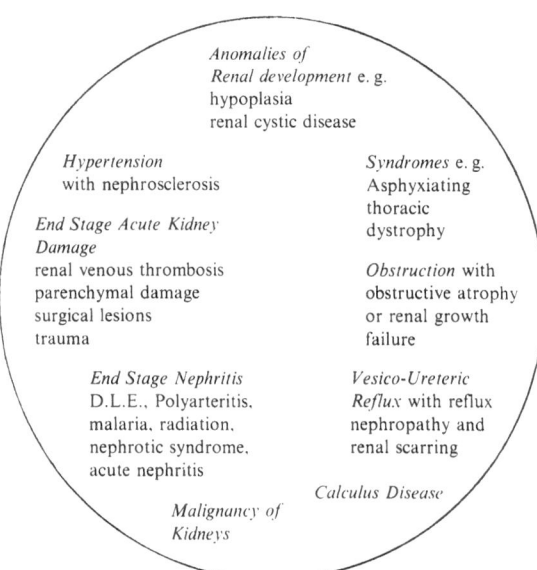

the urinary tract and the most common of these is obstruction to urine drainage. When hypertension develops hypertensive nephrosclerosis may add to the renal problem. Measures taken to alleviate hypertension by pharmacological means may exacerbate renal failure.

1.3 Enuresis – Retention – Incontinence

An astute clinical evaluation is of paramount importance in evaluating the problems of enuresis, retention and incontinence. The reason is that patterns of normal development vary quite widely and these need to be distinguished from habits which persist, habits which are acquired and pathological conditions which manifest themselves in terms of vesical emptying problems.

In the normal infant urine is passed periodically and there is no volitional control over the act of bladder emptying. As training of the toddler proceeds the act of voiding is controlled during the day, but voiding continues to occur periodically during the night. Later in childhood, and usually by the age of 4 years, voiding occurs in a controlled way during the day and it does not take place during sleep.

Certain deviations from this pattern can be defined at a very early age. An infant or child who is persistently wet may have a neuropathic bladder or an ectopic ureter draining low into the urethra (below the proximal sphincteric zone) or into the vagina.

Diurnal enuresis is a form of delay in development and the act of voiding is not controlled during the day by that time in the child's life when it should be. In some children there may be a considerable delay before continence is established during sleep and at night. Once the pattern of not voiding at night has developed then it should be maintained throughout childhood. If this pattern breaks and the child has nocturnal enuresis, this may be a response to some "crisis" in the child's life, such as the conception of a sibling. However, enuresis must be distinguished firstly, from frequency (which may be caused by a urinary infection and cystitis), secondly, from the production of large volumes of urine the voiding of which the child can no longer control (as in for example, renal failure). When there is the slightest doubt about the functional nature of the child's problem investigation can be decisive.

Urine retention often occurs, very transiently, in young children whose play (or work) so absorbs their interest that they put off the moment at which they would ordinarily void urine. Unpremeditated and precipitate voiding may then occur, especially when, for some happy reason, laughter breaks out. Girls of a sensitive disposition may, when they start going to school, void infrequently and it might be held that this accounts for the incidence of urine infection in schoolgirls. Nevertheless, a sore perineum in a girl or a meatal ulcer in a little boy may lead to painful retention because the act of voiding is so painful in itself; a rather similar event can occur occasionally after removal of a catheter passed per urethram. In such circumstances the child will usually void easily when sitting in warm bathwater. Serious and painful retention of urine can occur in patients who have obstruction to outflow of urine from the bladder due to pelvic mass lesions.

Chronic retention may be a feature of the neuropathic bladder or a consequence of obstruction to bladder emptying. This is a painless form of retention and it is often accompanied by a dribbling incontinence of urine.

Incontinence may be a sequel to surgical operations. In some boys whose posterior urethral valves have been resected incontinence persists for a period, which may be several years, even though no obstruction remains and there is no retention or residual urine. Very occasionally and rather more commonly in girls than boys, incontinence follows surgical uncapping of an extensive ectopic ureterocoele. Finally, children with spinal dysraphism may unfortunately develop incontinence, despite surgical efforts directed to preventing the inexorable deterioration which is so predictable without operation.

Causes of Enuresis; Retention; and Incontinence

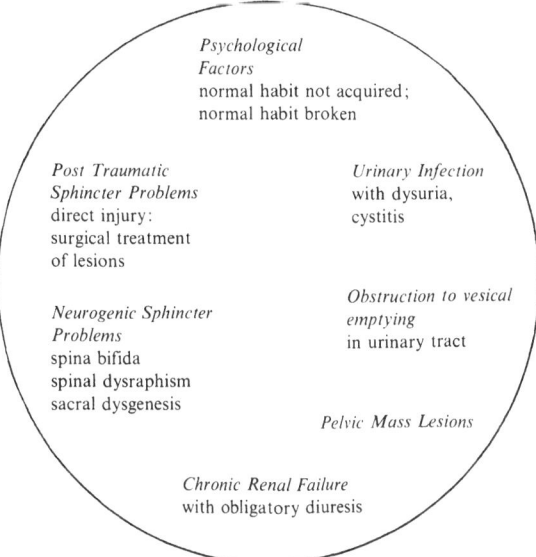

Psychological Factors
normal habit not acquired;
normal habit broken

Post Traumatic Sphincter Problems
direct injury:
surgical treatment
of lesions

Urinary Infection
with dysuria,
cystitis

Neurogenic Sphincter Problems
spina bifida
spinal dysraphism
sacral dysgenesis

Obstruction to vesical emptying
in urinary tract

Pelvic Mass Lesions

Chronic Renal Failure
with obligatory diuresis

1.4 Oliguria

In the first 1 or 2 days of life the normal infant may ordinarily excrete and void very little urine. [This is one very important reason for not undertaking intravenous urography (IVU) at this early stage – the contrast medium injected is not cleared in a predictable way and so there may be no meaningful outcome to the procedure]. However, in the normal infant normal volumes of urine are cleared and voided in the usual way subsequently. In infants with agenesis or severe hypoplasia of the kidneys the initial anuria or oliguria persists.

Shock states in the perinatal period may reduce cardiac output with a reduction of renal perfusion; oliguria then occurs. The reasons for such states developing are numerous and among them are hypoxia, diabetes in the mother, traumatic delivery and intracranial catastrophes in premature infants. If perfusion of the kidney is diminished for a long period the kidney may sustain damage and necrosis of the medulla or tubules. Young infants sustaining this type of kidney injury have a period of oliguria which may be quite short.

Older children who develop tubular necrosis have oliguria which lasts for several days, very much the pattern of events seen in adults with this problem. Both infants and children may suffer catastrophes in which the adrenal is affected and undergo either haemorrhage or infarction. Oliguria is a feature of such catastrophes.

Causes of Oliguria

"Normal" in first 24 hours of life

Renal Agenesis and Hypoplasia

End-Stage Renal Failure from any cause

Obstruction in Urinary Tract e. g. calculus disease

Dehydration vomiting, diarrhoea as in gastroenteritis, pyloric stenosis and colitis: seriously ill infants and children: meningitis, may be with renal infection

Shock States: as in severe illness, severe trauma, post cardiac bypass, intracranial catastrophes

Acquired Kidney Parenchymal Lesions
Acquired Kidney Parenchymal Lesions
Parenchymal necrosis (e. g. tubular necrosis): bilateral renal venous thrombosis: haemolytic uraemic syndrome: nephritis

However, foremost amongst all the causes of oliguria is dehydration. The balance of fluid intake does not meet what is needed to maintain an adequate urine flow. Everyone concerned with the care of infants and young children is aware of the need to maintain their state of hydration (and not overhydration) because of their distinctive and characteristic fluid compartments. The causes of dehydration are numerous and well known.

1.5 Polyuria

When the volume of urine cleared by the kidney is excessive polyuria is present. Very rarely in children polyuria is a consequence of compulsive and excessive water drinking which is psychologically based. Indeed this condition is so rare that in childhood it is virtually the diagnosis of last resort. Very much commoner are patients who have diabetes. Inadequately controlled diabetes mellitus is associated with polyuria, acidosis, and dehydration. Diabetes insipidus is characterised by polyuria and under the generic heading of diabetes insipidus lie specific entities: (i) there is a condition with a dominant pattern of inheritance which is vasopressin sensitive; (ii) a group of disorders lying in the vicinity of the pituitary and hypothalamus are associated with vasopressin-sensitive diabetes insipidus and they include conditions (which may have already manifested themselves in another way) such as craniopharyngioma, pituitary adenoma and histocytosis X; and (iii) nephrogenic diabetes insipidus is a condition which is not vasopressin sensitive and which has a dominant pattern of inheritance, most markedly expressed in males. In this last entity, nephrogenic diabetes insipidus, the abnormality is not vasopressin sensitive and polyuria is unremitting: and so the ureters tend to dilate slightly, the bladder is large, but it empties completely on voiding.

Polyuria, with a high fluid intake, is seen in infants and children with renal failure. This polyuria is a consequence of their obligatory diuresis and they are vulnerable to any restriction of fluid intake – such as might be contemplated (mistakenly) prior to high-dose IVU.

Kidney lesions associated with polyuria include the later stages of dysplasia of the kidneys and urinary tract, renal cystic disease (especially infantile polycystic disease and juvenile nephronophthisis), chronic pyelonephritis, obstructive atrophy and obstructiveuropathy, and chronic glomerulonephritis. Late in the history of a variety of diseases affecting renal parenchyma, polyuria occurs. Medullary necrosis is associated with polyuria because of loss of so much of the concentrating capability in the damaged medulla. Polyuria is also seen during recovery from acute tubular necrosis. In all these conditions bilateral kidney involvement must be present for polyuria to develop.

Causes of Polyuria

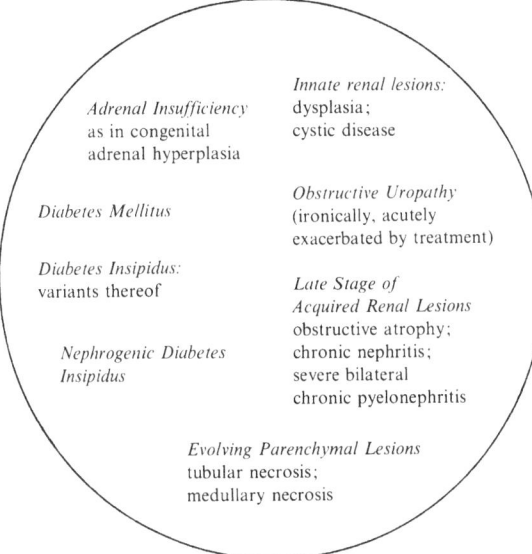

1.6 Haematuria

Haematuria originates in many sites and has many causes.

The classic picture of acute nephritis is one of haematuria with smokey urine, periorbital and generalised oedema, and following a streptococcal infection. Sometimes there is a frank haematuria and no clinically detectable oedema. In such circumstances changes on the chest radiograph can be helpful in furthering diagnosis. However, it is always wise to exclude a neoplasm as a cause of haematuria. This step can generally be delayed until frank haematuria has stopped.

Any acute urinary tract infection may produce haematuria but so can chronic conditions such as cystitis cystica, eosinophilic cystitis and tuberculosis. Overwhelming septicaemias with purpura, notably meningococcal infections, may be associated with haematuria. Low-grade septicaemic states are commonly associated with microscopic haematuria caused by focal infective nephritis.

Haematuria can occur in certain blood dyscrasias in which there is an abnormality of coagulation. Among these are haemophilia, thrombocytopenic purpura, aplastic anaemia and leukaemia; leukaemic infiltration enlarges the kidneys.

A kidney mass with haematuria may be due to renal venous thrombosis, nephroblastoma or a large hydronephrosis. Rarely adult type polycystic disease presents with haematuria in childhood and predominant enlargement of one kidney.

Angiomata may be localised within the kidney or may be part of a more generalised angiomatous malformation affecting the kidney, ureter, bladder and other body tissues: occasionally such an angioma will result in haematuria. Urogenital rhabdomyosarcoma may have haematuria as the presenting feature.

Traumatic renal injury can produce a renal mass and haematuria. The large hydronephrotic kidney or nephroblastoma is especially susceptible to trauma which results in haematuria: in these circumstances the traumatic episode may be slight or even not recognised. The adenomyolipomas of tuberous sclerosis very rarely cause haematuria in children.

Haematuria may be due to a urinary calculus. A foreign body introduced into the lower urinary tract can give haematuria. Very rarely a foreign body, such as a hair grip, is arrested in the duodenum and perforates the right renal pelvis to produce haematuria.

When comprehensive but unrewarded investigation into the patient with recurrent haematuria has been

Causes of Haematuria

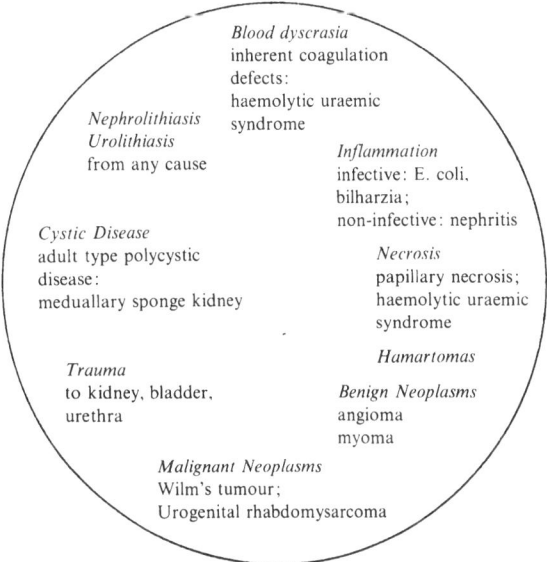

made a focal nephritis, diagnosed by renal biopsy, is not uncommonly held to be the causative lesion.

In summary when confronted by a patient who has haematuria, medical advisers should think systematically about possible sites and possible causes of blood entering the urine. The sites of bleeding start with the blood flowing in capillaries of the glomeruli and then lie distally in the nephrons, extend into the collecting systems of the kidneys and lie along the length of the urinary tract as far as the external urethral meatus. At virtually every site the causes may be encompassed as illustrated specific examples being given.

1.7 Urinary Infection

An acute urinary tract infection can be diagnosed when an uncontaminated specimen contains at least 100,000 organisms per millilitre and generally in fresh uncentrifuged urine 10 or more pus cells per cubic millimetre are also seen. *E. coli* is the common infecting organism in acute infection. Reinfections are common in paediatric practice and there is a change in organism type with successive episodes of infection.

Chronic infections, due to a variety of organisms, tend to be found in patients with a sizeable residual urine volume: these infections are frequently clinically silent but may result in increasing nephron damage. Tuberculosis of the urinary tract is now rare in many countries.

Even with an acute urinary infection, symptoms suggesting infection of the urinary tract may be in abeyance. For example in an acute infection, the infant or toddler may simply appear unwell and miserable and fever may be absent. Alternatively there may be anorexia, vomiting and diarrhoea or features of a respiratory infection. Severe urinary infections can precipitate renal failure especially when kidney function has already been compromised by an underlying abnormality. In very young infants a concurrent septicaemia may produce jaundice.

Acute urinary infection in older children is associated with a more distinctive symptomatology, namely dysuria, frequency and pain and discomfort in the suprapubic region. Pain in the loin, a tender slightly enlarged kidney and fever suggest acute pyelonephritis.

In the first year of life the incidence of urinary infection is about the same in the two sexes but in childhood girls are very much more commonly affected than boys. Surveys in children have shown a high incidence of urinary infections, as many as 1 in 20 girls being affected in their years at school.

Many patients who develop urinary infection have no radiologically demonstrable pathological changes in the kidneys, ureters or bladder; however, many patients do have primary developmental abnormalities which predispose to infection.

Urinary calculi are commonly associated with urinary infection. Recurrence of infection in a patient who has had a calculus or calculi removed is frequently a sign of recurrence of calculus disease. Children who have a compromised immunological status (for example children with leukaemia under treatment) may develop urinary infection. Sometimes such infections are by uncommon pathogens such as *Monilia* or *Actinomyces*.

1.8 Pain

Evaluating pain in children is complex; it requires a careful assessment of the clinical history, observation of the infant or child and clinical examination. Infants are incapable of saying they are in pain and toddlers have difficulty in communicating how they feel. Pain may be associated with crying, vomiting and pallor. Despite these difficulties certain patterns of pain associated with underlying problems in the kidney and urinary tract can be reasonably well defined.

Acute pyelonephritis so often produces pain in the flank in a child, but in infants such a continuing pain is impossible to assess. Pain may not be a particularly distinctive feature either of renal abscess or perinephric abscess – indeed the very absence of pain in these conditions can be misleading to the unwary. Dysuria may be a feature of urinary infection in a child. Male infants may cry on voiding if they have a meatal ulcer and, if there is soreness in the perineum of a girl, voiding concentrated urine can be painful. Pain on micturition does not necessarily point to urinary infection being present.

Protracted obstruction in itself is not painful unless some complication has arisen. However, acute obstruction is almost always painful whatever the cause; intermittent pelviureteric junction obstruction, ureteric colic due to either calculus or blood clot and acute retention all cause pain. Localization of the level and side of acute obstruction is important; when renal involvement is suspected it is often best to investigate during the acute episode of pain if this is otherwise reasonable and possible.

1.9 Complexes, Syndromes and Conditions of a Generalised Nature

As a very broad generalization maldevelopment somewhere may be associated with maldevelopment elsewhere. Congenital heart disease, oesophageal atresia, anorectal anomalies (Fig. 1.1) radial bone hypoplasia (Fig. 1.2) and vertebral anomalies can have concomitant renal problems. In congenital heart disease a post-angiocardiographic film of the urinary tract will show most lesions. Anorectal anomalies are associated with a higher incidence of fused crossed ectopia and single kidney quite apart from fistula to the lower urinary tract. Radial hypoplasia is associated with duplication of the kidney. A single umbilical artery is associated with urinary tract problems, but it is doubtful if it is worth ever considering investigating infants solely because of this feature. Patients with chromosomal abnormalities tend to have a specific predilection for abnormalities of varying degrees of severity in many systems (Fig. 1.3).

Patients with certain syndromes also may have urinary tract anomalies. The range is almost infinite. Ehlers-Danlos syndrome is associated with mega ureters; Laurence-Moon-Biedl syndrome has a high incidence of renal dysplasia (Fig. 1.4). Klippel-Feil syndrome is quite commonly found with renal agenesis or other anomalies; the short rib polydactyly syndromes, including the Ellis van Crevald syndrome, are associated with renal dysplasias, as in Jeune's asphyxiating thoracic dystrophy; Fanconi's syndrome is seen with a variety of renal malformations (Fig. 1.5); Meckel's syndrome and the Beckwith-Weidemann syndrome are both characterized by cystic disease of the kidneys; Bechet's syndrome is noted for late veno-occlusive disease which may involve the kidneys. Further details of

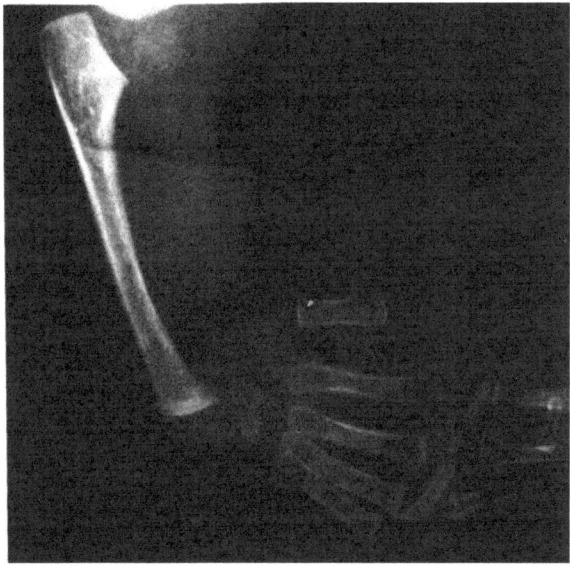

a

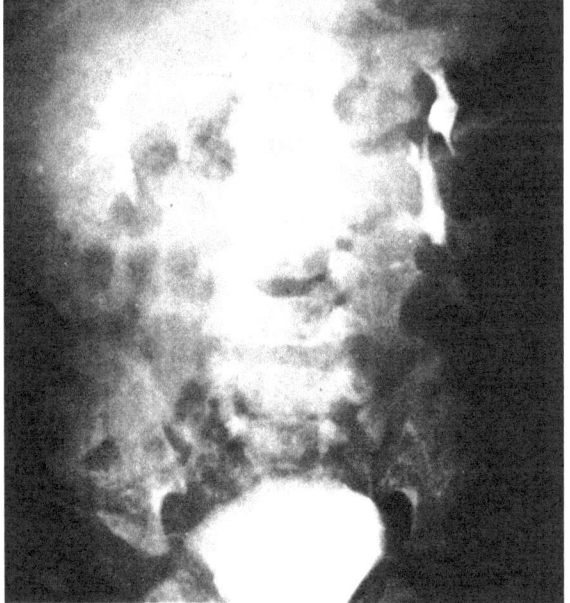

b

Fig. 1.1. Anorectal anomaly. At IVU there is a large solitary left kidney present. Fused crossed ectopia is also a quite common anomaly found with anorectal anomaly. Very frequently there is an absence of the lower part of the sacrum and vertebral anomalies, as shown here, higher up the spine. At micturition cystourethrography vesico-ureteric reflux may be shown

Fig. 1.2 a, b. Thrombocytopenia – absent radius syndrome (TAR syndrome). **a** There is an absent radius but no associated absence of the thumb. The forearm feature was bilateral. **b** IVU shows a duplex left kidney but also a hip dislocation – another a feature of the TAR syndrome

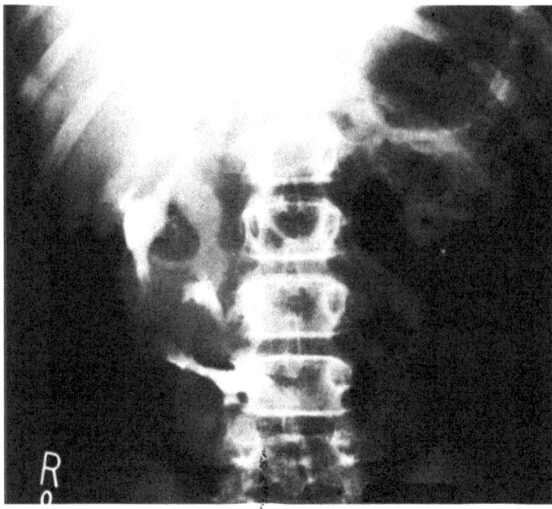

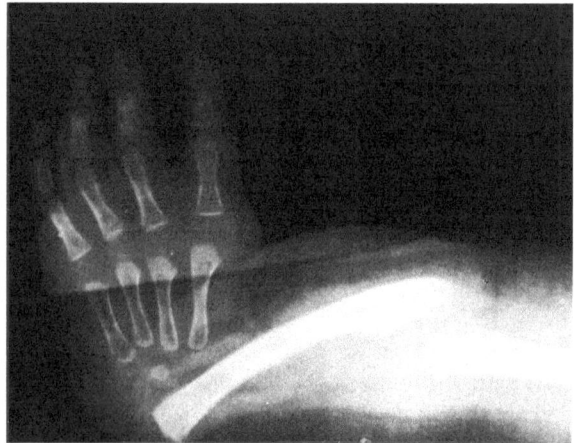

a

Fig. 1.3. Turner's syndrome. The IVU in this child shows fused crossed ectopia. Abnormalities of development in this condition are recognisable on clinical examination and there is a multiplicity of skeletal anomalies which are present in varying number and degree

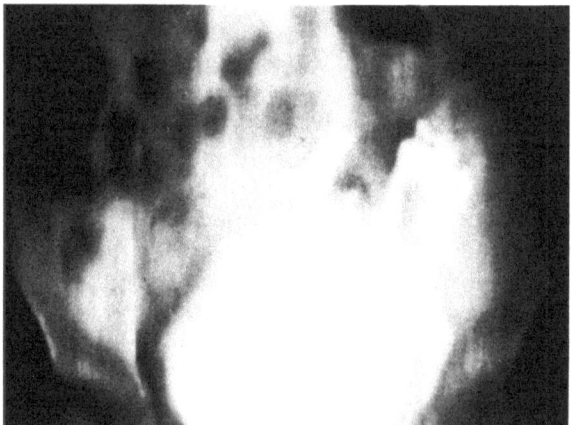

b

Fig. 1.5 a, b. Fanconi's anaemia. **a** In the forearm there is an absence of the radius and the thumb. This anomaly affected both forearms. **b** IVU in same patient shows on this tomographic cut two pelvic kidneys, which is but one anomalous variant affecting the urinary tract in Fanconi's anaemia

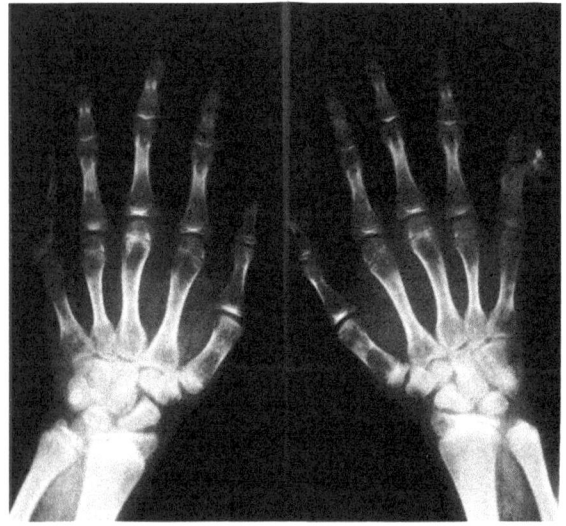

Fig. 1.4. Laurence-Moon-Biedl syndrome. In this obese child there are characteristic changes in the hands with bilateral post-axial polydactyly. At IVU the kidneys showed dysplastic changes

these and other conditions may be found among the suggested reading list.

Many conditions are characterized by a disease process which may affect the kidneys. Polyarteritis nodosa may show a concomitant nephritis, renal arterial stenoses, or a perinephric haematoma. Systemic lupus erythematosus may evolve to a nephritis or nephrotic syndrome. Neurofibromatosis may affect the kidneys and urinary tract in a variety of ways; for example, it may produce renal artery stenosis, it may infiltrate the bladder or ureteric wall or it may produce enlargement of genital structures. Tuberous sclerosis can be complicated by hypertension with angiomyolipomata or cystic disease of the kidneys. Amyloidosis with renal enlargement and rather rigid ureters is a late sequel in protracted sepsis (very rare these days), juvenile rheumatoid arthritis or familial Mediterranean fever. Thalassaemia may precipitate renal papillary necrosis. Of the parasitic diseases, hydatids notably infect kidneys (and the liver and lungs) and bilharzia affects the bladder wall and lower ureter; malarial disease affects kidneys in one of three ways – *Plasmodium falciparum* infection interferes with the microcirculation producing oliguria and anuria, and glomerulonephritis and the nephrotic syndrome may be sequelae to malarial infection in children. Caffey's infantile cortical hyperostosis may be associated with vesico-ureteric reflux, but it is seldom worth looking for this feature unless there are further reasons to indicate this should be done.

Two final conditions are important and worthy of mention. Pneumothorax is quite a common incidental radiographic feature in the newborn; but if a pneumothorax is severe it will in itself precipitate investigation of the chest and in these circumstances it is important to consider that, in the male, posterior urethral valves could be present. In radiographic studies of the urinary tract it is always important to scrutinize the entire radiograph; Perthe's disease of the hip can be found together with a wide variety of urinary tract lesions.

1.10 Conclusion

This presentation of the clinical context is inevitably a sketch of salient and relevant features, of a very wide variety of conditions. Nevertheless it is important to have an outline to begin with and we give a list of general reference texts which may be used to complete the picture of the clinical detail. However, in general, presenting features discussed in this section should be sufficient to begin the analysis which leads to the most appropriate lines of investigation.

References

1. Bloom, H. J. G., Lemerle, J., Neidhardt, M. K., Voûte, P. A. (eds.): Cancer in children. Berlin, Heidelberg, New York: Springer 1975
2. Eckstein, H. B., Hohenfellner, R., Williams, D. I.: Surgical pediatric urology. Stuttgart: Thieme 1977
3. James, J. A.: Renal disease in childhood, 3rd. ed. Saint Louis: Mosley 1976
4. Marsden, H. B., Steward, J. K. (eds.): Tumours in children, 2nd ed. In: Recent Results in Cancer Research. Vol. 13. Berlin, Heidelberg, New York: Springer 1976
5. O'Grady, F., Brumfitt, W.: Urinary tract infection. London, New York, Toronto: Oxford University Press 1968
6. Royer, P., Habib, R., Mathieu, H., Broyer, M.,: Pediatric nephrology. Philadelphia, London, Toronto: Saunders 1974
7. Rubin, M. L., Barratt T. M.: Pediatric nephrology. Baltimore: Williams & Wilkins 1975
8. Williams, D. I., Barratt, T. M., Eckstein, H. B., Kohlinsky, S. M., Newns, G. H., Polani, P. E., Singer, J. D.: Urology in childhood. In: Handbuch der Urologie. Andersson, L., Gittes, R. F., Goodwin, W. E., Lutzeyer, W., Zingg, E. (eds.), Vol. XV Suppl. Berlin, Heidelberg, New York: Springer 1974

2 Investigatory Techniques

2.1 Introduction

The techniques employed in radiological examination of the kidney and urinary tract in children produce the information for diagnosis. In the vast majority of patients the studies can be performed without either sedation or anaesthesia. A successful outcome to a procedure is related in part to the level of co-operation from the child. It is wise to accept that most children embark on a study without really wanting to do so.

In order to establish contact with the parent and child it is essential to talk to them from the outset and throughout the procedure. Some of this conversation is devoted to describing, in limited detail, what a procedure entails as far as the child is concerned. When the child is able to understand reasonably well (from the age of 5 years or so upwards) it is best to talk directly with the child. After all he is to undergo the procedure and it is his co-operation that is required. Much of the conversation can be diversionary and about interesting events in a child's life such as birthdays, holidays, play, books, television programmes and so on. In the present climate where marriages are no longer like a pair of working boots, durable but sometimes uncomfortable, it is wise not to talk in a direct way about the family situation. It is also best to avoid all discussion of school life, which can be a very sensitive subject.

From time to time it is good policy to tell the child and his parent how well the procedure is going. It is important to emphasise success for this gives encouragement and reinforces the motivation to succeed further. After a procedure has been completed a child needs to be reassured and indeed congratulated on the way he has helped. Many children react visibly with a sense of pride and achievement. This is important because examinations of the same or related type may have to be repeated.

Initial fears, self doubts and lack of confidence on the part of the child need to be replaced as the procedure goes forward by a sense of success in overcoming them. In no circumstances must a radiologist or his assistants display any anxiety about the future course of events, no matter what may be felt inwardly. A sense of anxiety or despair is rapidly and often imperceptibly communicated to the child and his parent. A smiling face and eye-to-eye contact are a great source of reassurance to a child and his parent. A pompous authoritarian manner is prejudicial to success.

Modern medical technology has provided an ever widening range of techniques for investigation. It is important to think rationally and incisively about the indications for using a particular technique and the information which is likely to accrue from a particular procedure. It is preferable for a clinical question to be formulated and an answer sought, rather than embark on a certain investigation which may have been vaguely requested and thought of in terms of something to do. It should not be difficult to think of the most appropriate investigation if there is a clinical question which needs to be answered. At all times it is essential to employ the technique which is most likely to be decisive in furthering clinical management of a child's problem. Some knowledge of probabilities is helpful but although cases may have similarities they also have differences and so a routine type of approach is often not wise. Each case must be assessed on the basis of a sensitive examination of the facts and there must be a clear-cut clinical indication for a study.

2.2 Intravenous Urography (IVU)

2.2.1 Preparatory Details

In infants and children, because an injection of contrast medium commonly produces transient nausea the stomach should be empty at the start of the procedure. However, young patients tend to develop hypoglycaemia rather easily. It follows that in infants it is best to plan the urogram for a time when a feed is due and only delay the feed for a short period after injection. In children a period of abstinence from solid food of about 5 h is sensible in most instances.

Dehydration is not an objective in any part of this regime and indeed an adequate state of hydration is essential in young infants because the injection of contrast medium represents a considerable solute load and it has a sharp diuretic effect.

Shortly after the contrast medium has been injected it is usual to give a feed to an infant or a fruit flavoured drink with added glucose to a child. The presence of some gastric content often makes it easier to demonstrate the kidneys during excretion of the contrast medium.

In general there are two sets of circumstances in which it is important to be especially careful about the status before and after injection. The problem in diabetes mellitus is one of maintaining an adequate control over the clinical situation when there has been a limited calorie intake. In severe diabetics it is best to err on the side of a hyperglycaemia, even with mild acidosis, because diabetic coma and dehydration take a considerable period of time to develop. It is preferable to omit or diminish and certainly delay a dose of insulin and plan to carry out the urogram at the start of the day. Failure to alter the insulin dosage combined with abstinence from food may result in hypoglycaemic coma of rapid onset. The second set of circumstances is when kidney function is such that there is uncontrolled loss of

water and cations. For example, many children who either have incipient or developed renal failure are in such a state, and, in children with nephrogenic diabetes insipidus there is an obligatory water loss; it is crucial in these circumstances to maintain an adequate fluid intake before the urogram and to resume fluid intake as soon as possible after the contrast medium has been injected.

In all children it is helpful to have the colon empty of faecal residues to improve the chances of achieving a good excretion series of radiographs. A dose of a mild purgative on the evening before the study can help. However, improved imaging techniques have meant that there is no need to be obsessional about this aspect.

2.2.2 Injection of Contrast Medium and Radiographic Techniques

2.2.2.1 Preliminary Film

Radiographs of the abdomen and pelvis are taken before the injection is carried out. Fast screen-film combinations, such as the rare earth intensifying screens with their matching film, reduce the radiation dose. The gonads in the male can be directly protected. This is not possible in girls and so it is wise to use about 85 Kilovolts (KV) when radiography of the pelvis is being carried out because the gonad dose is reduced at a high KV. However, such a style of work does demand a flexible control of exposure factors. It is important to scrutinise all details on preliminary films. Spinal lesions are especially important in urology and findings on the antero-posterior projection such as dysraphism. spina bifida, sacral agenesis and invasive posterior abdominal wall lesions such as neuroblastoma may necessitate lateral radiographs at this stage.

2.2.2.2 Injection of Contrast Medium

An intravenous injection of contrast medium must be obtained. The veins of young patients can present problems. The back of the hand and the dorsum of the foot often have veins which are easily seen and can be used. It is helpful to inject the contrast medium through a standard scalp vein needle because minor movement of the extremity after the injection has started does not then result in the needle coming out of the lumen of the vein. If, once the needle has passed through the skin surface, an assistant gently pulls back on the syringe which contains the contrast medium and which is connected to the scalp vein needle, blood enters the plastic tube the moment the needle enters the lumen of the vein. It is usually best to use a small elastic tourniquet to produce venous congestion in the extremity rather than the uncertain hand of an assistant around the child's limb.

If neither the hand nor foot carry a suitable vein then it is possible to resort to a vein in the antecubital fossa; the brachial artery must be avoided and the venous channel leading to the cephalic vein is usually the easiest to enter. In very young infants the veins of the scalp are excellent alternatives. The external jugular vein can be used but carries a risk of pneumothorax. The femoral vein must be avoided because cases of septic arthritis of the hip may tragically follow the use of this site.

The dose of contrast medium to be injected depends on the age and size of the patient and the clinical circumstances. However, in young infants little if any advantage ever accrues from doses in excess of 15 ml of 45% Hypaque (sodium diatrizoate) when the weight is 3 kg. For smaller infants doses less than this are appropriate. Iodinated salts have a high osmolality [1, 2], but a non-ionic contrast medium such as metrizamide has theoretical and practical advantages for it reduces the solute load for a young infant. Above 5 kg doses based on a schedule of 3 ml/kg of body weight may be given. Sometimes, because of technical problems with the injection, only a very few millilitres of contrast medium may be given, but it is always worthwhile taking a radiograph subsequently because an adequate urogram may be obtained. Doses of contrast medium given in excess of this scale have produced serious sequelae. However, in an older child higher total doses of contrast medium can be given and it is important to do this when there is an element of renal failure present if a satisfactory urogram is to be obtained. Doses at a rate of between 2 and 3 ml per kg can be given with safety. It is not necessary to use such high doses in ordinary circumstances when between 20 and 40 ml of 45% Hypaque generally suffice. Intravenous infusions of contrast medium are not needed and a single rapid direct injection brings this phase of the study to a prompt conclusion and this is welcomed by all children.

Abnormalities of the urinary tract are sufficiently common to make it worthwhile using the renal clearance of contrast medium injected primarily for other purposes. A radiograph of the abdomen and pelvis after angiocardiography or intracranial angiography or CT scanning can be very revealing.

2.2.3 Cavography

If a mass is palpable in the abdomen, especially if it is suspected that the mass may be malignant and associated with renal venous thrombosis, then opacification of the inferior vena cava can be helpful [3]. It will show its position, patency, or extension into the lumen of any thrombus or tumour.

A cavogram may be obtained by exposing a radiograph placed under a young child as contrast medium is injected into the vein of a foot. For this procedure to be successful the child must be breathing quietly and not breathholding or crying. These last activities prevent free flow of contrast medium up the cava and into the thorax. A tourniquet should be placed on the opposite thigh to reduce the dilution of contrast in the inferior vena cava.

2.2.4 Timing of Radiographs

In studies of the urinary tract in children there is no such thing as a routine study. Each child's examination must be dictated by the indications for the study and the ease with which the examination proceeds. It is best when carrying out the first IVU to secure a study which provides good detail and which is definitive.

2.2.5 Radiographs of the Kidneys

Contrast medium injected intravenously is normally cleared through the glomeruli and when the filtrate passes down the tubule water is resorbed [4]. And so as the contrast medium enters the collecting system of the calyces it produces the density necessary to give the anatomical delineation [5].

In the early phase of the urogram the kidney parenchyma is most heavily opacified. This nephrographic phase is useful for defining the contours of the kidney, its size and any abnormalities of shape and position. The nephrogram is especially important in the study of patients who have haematuria which may be due to a tumour. A relatively diminished nephrographic density may be a feature of a diminished renal blood flow in a child with unilateral renal disease and hypertension. The best nephrographic film is obtained some 2–3 min after completing injection of the contrast medium. The nephrographic phase occurs whilst there is still an exceptionally high level of contrast medium in circulation. In young infants cystic lesions in the abdomen are not opacified and vascular lesions such as angiomas are heavily opacified, relative to other structures such as the liver: these are the two aspects of the total body opacification effect [6]. It follows that when a mass lesion is present some indication as to its content may be obtained by exposing a radiograph within the first 2–3 min after injection of the contrast medium. This feature of a urographic study is only of use in young infants: simple radiography in older children will not demonstrate the phenomenon. However, this phenomenon is used consistently in image enhancement in CT scanning.

About 5 min after completing the injection of the contrast medium the calyces and pelvis, when of a reasonably normal size, begin to opacify. If gut overlies and obscures the kidney and calyx detail, then it is usually important to take steps which minimize this problem. The renal window view does

this by imaging the kidneys against the relatively homogeneous background of the liver, heart and the upper part of the stomach which can usefully be filled by a drink of water. The X-ray beam is centred on the xiphisternum and angled towards the feet of a supine patient at about 30°/35° degrees to the vertical (Fig. 2.1). It is necessary to increase the KV for the renal window view exposure (by about 15–20 KV) in order to penetrate the additional tissue mass. The reverse of this view can be taken when the patient is prone and the beam is angled cephalad to a similar degree. The distortion of the kidney and its

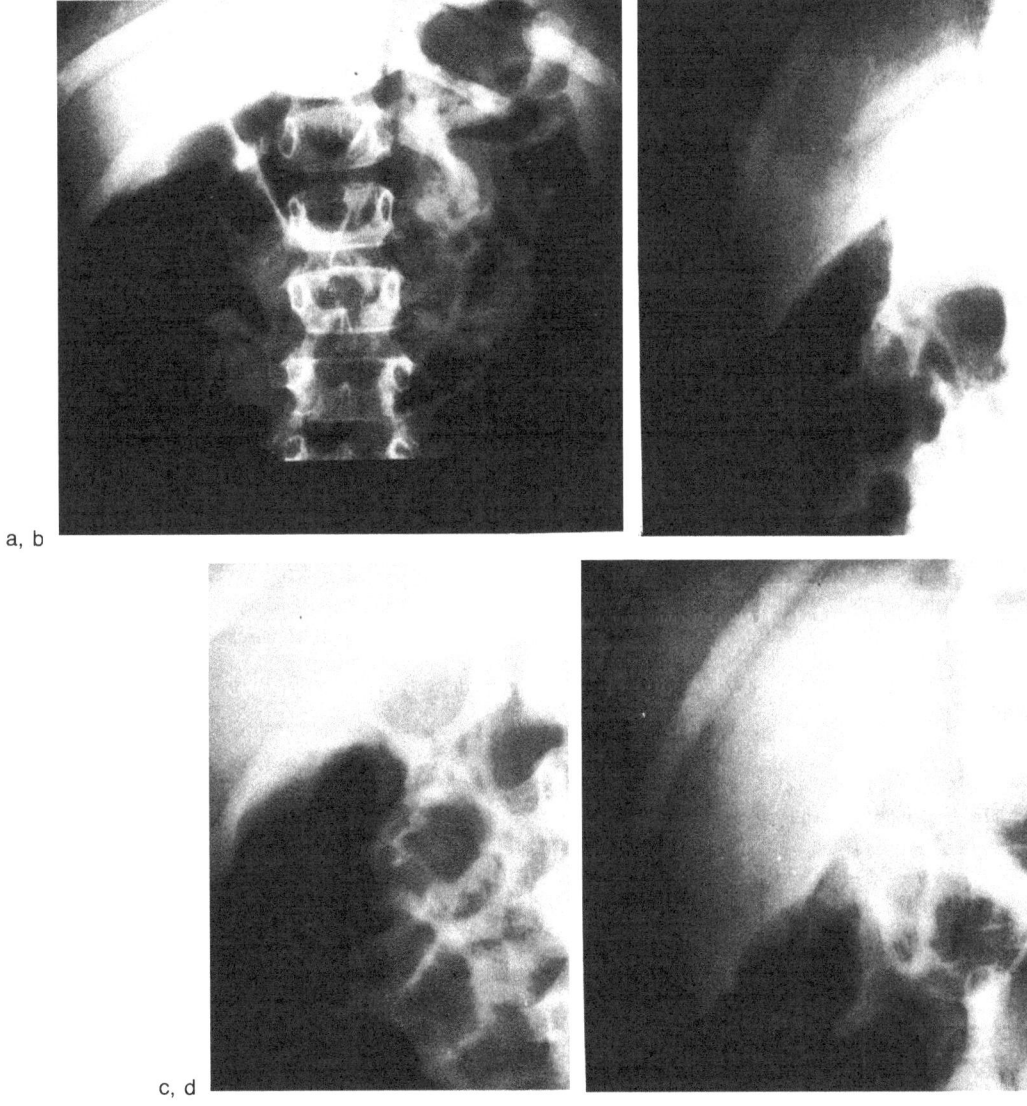

a, b

c, d

Fig. 2.1. a The problem of gas in the gut. Preliminary film shows the renal areas obscured by gas. **b** Renal window view with beam directed caudad shows a calculus in the vicininity of the right kidney. **c** IVU, antero-posterior projection, presents the same problems as in **a**. **d** IVU renal window view shows no calculus visible. The contrast medium cleared through the kidney produces a similar density to that of the calculus. The inference is that the calculus lies in the colecting system of the small right kidney

structure is not so great as might be expected because the long axis of the kidney normally lies obliquely in the posterior abdominal wall.

The second step which can be taken to minimize the effect of gut overlying the kidneys is tomography. For this it is best to use a narrow arc of swing of about 15° when using a linear tomographic unit. Although in theory it is essential to have no movement during tomography, a skilled radiographer can usually obtain entirely satisfactory results in infants and children. Three well-selected cuts at intervals of 1 cm generally provide adequate detail.

Oblique views of the kidneys can sometimes be helpful in detecting localised scars or kidney masses. The X-ray beam can be used in a vertical projection or with an angulation similar to that of the renal window view. Prone and erect projections may also be helpful (Fig. 2.2).

Calyces may not be identifiable in end-stage kidney failure from any cause and the kidney may not function in extensive and severe renal venous thrombosis, Wilm's tumour and traumatic injuries to the vascular pedicle. When the calyces are grossly dilated, as in severe obstructive uropathy, their opacification may be very faint and it may take a long time (several hours) to develop. If the calyces and pelvis are not opacifying rapidly this is a good reason to transfer the patient to the ultrasound table. Ultrasound may resolve the morphological problem and the subsequent radiographic approach appropriately modified.

In post-operative or repeat IVU studies a very limited examination is often appropriate. One radiograph taken some 10–15 min after the injection of contrast medium will often demonstrate all that is necessary to show an unchanged or improved status in the urinary tract.

When contrast medium is not cleared by the kidneys then it is cleared vicariously through two routes. The liver is the more important and the biliary tract may opacify several hours after the injection. This feature may be striking in cases of acute urinary tract

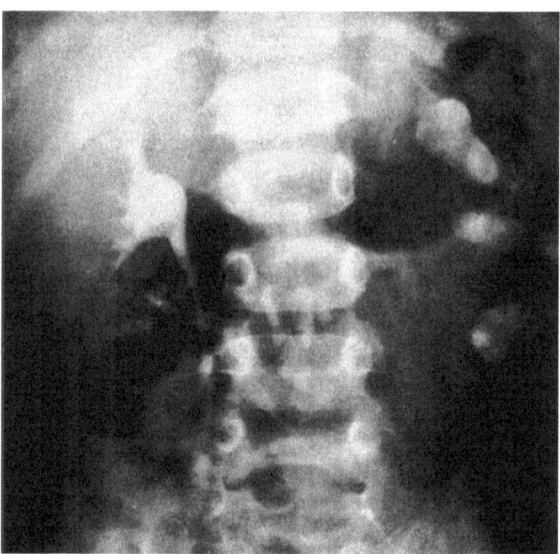

a

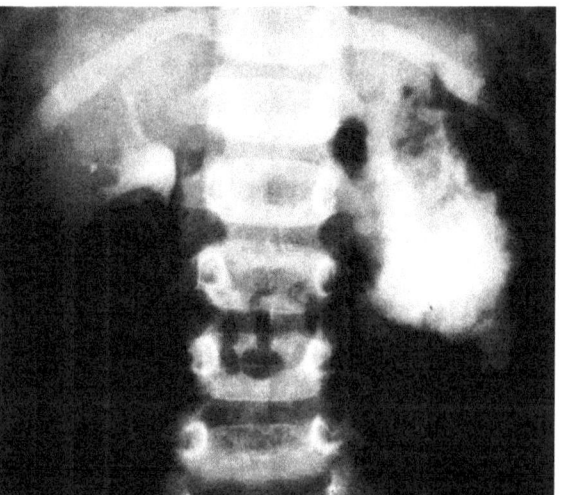

b

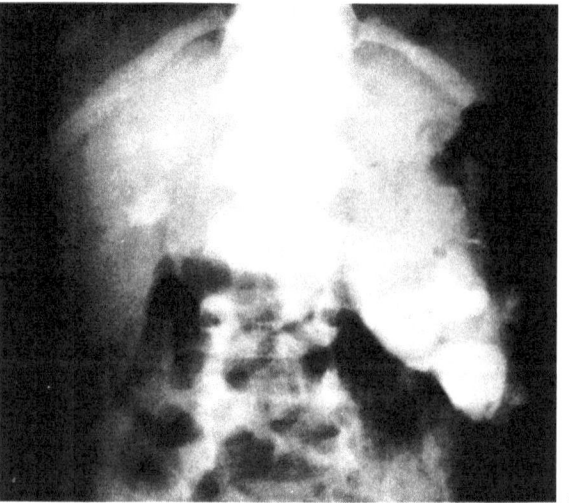

c

Fig. 2.2. a Follow-up urogram in a child referred for study following previous pyeloplasty. The radiograph at 5 min after start of injection of contrast medium shows a normal right kidney and collecting system. On the left side dilated calyces are beginning to opacify. **b** Radiograph with patient prone shows the left pelvis opacified but no opacification of the ureter distally at 25 min. **c** Erect radiograph at 35 minutes shows much of the contrast medium has cleared from the right pelvicalyceal system. On the left side there is layering of contrast medium in the lower calyces and contrast medium opacifying the pelvis. In a previously unoperated situation it would be reasonable to infer that pelvi-ureteric obstruction is present. However, post-operative study like this raises the additional question – is there simply residual dilatation in the upper tract? See Fig. 2.15, same case

obstruction even when this is unilateral. In young infants the wall of the gut may sometimes opacify early in a urogram and it is likely that this provides the second route for clearance. Contrast medium in the large intestine can be seen between 12 and 24 h after injection in some children with renal failure.

2.2.6 Imaging of the Ureters

Ureteric opacification begins as contrast medium passes into the ureters from the renal pelves and calyces. If it is important to see ureters throughout their length then a relatively high dose of contrast medium must be given. Normal calibre ureters may be studied for displacement by antero-posterior, lateral and oblique views covering the whole length of the ureter. Such studies are useful in defining posterior abdominal wall and pelvic lesions. In children with duplications of the urinary tract where there is a possibility of ureters joining at some point before reaching the bladder a limited fluoroscopic study with spot films can often localize the point at which they join. A very large dose of contrast medium will produce a mild dilatation of ureters which are then filled throughout their length. A slight increase in size of the calyces and pelves can also be seen in these circumstances. A ureter filled throughout its length can sometimes be a feature of vesico-ureteric reflux or diabetes insipidus. Widening of the ureter occurs when a ureter is obstructed distally. Peristalsis in a wide ureter can be observed at fluoroscopy which can show the peristaltic wave is less able to obliterate the ureteric lumen as it progresses distally towards the point of obstruction. Such ureteric incompetence is seen in a single ureter. When two ureters in a duplex system join above the bladder the two limbs may dilate and the single ureter distally remains undilated – peristalsis in one limb of a double ureter results in filling and distension of its companion, this being inter-ureteric reflux.

2.2.7 Lower Urinary Tract

Radiographs of the lower urinary tract are generally taken considerably later than those for the upper urinary tract, often at about 10–15 min after injection ceased. At this time the bladder is usually well opacified. If the child has remained quiet in the supine position urine carrying contrast medium tends to produce a layer posteriorly in the bladder cavity. It is important not to infer too much about bladder capacity in these circumstances. Nevertheless intravesical lesions such as polyps, tumours and ureterocoeles can be well shown. Lateral projections of the bladder can be important in differentiating such intravesical lesions from gas in the rectum which can produce a deceptively similar appearance. Usually the low density of the image produced by contrast medium in the bladder prevents useful views of the urethra being obtained when voiding during a urographic series. A post-micturition film is often not a necessary feature of a urogram in a child. When haematuria is present as a dominant clinical feature a post-voiding radiograph of the bladder is important for intra-vesical lesions such as polyps and non-opaque calculi may be evident only on such a projection.

2.2.8 Reactions to Contrast Medium

These may be trivial such as transient vomiting, sneezing, sensations of warmth, conjunctional reddening and mild discomfort along the limb as contrast medium is being injected.

Rather more serious is urticaria which develops both in those with a background of sensitivity to foods and drugs and other potential allergens and in those who have no antecedent history of sensitivities. Usually a few urticarial spots disappear spontaneously. If urticaria is more extensive and distresses the child chlorpheniramine injection (10 mg in 1 ml) may be given intravenously or intramuscularly at a dose of up to 5 mg up to 2 years of age and up to 10 mg at ages ranging to 10 years and above.

Reactions to contrast medium may be of a different and more serious character and even threaten life. Cardiac arrest may occur and this is treated by a sharp blow on the chest followed by external cardiac massage with oxygen administered and an open airway maintained. Additional help from a resuscitation team must be obtained quickly.

Severe vasovagal inhibition may develop even when the patient is supine ("faint on the flat"). Such an episode may be protracted and the best plan is to place the patient on to a tilting table in the Radiology Department and then incline the table top so the head is downward and venous return from the lower lims and trunk is improved. For a serious vasovagal attack following an injection of contrast medium it is possibly not wise to give intravenous atropine. Do not return the child to the horizontal or erect position before it is clear he has fully recovered from his vasovagal attack; this can take quite a long time. The third form of serious reaction is the onset of severe airways obstruction. This may be due to laryngospasm as a part of angioneurotic oedema or it may be caused primarily by bronchospasm. There may be no audible wheezing because air entry is very severely limited indeed. Rapid onset of laboured breathing with pallor and central cyanosis can be the most important clinical observations to be made. These features may occur during, immediately following the injection or sometimes after injection of contrast medium. Treatment is an urgent matter. Oxygen delivered at a high rate of flow is essential throughout. Isoprenaline given intravenously is a potent bronchodilator and vasopressor and general antagonist for such a sensitivity reaction. Intravenous chlorpheniramine and hydrocortisone can usefully follow the isoprenaline if relief is not rapid. Finally, there is much to be said for giving aminophylline (3 mg/kg) by *slow* intravenous injection for a child with bronchospasm; the side-effects of this drug are not usually a problem and in addition to its bronchodilator characteristics it also improves cardiac output.

Many of the foregoing details suggest it is wise to set up an intravenous drip in a patient who has a reaction to contrast medium and it is better to do this sooner rather than later. This step obviates the need to search repeatedly for veins which can become increasingly difficult to enter if the reaction progresses.

One of the facets of reaction to intravenous injections of contrast medium for IVU is that their onset is completely unpredictable. The most serious reactions, fortunately very few, have in our experience occurred in children with no history of sensitivity in themselves or in their family. It is logical to deduce that no system of testing for sensitivity to contrast medium or desensitization regimes will be of value.

Many children who undergo intravenous urography or any other procedure in a Radiology Department have dilatation of the pupils. This probably reflects the fear which they experience. It is noteworthy that two groups of patients seldom experience reactions to contrast medium – the very young infant and patients undergoing angiography who are either very heavily sedated or who have a general anaesthetic. Perception of events and fear are frequently the trigger for the onset of reactions in a child. Certain studies in adults support this view [7, 8].

It is current practice, therefore, to avoid anything which might increase apprehension on the part of the child or the parent. In particular no enquiry is made about sensitivities and no description of possible side-effects is made to either parent or child before the IVU. When a minor reaction occurs it is best to reassure the child and the parent and indicate

that the unpleasant episode will rapidly pass off. It is wise to stay with the child and parent and chat in a superficially lighthearted way with the child and parent until it is apparent which way events are moving; an astute perceptive observation is essential if serious events are to be recognised sooner rather than later.

If a child has atopy and has asthma it is important not to undertake an IVU when there is bronchospasm. Clinical colleagues must make every effort to control airways obstruction beforehand. Such children often seem especially apprehensive and some sedation can be a helpful adjunct. Consideration should be given to the possibility that the clinical question can be answered by another investigation without the need of intravenous contrast agents.

2.3 Micturition Cystourethrography (MCU)

Contrast medium may be introduced directly into the bladder via a urethral catheter, a suprapubic catheter, a suprapubic needle puncture and from the upper tract via a nephrostomy tube or similar diversion intended primarily for drainage.

Urethral catheterization is the most widely practised of these methods. A 6 FG Jacques catheter is passed through the urethra with the strictest aseptic methods possible. The advantage of a catheter of this size is that, when lubricated with a jelly containing local anaesthetic, it will pass through the sphincteric zone of the urethra with little discomfort even though the voluntary muscle is contracted. If in boys the catheter does not pass easily because of voluntary sphincter spasm, a few seconds pause in the procedure is sufficient for the muscle spasm to abate. The catheter then moves easily into the bladder: voluntary perineal muscle contracture cannot be maintained for more than 10 s or so. It is imperative to be as gentle as possible when introducing catheters into the bladder; firstly, it is kinder for the child and secondly, the chance of obtaining good co-operation during voiding is enhanced.

Suprapubic puncture has its devotees [9]. It has the advantage of being a sterile procedure. Urine samples appropriate for bacteriological study can be obtained before beginning the radiological survey. Abdominal wall tissues in the midline and anterior to the bladder are infiltrated with local anaesthetic. The needle required for introducing the contrast medium is then passed through the anaesthetized zone into the vesical lumen. Fluoroscopic control of the procedure can be used and the bladder lumen can be localized by contrast medium given previously at urography. A better alternative is to use ultrasonics to define bladder position and volume.

In some young patients temporary drainage by suprapubic catheter may have been instituted by clinicians and obviously the bladder can be filled through such a drain or by a drainage tube introduced into the upper tract. In these circumstances there is knowledge of obstruction in the urinary tract before cystography is undertaken.

The bladder may be filled by a freely running drip system like that used in general intravenous work. Alternatively it may be filled from a 50-ml syringe which is repeatedly recharged. Dilute contrast medium is used and 17% Hypaque is reasonably non-irritant when voided; a catheter lubricated with local anaesthetic desensitizes the urethra to some degree. The filling procedure is controlled by intermittent fluoroscopy.

2.3.1 Radiological Technique at MCU

The capacity of the bladder should be recorded. There are no satisfactory normal values of capacity at different ages, but it soon becomes clear if the bladder has an excessively large capacity or a particularly small capacity.

The bladder normally has a smooth contour when full. Irregularity caused by trabeculation and the presence of many small saccules are features of detrusor hypertrophy. By rotating the child into oblique and lateral positions saccules and diverticula lying posteriorly and in the vicinity of the uretero-vesical junction may be seen. These may either obstruct a ureter or be associated with vesico-ureteric reflux. They may become evident only when micturition takes place.

As vesical filling proceeds the moment when voiding is about to start is approached and the most proximal part of the urethra then opacifies with contrast medium. Vesical distension leads to inhibition of the most proximal part of the sphincter. If proximal urethral filling occurs early in the vesical filling this suggests a neuropathic bladder may be present. In the ordinary way, however, proximal urethral filling together with curling of the toes are signs that micturition is about the begin. If the patient is old enough he should be encouraged verbally to begin to void. When this starts a urethral catheter can be gently withdrawn without discomfort. In young infants the act of micturition can frequently be precipitated by removing a dummy from the mouth.

There are many instances, however, when the child is unable to micturate immediately after the catheter has been withdrawn. It is then essential to be extremely kind, patient and optimistic and to induce an atmosphere which is unhurried. A child given a drink will often relax quickly. An infant who is fed will often void soon after starting his feed. If little children can play with toys floating in water in a washbasin, the urge to void often becomes irresistible.

During voiding, views of the urethra must be obtained when there is a rapid outward flow of contrast medium (Fig. 2.3). This is essential if a possible urethral obstruction is not to be missed. A ureter draining ectopically into the urethra may fill by reflux when micturition occurs and this may be the only time when such a ureter is seen. In boys the various components of the genital tract may opacify and this is always abnormal. As micturition comes to an end, there may be an undrained vesical residue – this is not necessarily abnormal in nervous sensitive children. Most infants, once micturition has started, empty the bladder completely. The bladder may

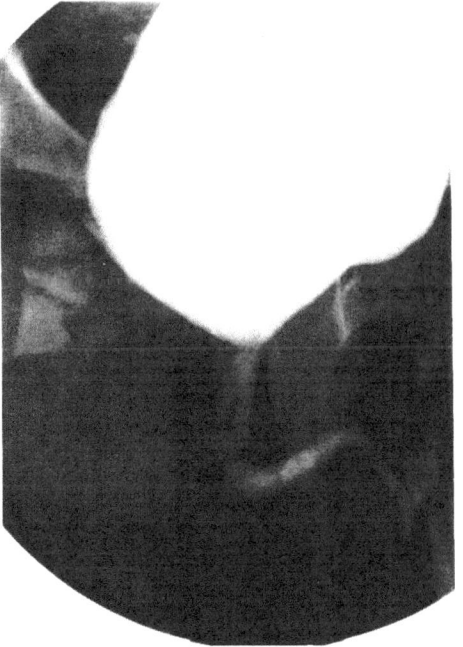

Fig. 2.3. Voiding cystogram in a boy. The bladder is emptying rapidly. The most proximal normal feature of note in the urethra is the negative image due to a prominent verumontanum. Sphincteric relaxation occurs at many levels during voiding and when inhibition is complete rapid flow of contrast medium through the sphincteric zone permits full urethral opacification. Note that, at the level of the pelvic floor there is a transverse impression in the contrast medium, a normal feature

contract asynchronously to produce a contraction ring as emptying proceeds (Fig. 2.4).

Vesico-ureteric reflux is a common but abnormal event. During cystography local abnormalities such as saccules in the vicinity of the ureterovesical junction must be sought. If reflux does take place it is important to observe the extent of ureteric filling and if calyx opacification occurs a radiograph of the event should be taken. Local views of the kidney may then show intrarenal reflux.

Although fluoroscopic control of cystography is not practised in all centres we believe that it has a most important role. However, fluoroscopy must be carried out intermittently and restricted to that which is strictly necessary; fluoroscopy can represent an important fraction of the total radiation dose incurred. A high-quality videotape recorder minimizes the need for films Film records, of either fluorographic or X-ray film type, should be limited to the positive findings in a study. Fast screen/film combinations must be used to reduce radiation dosage.

2.3.2 Equipment

If there is a choice of equipment a system with an overtable X-ray tube and an undertable intensifier is to be preferred. With such a system one can see and talk to the patient throughout the procedure. The standard overtable intensifier is a terrifying piece of equipment for a child: this is because the intensifier comes close to the child (often nearer than the near point of vision) and it produces acute sensory deprivation. Fluoroscopic units specially designed for work with children have an overtable X-ray tube, but the small size of such a table can restrict the patients who can be studied to those who are young and small.

2.3.3 Sedation and Anaesthesia

In especially anxious children sedation may be employed. But it is only the very exceptional child who is unable to co-operate to a degree which precludes any useful information being obtained. In these circumstances it may be necessary to resort to general anaesthesia: the bladder may then be filled easily. Under quite deep anaesthesia pressure by a protected hand on the bladder will express contrast medium down the urethra. Occasionally when posterior urethral valves are suspected in a young boy an elective study of the bladder and urethra may be carried out under anaesthesia. Diathermy of the valves can then follow under the same anaesthetic. For this and other types of procedure requiring a general anaesthetic it is best to have a special room in which fluoroscopic facilities and allied image recording techniques are available.

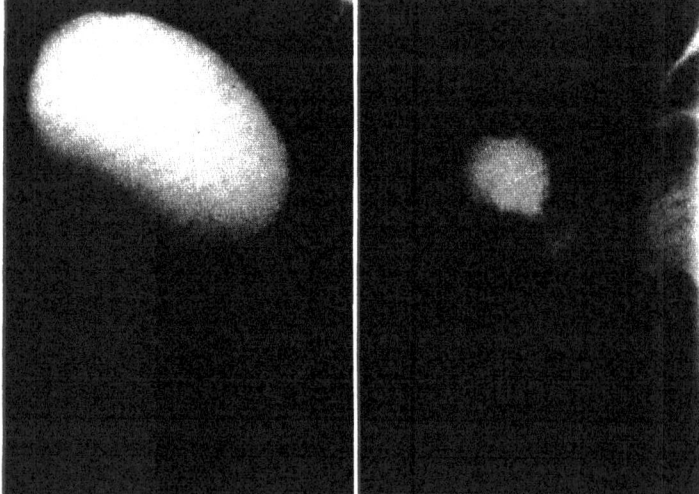

a, b

Fig. 2.4 a, b. Vesical contraction ring. **a** At MCU at the start of voiding the bladder contour is smooth and round. The urethra is normal. **b** As voiding proceeds a contraction ring develops. There is narrowing of the lumen of the bladder with an upper, densely opacified larger component and a smaller, less densely opacified lower component, between which lies the contraction ring. At a superficial glance, these features might give the impression of some sort of deformity of the bladder base and proximal urethra. The key to avoiding any such error lies in defining the vesico-urethral junction; this information can be derived from **a**

2.4 Injection Urethrography

The role of such studies is *very* limited in paediatric uroradiology. Urethrography is used to define strictures in the male urethra. Almost invariably such strictures originate from a traumatic episode or arise as a complication following some form of urethroplasty in a male.

An *end-hole* catheter of appropriate size (6 FG) is introduced into the urethra and warm viscous medium (e. g. Umbrodil viscous) or Hypaque may be injected slowly into the urethra (Fig. 2.5). Radiographs of an anterior urethral stricture are obtained and its site and length determined by this method. Some of the injected contrast medium may enter the bladder.

Injection urethrograms are generally not appropriate for the investigation of the many causes of obstruction which may affect the urethra in infants and children.

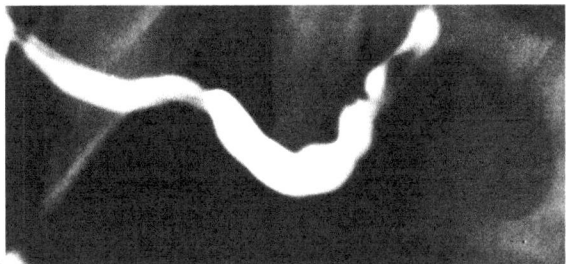

Fig. 2.5. Injection urethrogram showing the prominent verumontanum. There is a change in urethral calibre in this boy at the level of the pelvic floor; this is a normal feature which may also be visible at MCU

2.5 Retrograde and Descending Contrast Medium Studies by Injection

Contrast medium, diluted as for cystography, may be injected into the upper urinary tract. Nephrostomy, pyelostomy and ureterostomy all provide routes for injection. Direct puncture into the kidney calyx in hydronephrosis under heavy sedation or anaesthesia may also be carried out − the so-called antegrade pyelogram. Retrograde pyelograms are an exceptional event these days and for these contrast medium is injected through a catheter passed into the ureter (Fig. 2.6).

The purpose of such injections can be to (i) define structures which otherwise are not shown (e. g. hydrocalicosis), (ii) demonstrate levels of obstruc-

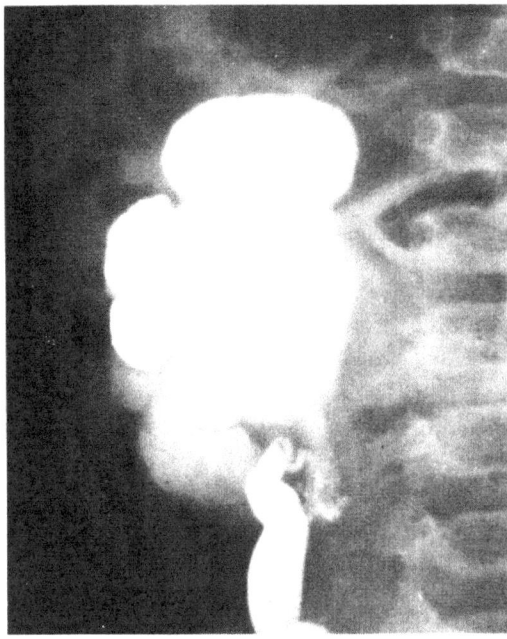

Fig. 2.6. Retrograde pyelogram. The injection of contrast medium into the ureter has slightly dilated the ureter, but at the pelvi-ureteric junction and immediately below there is extreme narrowing. Proximally the pelvic and calyx dilatation is show, indicating obstruction. Note ureteral trauma and leak

tion, and (iii) study urine flow patterns and ureteric peristalsis as part of a urodynamics study of the upper tract.

2.6 Ultrasonography

2.6.1 Preparation

Special preparation for a child undergoing its first urinary tract ultrasound examination is not necessary. This gives echography one of its supreme advantages: as soon as the radiologist or clinician has decided to use ultrasound the only limiting factor is the availability of personnel and equipment. The child does not have to be fasted or wait for appropriate radiopharmaceuticals to be obtained.

The renal areas are always amenable for echographic review and at the same investigation one can examine the bladder. If this is not full enough for adequate examination, and the clinical situation permits, the child can be given fruit-flavoured water to drink and re-examined after an appropriate wait in the department. The use of an ice-cold drink facilitates rapid filling of the bladder.

During the first examination the entire abdomen can also be scrutinised and if satisfactory visualization cannot be achieved either because of interfering bowel gas, barium in the gut or lack of co-operation, the child can be re-examined at some future time and appropriate preparation such as fasting arranged. In ideal practice such children should be re-examined before their breakfast the following day, to make use of the natural overnight fast and lessen discomfort for the child and its attendants.

Older children with bladder control can be asked not to empty their bladder before coming to the department, and in addition they may be given drinks beforehand.

2.6.2 Sedation

At the Hospital for Sick Children we make a point of not sedating children, and we have found that diagnostic scans can be obtained in most cases at the price of having to bring the child back to complete the examination on a separate occasion.

The option of sedation is always available however in those few children in whom the ultrasonic information is crucial, and this can be discussed and arranged with the clinical team.

Every child is accompanied by a parent, other relative, or nurse known to the child. This personal source of comfort and confidence facilitates the examination.

2.6.3 The Room

It goes without saying that the equipment should if possible be placed in a warm quiet room *which is adequately lit*. Undoubtedly entering a darkened room or being plunged into darkness is not conducive to tranquillity in young patients.

An overhead heating apparatus will be necessary for the study of small babies.

2.6.4 Equipment

Size. The ultrasound apparatus should in preference be small, or in particular that part of the apparatus applied to the child and hanging over the child should be small and unintimidating.

TV Monitors. It is essential to have the diagnostic monitors placed at a height which is comfortable for the operator who is looking at them and it is helpful if one of the monitors can be seen by the child and

parent. Older children may appreciate the customary familiarity of "watching the telly" and their curiosity may encourage co-operation. The parent's ability to see what is going on, despite the probable meaninglessness of the images, can increase their feeling of involvement in the child's management.

Image Polarity. There is no accepted convention with regard to presentation of echograms with echoes being represented as black dots on a white ground or white dots on a black ground. It is easier to see black dots on a white ground in a brightly lit room, but the human eye can see *small* low-amplitude echo differences better if dots are white against a dark ground. We have covered this problem by having two diagnostic monitors with the image in opposite polarities on each screen.

This speeds the examination as it reduces the necessity to enhance images during scanning to bring out differences at the high or low end of the amplitude range.

Transducers. For paediatric ultrasound it is essential to have a wide range of transducers, ideally differing not only in frequency and diameter but also in depth of focusing. We do not favour the use of biopsy transducers for aspiration and biopsy purposes.

Waterbaths. Waterbaths are essential for ultrasonic examination of other organs such as the eye and thyroid gland. Occasionally they may be useful in the study of the urogenital tract. This is especially so when examining infants and neonates in whom the spinal flexion reflex is so strong that adequate examination of the kidneys in the prone position is not possible, and also in those situations where there is a painful wound or incision overlying the area of interest.

Coupling Agent. We use ordinary vegetable oil of the cooking variety. This produces excellent coupling and is easily cleaned off the skin and clothes (patients' and ultrasonographers'!) Mineral oil runs off the skin more readily and is difficult to remove. We do however use small vials of sterilized mineral oil for cases in which infection may be a hazard such as when working near a recent operative incision. Proprietary baby oils should not be used as they tend to increase skin resistance to diathermy pads, and in any child who may be undergoing surgery soon after the examination this could result in poor function of the diathermy probe and skin burns from the diathermy pads (personal communication Mr. Taylor, St. George's Hospital, London).

2.6.5 Real Time Ultrasound Systems

Single crystal/hand guided/Compound B scanners, at the moment of writing, give the best resolution for static images.

Real Time Sonography (RTS) is bound to improve, and at the moment tends to take second place in abdominal echography. However, in paediatrics there are several distinct advantages:

(a) Difficult wriggling patients are more easily examined.

(b) Because of instantaneous image build-up, the examination is potentially more rapid and identification and alignments of blood vessels may be more readily identified.

(c) Vessel dynamics, tissue pulsations and responses to physiological manoeuvres which may be of diagnostic importance can be appreciated.

(d) Biopsy, diagnostic aspiration and catheter drainage can be performed, for it is possible to see clearly the needle entering the desired target. There is *no other method* which can give accurate placement of a *mobile* and *moving* organ such as the kidney in all three planes at one moment in time.

(e) The application of echographic diagnostic techniques may be more readily learned by those relatively inexperienced in its use and so they may provide diagnostically valuable information at an earlier stage of their training.

Ideal Characteristics of RTS for Paediatrics. There are several designs of RTS, the most widely available of which at the moment is the linear array system; however for paediatric use the ideal qualities are:

(i) The probe should be capable of looking through a small acoustic window.

(ii) It should provide for minimum disturbance for the child – this feature is a special consideration when contemplating units using mechanical principles.

Technique. In adult ultrasound examination it is normal to scan the kidneys with the patient in the prone position. However with children a different technique must be applied. Generally we start with the child supine and steadily attempt to complete a routine which should reveal as much information about the urinary tract as can be obtained. This routine is as follows:

1. Supine longitudinal scans. Upper abdomen.
   Starting near the midline a few sweeps quickly establish whether the aorta, I.V.C. and upper retroperitoneum are normal. This is the easiest spot of the paediatric abdomen for echographic

examination. There are no intervening bony structures and the child is not ticklish over the abdomen. The child soon realises that this examination is unlikely to be painful and loses apprehension, and the ultrasonographer can use this period to concentrate on the adjustment of factors and chatting to the child. The probe is then shifted to the right and longitudinal scans of the right kidney through the right lobe of the liver are obtained (Fig. 2.7). The particular information that may be obtained is:

(a) Relative size of liver and kidney.

(b) Relative echo texture of hepatic and renal parenchyma.

(c) Renal parenchymal structure – often this is the only position in which relatively clear distinction of the renal lobules can be made.

(d) Good visualisation of the upper pole of the right kidney. (There may be in rib shadow in the prone position.)

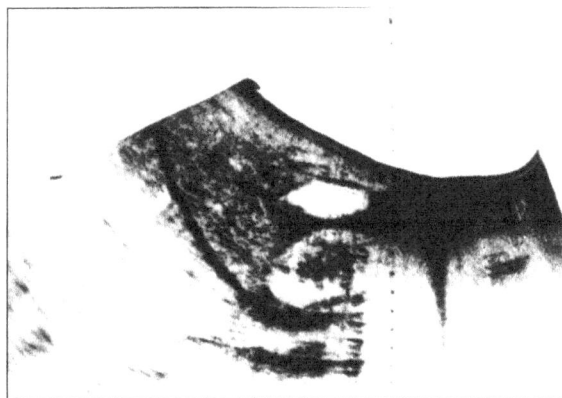

Fig. 2.7. LS supine echogram of a 4-year-old showing the upper pole of the right kidney, right lobe of liver and gall bladder

2. Supine longitudinal scans of the pelvis (Fig. 2.8). To demonstrate:
   (a) Bladder volume
   (b) Bladder wall thickness and any vesical sacculation
   (c) Intraluminal and extravesical masses
   (d) Abnormal ureters

3. Supine transverse scans of the pelvis (Fig. 2.9). To demonstrate:
   (a) Bladder volume [with 2 (a) above this can be calculated];
   (b) Ureters. These are best demonstrated in this position if care is taken to reduce sensitivity so the ureters are not masked by a shower of echoes.

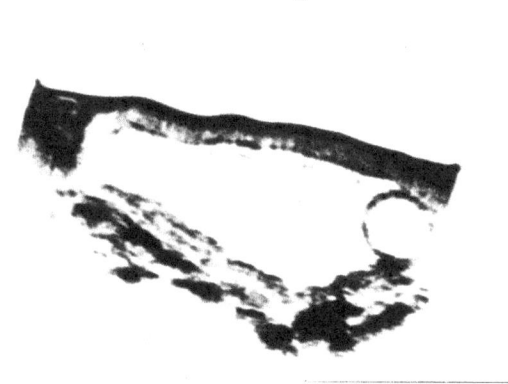

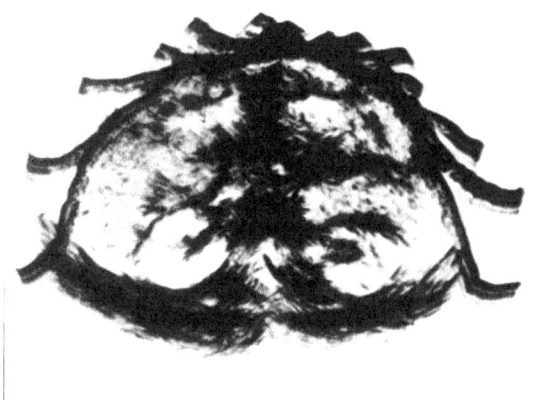

Fig. 2.8. Age 8. LS supine echogram of the bladder showing bladder wall thickening. The baloon of a Foley catheter can be seen at the bladder base. Despite drainage this neurogenic bladder was incapable of contracting further

Fig. 2.10. Age 14 months. TS supine. Unusual view of both kidneys from the front. In this child the bowel was fortuitously empty of gas

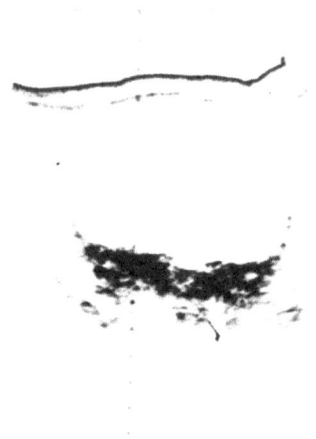

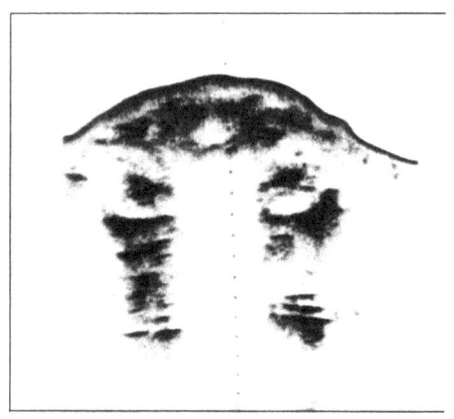

Fig. 2.9. TS supine view of the bladder, demonstrating normal ureters

Fig. 2.11. Age 4. TS prone echogram showing both kidneys, on either side of the spinal acoustic shadow

4. Supine transverse scan of the abdomen (Fig. 2.10).
   In this part of the examination the relationship to the spine is demonstrated of the right kidney and often some of the left kidney is shown. This is a particularly useful view for:
   (a) Retroperitoneal extravasation
   (b) Urinary ascites
5. Prone transverse scan of the renal areas (Fig. 2.11).
   Several cuts will show the relationship of the kidneys to the spine, their relative sizes, and any displacement or rotation.
6. Prone longitudinal scans (Figs. 2.12 and 2.13).
   These should be started in the parasagittal plane but obliques give better long axial views of the kidneys.

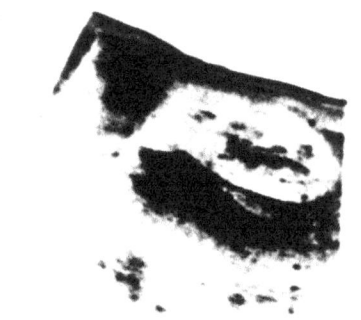

Fig. 2.12. Age 10. LS prone view of the left kidney. The relatively echolucent mass abutting on the upper pole is probably the normal left adrenal. The small mass deep to the kidney is the pancreatic tail

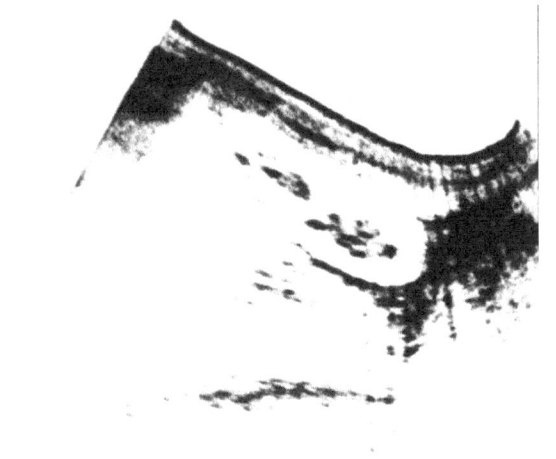

Fig. 2.13. Age 7. LS prone echogram of the right kidney. This girl has a duplex kidney with cortical thinning of the upper pole

This position usually provides the best views of the left kidney. Tilting the probe may also be necessary to "see" under transverse processes.

With small infants it is often easier to lay them on a pillow on the ultrasound couch and rotate the infant from longitudinal to transverse rather than moving the apparatus.

Using the above technique should provide good coverage of the urinary tract but often there are areas which are difficult to demonstrate; these are, particularly, the area of the mid-portions of the ureters and the upper pole of the left kidney.

It is sometimes possible to obtain supplementary information on the left kidney by either (a) coronal views (lateral decubitus position) and (b) erect views in which the kidney may drop into a lower position (Fig. 2.14).

The Future. Ultrasonic developments promise several potentially useful advances for renal echo-

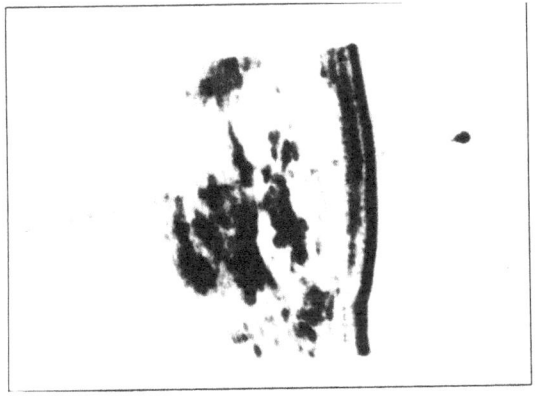

Fig. 2.14. Age 10. LS erect echogram of the right kidney

graphy. Improved resolution and focusing will result in better parenchymal detail. The advent of digital scan converters promises to allow objective quantifications to changes in the progress of a disease or its response to therapy may be better assessed. Development of combination B scan and doppler systems may provide non-invasive methods of estimating renal blood flow, perhaps even renal vessel flow. Already, echography is one of the most dynamic influences in investigation [10, 11, 12].

2.7 Radioisotope Studies

Technetium 99 m is a pure γ emitter with an energy of 140 KeV and this makes it an ideal radioisotope for paediatric purposes in conjunction with gamma camera studies. The isotope is eluted from a Molybdenum 99 generator and may then be labelled to a variety of different preparations often available in kit form. These radiopharmaceuticals allow very specific organ and cell types to be studied. Since the isotope is a pure emitter and has a half-life of 6 h, the radiation dosage to the whole body and to the specific organ is low when dosage schedules appropriate to the paediatric age range are used.

2.7.1 Kidney Scans Using DTPA

The 99 m-Technetium from the generator is labelled to the chelate, diethylene triamine pertecactic acid to produce 99 m TcDPTA. The labelling efficiency is high and the amount of free pertechnetate is very small. DTPA injected in a bolus intravenously is cleared by glomeruli with neither tubular absorption nor tubular excretion occurring to any significant degree. Therefore, clearance of DTPA closely reflects, glomerular filtration [13, 14].

Because DTPA has these characteristics it can be used to assess differential renal function; this can be done by comparing function in one kidney against function in the other. Renal plasma flow, glomerular filtration and renal clearance of DTPA may be derived from studies using this isotope.

Certain morphological information also accrues from such studies and this can, in broad outline, be presented as kidney size, considerations of the local contribution to overall kidney function of a part of a kidney, and by inference its local functional significance in the context of renal disease.

As the isotope passes down the collecting system into the ureter these structures are delineated and the rate at which the isotope disappears from them can be studied.

Thus DTPA evaluations yield information about overall renal function (the dynamic renal scan), specific localised deficiencies of renal function, and, sequential information about the way in which a kidney drains its urine through the ureters into the lower urinary tract.

2.7.2 Kidney Scans Using DMSA

For this type of study the 99 m-Tc is labelled to dimercaptosuccinic acid to produce 99 m-Tc DMSA. This complex has a high affinity for renal cortex. Within 6 h of injection some 60%–70% of the activity lies within the cortex, principally in the tubules.

DMSA is bound to plasma proteins, mainly albumin and α 1 globulins. Activity in the blood decreases from its peak to 20%–30% some 10 min after injection and declines further to some 2% after 24 h. Of the total injected dose between 2% and 5% is excreted in the urine.

The characteristics of this radiopharmaceutical carry, implicitly, the potential for accumulating data of a rather different type from that commonly obtained from a DTPA study. Imaging with DMSA yields a high level of renal detail; some 2–4 h after injection structural parenchymal changes may be identified with clarity and this may occur despite very poor renal function [15, 16, 17]. This makes DMSA scans especially appropriate for studying renal morphology, localizing small amounts of renal parenchyma (as in severely dysplastic kidneys which may have ureters draining ectopically) and identifying malpositioned kidneys which may possibly present as mass lesions on clinical examination. Nevertheless differential renal function studies may also be derived from the DMSA scan, but in this respect the DTPA scan generally yields the necessary information more quickly and without the higher radiation dose entailed in the DMSA scan.

2.7.3 Technique

All infants and children are examined with the camera face placed beneath the patient. Infants and most children under 2 years of age may be placed directly on the camera face. By examining young patients in this way the fearfulness induced by placing the camera directly over the young child is avoided.

Only very exceptionally is it necessary to sedate a child. In general it is possible to create a happy atmosphere in a brightly coloured room with the help of the accompanying parent or the nurse whom the child has come to know. Young infants will normally lie peacefully and quietly on the camera if they are kept warm and given a dummy coated with honey to suck.

To obtain a satisfactory intravenous injection of the isotope a scalp vein needle with its associated length of plastic tubing is introduced into a vein. Once this has been done and the needle is in position there is no pain and an atmosphere of quiet, so essential to the procedure, descends upon the scene. A three-way tap connected to a syringe containing saline allows the operator to be certain the needle is truly in the lumen of the vein and then injection into the vein can be achieved. A clean absorbent, disposable paper pad with a plastic back is then placed under the tap and syringe and the syringe containing the measured isotope connected into the system. The bolus injection of isotope is obtained by injecting first the isotope, rapidly followed by several millilitres of saline. There must be no constriction proximal to the injection site as the isotope and saline are given sequentially.

If an abdominal mass is present or if renal venous thrombosis is suspected the isotope is injected into a vein in the foot so that its transit up the inferior vena cava can be recorded and abnormalities of position or even of occlusion of the cava noted.

When the procedure is carried out in this way there is very rarely any need to restrain a child. The isotope injection itself is very brief, painfree and it has none of the minor systemic side-effects which cause a child undergoing intravenous urography to feel unhappy. Furthermore, there are no serious side-effects such as the severe reactions encountered from time to time with IVU procedures. These features and the low radiation dosage of isotope studies must be a constant encouragement to ever widening the scope of this type of examination and diminishing the use of the intravenous urogram. When taken in conjunction ultrasonics studies and radioisotope studies must be vigorously directed to this end.

2.7.4 Dose of Radiopharmaceutical

As yet there are insufficient data for dosage schedules to have been universally adopted and accepted [18, 19]. Our current practice is as follows:
(i) The child's body weight is known and using standard nomograms the surface area is ascertained.

(ii) A linear graph giving the surface area against dose is then used and this incorporates the adult dose and surface area – the principle then followed is to give the infant or child the dose indicated as being appropriate on the graph for that individual child's surface area.

(iii) For DMSA static scans only one adult dose is used for the calculation of the paediatric dose.

(iv) For DTPA dynamic scans three adult doses are taken into consideration depending on the known clinical context and these are
 – dose for when renal function is normal,
 – dose for when renal function is slightly to moderately impaired,
 – dose when renal function is severely impaired.

2.7.5 Pictorial Data

The human eye and perception can give rather a good estimate of renal function and a very good estimate of renal structure on images derived from γ camera isotope studies. If these estimates are taken in conjunction with other studies of total renal function then they gain further in significance. However, it is essential to obtain these images in a systematic way.

2.7.6 DTPA Scan (Fig. 2.15)

A bolus injection of the isotope is made. Images are recorded on nuclear medicine radiographic film (or other film) from 0–30 s. At 1 min after the injection an image of the kidneys is obtained by accumulating 200,000 counts and time needed is recorded. Subsequently, images of the kidney starting at 5 min, 15 min and 30 min are obtained over the duration of time as was needed for the imaging starting at 1 min. These images obtained in sequence are then inspected and an impression of renal function and

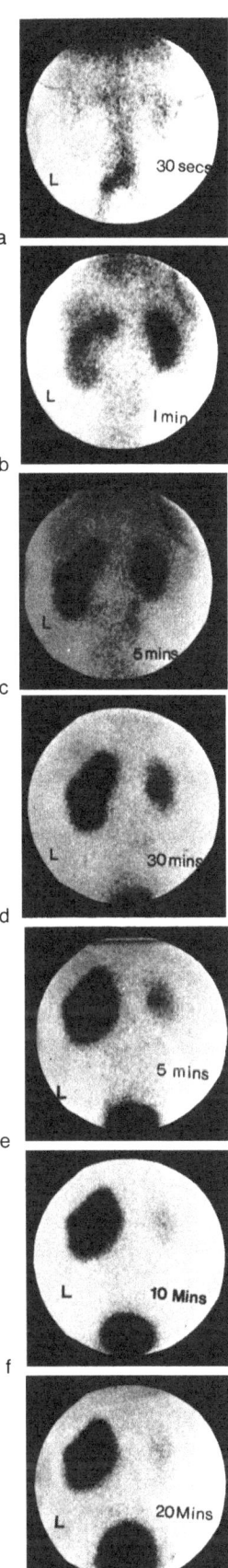

Fig. 2.15 a–g. Sequential scintigrams in DPTA study.
a At 30 s, vascular phase. **b** At 1 min, scintigram shows slower accumulation of activity with fewer counts in left kidney by comparison with the right kidney. **c** At 5 min, activity is seen in the right kidney, its pelvis and ureter, but on the left side the isotope lies in the parenchyma and the dilated calyces only. **d** At 30 min, activity is diminishing on the right side by comparison with the high overall activity on the left. Frusemide was therefore injected. **e** At 5 min after injection of Frusemide there is a reduction in activity on the right side, but on the left side overall activity remains high. **f** At 10 min, further reduction in activity on the right and no perceptible change on the left. **g** At 20 min, continued high level of activity on the left side with further clearance on the right: obstruction of left kidney in vicinity of pelvi-ureteric junction confirmed. (Same case as Fig. 2.2)

structure obtained. In the later images the way in which the isotope is cleared through the upper tract may be assessed. Certainly, by 30 min a bladder image must be recorded if it has not already appeared on the preceding images.

If there is accumulation of isotope progressively in either kidney or the ureters then a delayed image at 2–3 h is obtained. This will help in assessing the severity of any possible dilatation and, by inference, possible obstruction.

Should it be known the collecting systems are already dilated (say, from previous IVU study) then the significance of the dilation may be assessed, remembering that not all dilated ureters are obstructed. In general it is most likely that obstruction is not present if the isotope can be shown to clear on images recorded 2, 4 und 10 min after I.V. injection of frusemide. However, if dilatation is gross, caveats about interpretation have to be made.

2.7.7 DMSA Scan

Between 2 and 4 h after the injection a posterior image of the kidneys (200,000 counts) is obtained. An anterior image is obtained with the preset time needed for the posterior imaging. As with the DTPA scan an estimate of the functioning renal parenchyma can be derived simply by inspection of the images. If a structural abnormality is suspected pinhole collimator views of each kidney may be taken.

2.7.8 Anaylsis of Function by Isotope Study

An isotope complex such as DTPA can provide the basis for semi-quantitative and quantitative studies of kidney function, since it is rapidly cleared through the glomerulus [14]. DMSA although primarily used for imaging kidney parenchyma, may also give a similar yield of information but in a rather different way because it is handled by the kidney in a manner dissimilar to that of DTPA. And so for functional studies DTPA is generally the isotope of choice.

A rapid bolus injection of this isotope enters the circulation and arrives in the renal arteries, passes through the capillary bed and any of the isotope not cleared through the glomerulus enters the renal veins. This transit through the kidneys represents the vascular phase and may be equated with renal perfusion. A renal perfusion index can be calculated by assessing activity in the kidney in the earliest stage (1 min) following injection and comparing this with that in the aorta or iliac vessels. This perfusion index has proved most useful in sequential studies, for assessing events after renal transplantation and ascertaining if early rejection is occurring.

DTPA is cleared through the glomeruli. After measuring accurately the total dose of isotope injected (by assaying activity in the syringe before and after injection) the decline in radioactivity in the blood may be estimated 2 h and 4 h after injection. The overall glomerular filtration rate may then be estimated along the lines used in Cr^{51} EDTA studies – a method which has been well validated [20, 21]. To assess the contribution of each kidney to this overall total of glomerular filtration it is essential to select the appropriate renal areas of interest and the background levels of activity; background areas which are appropriate are those lying around the kidney bed.

After clearance by glomeruli the isotope DTPA is transported across the kidney and then it passes into the pelvicalyceal systems.

The form of activity registered in the renal areas as representing the vascular phase, the glomerular filtration and transport and the clearance into the collecting systems is represented in histogram form as shown:

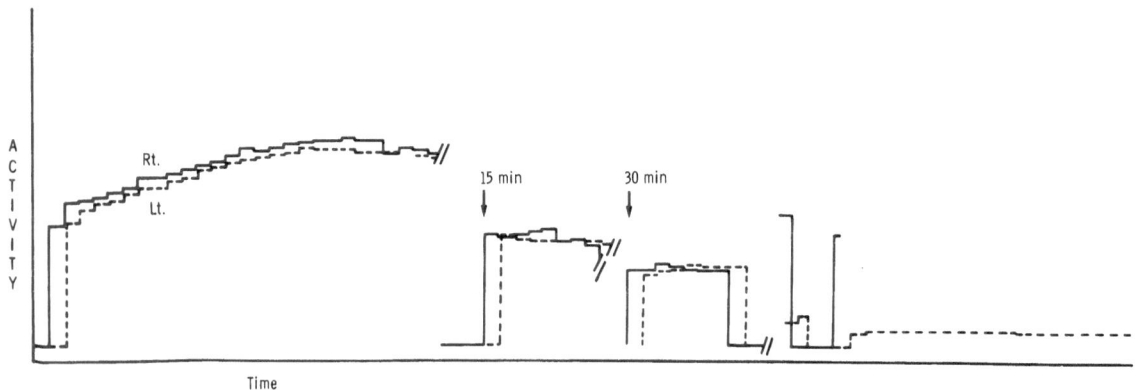

Fig. 2.16. Activity/time histogram in DPTA scan. *Rt.*, right; *Lt.*, left

Such data may be accumulated and analyzed by a variety of data processing systems [22, 23, 24, 25]. These may be programmed to give mathematically orientated data relating to the function of each kidney. This information and its form of presentation, whilst it is related to the system used, may be very helpful in assessing kidney function, especially in sequential studies. However, functional information of this type is also important in assessing status prior to operation and possible nephrectomy. Obviously, if the performance of one kidney is excellent and there is a clinical case for nephrectomy on the contralateral side functional isotope studies can be very important indeed. Provided quantitative assessments are made it would appear that no significant surgically operable lesion is likely to be missed by a dynamic renal isotope scan [49].

2.7.9 The Problem of the Dilated Upper Tract

In the presence of dilated collecting systems the presence or absence of obstruction may be difficult to substantiate. In such cases frusemide 20–40 mg IV may be given 30 min after the DTPA. A continual video recording can then be made for 10 min; images are obtained during this period at 2, 4, 6, 8 and 10 min with the same settings as previously described. A decrease in intensity of the renal images excludes obstruction. If no significant change is seen then no inference can be drawn since, in the presence of renal insufficiency, the kidneys may be incapable of responding to IV Frusemide.

During the procedure and the accompanying diuresis quantitative assessments of activity are needed if the significance of a dilated upper tract is to be determined in terms of whether or not it is obstructed.

2.7.10 Radioisotope Cystography

Since so much of the work in the field of paediatric urology is devoted to the study and surveillance of infants and children who have urinary infection and vesico-ureteric reflux, isotope cystography has been developed [27]. It gives a low radiation dose method of assessing these problems and is therefore potentially very useful for such long-term studies.

In radioisotope cystography the bladder is catheterized and drained of urine and 99 m pertechnetate is instilled into the bladder with the child lying supine, the gamma camera face being beneath the child. The bladder is then filled with sterile water to a point where the child wishes to micturate. In older children the camera face is been brought into the vertical position and the child repositioned. Boys stand and void directly into a receiver and girls may sit on a toilet seat with the receiver below. In the younger child (below 3 years of age) a plastic bag is placed over the genitalia so that all voided radioisotope is retained within a container.

Alternatively late in a DPTA study [29] the isotope may have been completely cleared from the upper tract and accumulated in the bladder. The child may then be asked to void and reflux is then assessed.

As vesical filling and micturition take place the events can be studied directly on the persistence monitor and recorded. Isotope appearing in the upper tract indicates reflux and the volume of reflux may be quantified because the amount of isotope and sterile water used is known.

Isotope cystography correlates fairly well with conventional micturition cystourethrography in assessing vesico-ureteric reflux [29]. The low cost and low radiation dose make it a preferred method for follow-up studies. Some authors [30] have used 99 m-Tc sulphur colloid particles (instead of 99 m pertechnetate) in the belief that such particles simulate more accurately the behaviour of bacteria in the urinary tract. However, the real relevance of this belief in terms of assessing vesico-ureteric relfux remains uncertain.

2.7.11 Imaging of the Adrenal Glands

99 m-Tc polyphosphonates are used in the study of bone lesions. Adrenal neuroblastoma may accumulate this isotope shortly after injection [31]; if a study for suspected bone metastases of unknown origin is being performed, then imaging the posterior abdominal wall structures may yield the gratuitous information about cause if a neuroblastoma is present. Similarly, because the kidneys have an affinity for radio-isotopes used in bone scanning a bolus injection followed by evaluation of the kidneys may show a previously unsuspected renal lesion [32, 33].

The adrenals have a proclivity for accumulating cholesterols, and labelled cholesterol derivatives may be used to image the adrenals directly [34, 35, 36]. This permits the study of adrenal hyperplasia such as may occur in Cushing's syndrome or the study and localization of an adrenal tumour. The tumour tissue itself may not take up the labelled cholesterol, as in the case of phaeochromocytoma, but the site of the lesion may nevertheless be determined by the change in size of the affected adrenal.

2.8 Angiography

2.8.1 Arterial Studies

Angiographic studies in infants and children with renal and urological problems are indicated in a fairly circumscribed set of circumstances. Paramount among these are the investigation of systemic hypertension and the study of recurrence of Wilms' tumour. At all ages the Seldinger technique via the femoral artery provides the method of choice for introducing the catheter into the circulation. Since the size of patients is so variable the type of catheter must be chosen to match the patient's artery size [31, 38]. *Radiplast* of Uppsala, Sweden, manufacture a range of catheters which come in complete kit form and are γ ray sterilized; these catheters are ideal for use in the paediatric age range.

For angiographic studies the patient may be either sedated or have a general anaesthetic. In any particularly nervous child anaesthesia is preferable and indeed, if the skills of a paediatric anaesthetist are readily available, general anaesthesia can shorten the time of an angiographic procedure.

Infants and children are of course small and their arteries are of corresponding size [39]. The detail needed in the image at angiography cannot be guaranteed to be of the desired quality if cinefluorographic filming is used. It is therefore important to use a cut film changer which produces the image on sheet radiographic film or 100 mm^2 indirect fluorographic film.

2.8.1.1 Injection Technique

The smallest possible catheter adequate to demonstrate the arterial tree is chosen. In infants and children under 2 years a catheter with external diameter 1.22 mm is used. In children between 2 and 15 years the external diameter measures 1.57 mm. Using a straight catheter with side and end holes a free flush aortogram is carried out. The tip of the catheter is placed at D.12/L.1 disc space. A rapid sequence of films is obtained (4 per second for 3 s then 2 per second for 4 s).

The catheter is changed and a preformed single end hole catheter is introduced. The renal arteries are then selectively catheterized. The sequence of exposures is less rapid (e. g. 2 per second for 4 s then 1 per second for 5 s). A hand injection is made for selective studies.

The contrast medium for the aortogram is sodium iothalamate (Conray 420) and the dose rate is 1 ml per kg. For the selective injection sodium diatrizoate

Hypaque 45%) is used and the volume of contrast varies with the kidney size and with the patient's age. For those under 2 years old between 2 and 4 ml is often adequate, but in the bigger child the dose may be increased up to 5–9 ml.

2.8.1.2 Control of the Examination

It is of great value to have a second experienced radiologist to review the films as they are processed so that the radiologist carrying out the catheterization is free to remain totally involved in the technical side of the procedure. When the procedure is finished, the catheter is withdrawn and the operator compresses the femoral artery continuously for 10 min, ensuring that there is a pedal pulse present during these 10 min. The child is not awakened from the anaesthetic until the radiologist has had an opportunity to observe the puncture site after compression.

2.8.1.3 Complications

The incidence of complications [40] varies with the following factors:
(1) Length of procedure: the longer the catheter is in the artery and the more often catheters are changed the higher the incidence of complications. (2) Age of patients: under 8 years of age there seems to be a higher incidence of complications compared to the over 8 year old. (3) Experience of the operator: the more experienced operator seems to have fewer complications.

2.8.1.4 Local Complications at Catheterization and Immediate Sequelae

1. *Haematoma.* If the catheterization has been carried out below the inguinal ligament (as it should be) any haematoma is readily visible at the site of the procedure. When a site above the inguinal ligament is used the blood can easily track retroperitoneally and so the bleeding is not obvious clinically until it either stops spontaneously or an emergency situation develops.
   The haematoma may be so large as to cause pain and even compression of the femoral artery, in such circumstances evacuation may be necessary.
2. *Obstruction to the Femoral Artery.* This may occur early and within 24 h of the procedure [40]. Uncommonly this complication occurs later. The signs are those of a threatened limb, namely, a cold white pulseless limb with a sensory loss. If there is no spontaneous improvement within 2–4

h, direct surgery on the femoral artery is mandatory to relieve the obstruction.

Late sequelae include the complications of limited limb growth and claudication associated with arterial thrombosis. An arteriovenous fistula has been reported following femoral artery catheterization. This must be a very rare occurrence.

3. *Other Complications.* Reactions to contrast medium are rare, possibly because most of these procedures are carried out under general anaesthesia. A subintimal selective injection may lead to infarction in the kidney supplied by that vessel. Clinically there is haematuria following the investigation, the patient is in discomfort and has back pain. The ESR and WBC rise and a mild pyrexia may develop. There is no specific treatment and therefore the operator carrying out the catheterization must be gentle, quick and develop an extremely sensitive touch. This is one reason why arteriography in paediatrics should be carried out by skilled operators.

2.8.2 Venous Angiography

Venous angiographic studies are of very limited use in investigating problems associated with the kidney and urinary tract. Inferior vena caval radiographic studies have been mentioned previously. However, the inferior vena cava is amenable to study with a very low or even no radiation dose by either pedal isotope injection or by ultrasonic examination. Catheterization of the venous circulation is needed to acquire blood samples for plasma resin assays in children with hypertension.

2.9 Urodynamics

2.9.1 Indications

The principal use of this procedure is to study the significance of dilatation in the urinary tract [41] – especially ureteric dilatation. In the vast majority of patients other techniques give sufficient information to allow a presumptive diagnosis of obstruction. This is not invariably the case however. Among those in whom a diagnostic problem remains are patients who have had some form of ureteric reimplantation procedure into the bladder and in whom upper tract distension remains and also those in whom a lower urinary tract obstruction has been

removed (e. g. posterior urethral valves) and yet upper tract distension persists or progresses.

2.9.2 Method

The objective is to perfuse the ureter at a known rate of 10 ml per minute (or less in the very young) and record the pressure response which develops at a known perfusion rate [42]. If no obstruction is present there is no rise in pressure as perfusion proceeds. When obstruction is present the pressure rises progressively to reach a plateau usually at about 20 cm of water. Obviously the perfusion fluid must be seen to cross the site of suspected obstruction and so this can be elucidated by putting contrast medium into the perfusion fluid (e. g. dilute sodium diatrizoate) and observing events by fluoroscopy.

The ways in which perfusion can be achieved are by using a surgical site of drainage, such as a pyelostomy or ureterostomy above the level of suspected obstruction. Direct puncture and cannulation of the dilated upper tract can be prior to an operative procedure and during operation, or as a separate investigation prior to a possible operation. With the appropriate apparatus the procedure is simple and straightforward.

There are, however, results which may mislead; if the urinary tract above a possible obstruction is very distensible there may be no rise in pressure as perfusion continues for quite a long time. What happens is that the upper tract distends progressively without transit distally of the perfusing fluid – this simply underlines the need to observe carefully at fluoroscopy the moment of transit of contrast medium through the site of obstruction and correlate this with the pressure profile during perfusion. Another misleading result can arise with possible obstruction at the uretero-vesical junction. After reimplantation and when there is marked vesical hypertrophy the characteristics of the intramural section of the ureter may change with variations in vesical capacity and there are two not uncommon variants: when the bladder is completely empty and its wall thickened there may be an obstruction present; and, when the bladder is considerably distended there may be a pressure gradient in such circumstances but none when the bladder volume is less. These findings suggest that in urodynamic studies for suspected obstruction at the uretero-vesical junction it is wise to know the bladder volume and pressure and these can be ascertained by catheterizing the bladder and filling the bladder in a controlled way from below. Cystometrogram studies lie outside the scope of this book [43].

2.10 Computed Tomography

The role of computed tomography [45, 45, 46, 47, 48] in the investigation of the kidneys, urinary tract and adrenals is probably very limited in diagnostic terms; if other cheaper and less radiation intensive modes of investigation are fully utilized the contribution of computed tomography is distinctly circumscribed.

However, it is almost certainly the case that CT scanning is uniquely able to provide, in a non-invasive way, information about any possible intraspinal extension of disease arising in the adrenals kidneys and the vicinity of the urinary tract. A second important role for CT scanning lies in the localization of pulmonary metastasis in malignancies associated with the urinary tract. The exceptionally complex problem, possibly arising in the course of follow-up evaluation, may occasionally suggest CT study could be helpful: in such circumstances the information of meaning and value which accrues can be disappointing in its paucity.

This may appear to some to be a severe criticism of the role of CT scanning. Nevertheless in terms of management of the individual child's problem it is, we believe, a realistic appraisal.

2.11 Strategy and Tactics in Investigation

2.11.1 General Comment

Careful clinical assessment of the individual child's problem will very often lead to the primary diagnosis. The subsequent sections of this volume are concerned with the way in which investigatory techniques can confirm the clinical impression. Quite frequently the investigatory technique is responsible for defining the nature of the pathological process from the outset; and so the final section of this volume is devoted to a recapitulation of certain findings which accrue directly from investigatory studies.

In reaching a diagnosis a deductive method of reasoning is used. However, before undertaking the next steps in management a further evaluation of the consequences for the individual child is necessary. This evaluation is concerned in part with the lesion itself but also with the structure and function of the kidneys and urinary tract as a whole. In conjunction with the management procedures this evaluation represents an inductive process and the need for continuing surveillance logically follows.

Thus, investigation covers diagnosis, evaluation and surveillance. Each clinical problem has these characteristics to a greater or lesser degree. In successive sections these problems are dealt with but at this stage three important topics of investigation must be discussed: these are investigation of the very young infant; acute renal failure in infancy and childhood, and haematuria.

2.11.2 Investigation of the Very Young Infant

In the very young neonate and within the first 48 h of life there is seldom any need to carry out intravenous urography. If such a study is carried out the findings, or absence of findings can be totally misleading. The contrast medium may not be cleared through the kidneys in the usual way at the usual time and so no meaningful radiographic evidence is gained. When an early assessment of the urinary tract is needed then abdominal ultrasound study is the first technique of choice. The indications for such a study can be suspected obstructive uropathy, mass lesions in the abdomen, suspected ascites and septicaemia from gram-negative organisms. Finally, ultrasound studies carried out prenatally may have suggested the need for post-natal check up in the newborn infant.

The principal lesions which lead clinicians to contemplate an IVU during the first day or two of life include multicystic kidney, suspected infantile polycystic kidneys, and obstruction affecting the upper tract and associated with a mass lesion. None of these conditions necessitates a urographic study in the first 24 h of life. Mesoblastic nephroma, being a primarily benign lesion with solid characteristics, should not precipitate an unduly premature IVU. Subsequently, examinations such as MCU, radioisotope studies and intravenous urography can be carried out after this preliminary echographic survey.

2.11.3 Renal Failure in Infancy and Childhood

The causes of renal failure in infants and children include the following conditions:
Renal agenesis
Severe bilateral renal hypoplasia
Dysplasia or hypoplasia in a single kidney
Bilateral renal cystic disease
End stage chronic pyelonephritis (reflux nephropathy) and nephritis
Obstructive uropathy (and obstructive atrophy)
Calculus

Acute parenchymal lesions such as:
   Tubular necrosis
   Haemolytic uraemic syndrome
   Bilateral renal venous thrombosis
   Acute pyelonephritis

2.11.3.1 Acute Renal Failure in Infancy

Young infants who have acute renal failure have developed or are in the process of developing serious fluid balance and electrolyte problems. An intravenous urogram with its high solute load simply adds to these problems and so it is best to avoid IVU if possible in the early stages of assessment and management.

Dilatation of the urinary tract, which is a feature of obstructive uropathy, can be assessed by sono-graphy. MCU will define lower urinary tract obstruction and its cause. Obstructing ectopic ureterocoele, which can be shown by MCU, will almost certainly have been shown at the ultrasound study. Urinary infection possibly with an associated septicaemia, may also be present in infants with urinary tract obstruction. Once the clinical situation is under control the IVU will give decisive information about the condition of the upper urinary tract.

Nevertheless early decisions about management are of cardinal importance. Central to such decisions lies the question – does the infant need surgical intervention or is the problem essentially one for medical management? After a plain radiograph of the abdomen has been taken echography can be carried out and analysis can proceed broadly along these pathways:

Findings at Echography in Infants in Renal Failure

A → *No calyx dilatation*   → bilateral agenesis/ hypoplasia
                                → multicystic kidneys – bilateral or unilateral with contralateral dysplasia
                                → infantile (neonatal) polycystic disease
                                → acute pyelonephritis
                                → tubular necrosis/medullary necrosis
                                → bilateral renal venous thrombosis
                                → haemolytic uraemic syndrome

B → *Bladder hypertrophy*
   Almost invariably with upper tract dilatation   → inference: bladder outflow obstruction → MCU (Fig. 2.17)

C → *Bladder dilatation*
   Usually with vesical residue and upper tract dilatation   → inference: possible severe primary reflux → MCU

D → *Calyx dilatation present*
Bilateral with two kidneys
Unilateral with one functioning kidney   → inference: obstructed kidney(s)
↓
Determine level of obstruction

Distal ureteric dilatation absent	Distal ureteric dilatation present
↓	↓
Inference: high obstruction (PUJ obstruction?)	Inferences: (i) Possible distal obstruction – ureteral or bladder outflow (ii) Severe reflux, maybe with distal obstruction ↓ MCU demonstrates bladder outflow obstruction or reflux – alone or in combination with obstruction

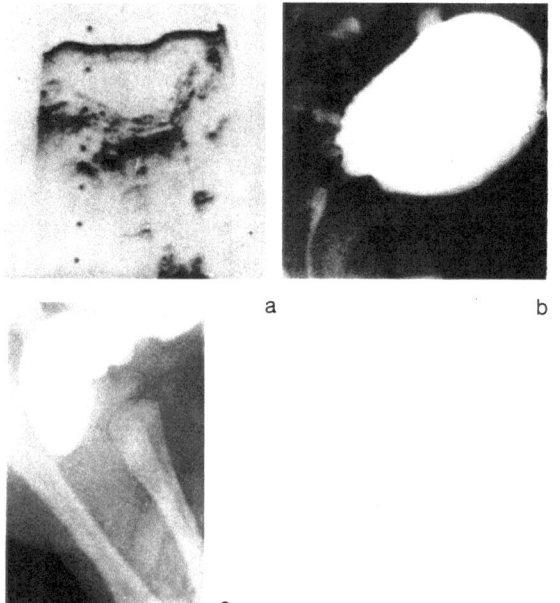

Fig. 2.17. a Echogram of bladder in a male infant with urinary infection and renal failure shows thickening of the bladder wall with no sign of sacculation. Inference: obstruction to bladder emptying. **b** Cystogram confirms the absence of very much irregularity of contour of the vesical lumen. **c** Voiding shows the presence of urethral valves obstructing vesical emptying

In group A and taken together with the clinical context the echonephrogram will often be decisive in itself and this is shown in subsequent sections. The clinical problem initially, will generally lead to appropriate medical management.

In groups B, C and D the possibility of surgical intervention must always be in the forefront of thinking even though preliminary resuscitative medical measures may be necessary. Frequently the clinical context is sufficiently suggestive – in infants with obstructive uropathy – for radiological studies such as MCU to be warranted as the first and most appropriate investigation.

2.11.3.2 Renal Failure in the Child

There is a group of children who develop renal failure who have a congenital anomaly of the urinary tract. This anomaly, but for the absence of urinary tract infection, would generally have presented in infancy. These children sustain kidney damage during their childhood years which is a consequence of the urinary tract anomaly which has passed untreated.

A major group of children in renal failure have had a urinary tract anomaly defined in early life. Remedial measures have been taken, but because of their limited efficacy or because the initial degree of kidney damage precluded satisfactory development of the kidney renal failure ensues. This occurs particularly as the child grows and the kidney does not, and so its function falls below that which is necessary to sustain further somatic growth.

A wide variety of innate abnormalities of renal parenchymal development – notably cystic disease of the kidney of various types – lead to renal failure as the years go by. This is because the potential for renal growth is not and never has been present.

Lesions of the kidney which are acquired during infancy and childhood may lead to renal failure. Frequently, hypertension is also present. Among such lesions are atrophic pyelonephritis, obstructive atrophy and end-stage nephritis. In common with many of the foregoing causes of failure the potential for renal growth has been compromised by preceding events.

Renal failure in children tends to develop slowly by comparison with the acute crises which are seen in infancy. The same principles of assessment as have been outlined for infants may be utilized in children. The inexorable progression of events in children under surveillance for known disease is, sadly, a continuing feature at the present time.

Bone disease is a consequence of renal failure in children and so periodic evaluation of bone status and development in children in renal failure must be maintained.

2.11.4 Haematuria

When considering how to investigate an infant or child with haematuria close attention to the clinical history, clinical findings and family history is essential. Bleeding may arise from any site from the kidney itself down to the urethral meatus. The causes may include neoplasm, inflammatory lesions (with or without infection), calculus disease and trauma. Very commonly indeed the cause of haematuria is defined by standard imaging procedures.

Given that there is no evidence of a blood dyscrasia, there is a group of children who have haematuria for which no cause can be defined by such procedures. In such circumstances biopsy of the kidney and endoscopy may be essential. It is often helpful to undertake less invasive investigation during an episode of bleeding, if it is a periodic phenomenon. Such timing of investigation may illuminate the cause and the level in the urinary tract from which bleeding is occurring, whereas at other times the studies may be unrewarding.

2.11.5 Objectives in Investigation

If it is the role of investigation to define the nature of a problem it is the purpose of management to secure as good as residuum of functioning renal tissue as possible. This renal tissue should be capable of sustaining life for the present and providing the potential for renal growth which the child's growth will demand.

When problems are not defined accurately then inevitably management is a risk business. The risk for the child is that he will be left unnecessarily vulnerable. The residuum of renal tissue may be inadequate for his present needs; it may compromise his prospects for the future.

Paediatric urology and nephrology are devoted to the protection and conservation of kidney tissue. None of this should be allowed to deteriorate or be sacrificed without good reason, but sometimes, unfortunately, innate problems of development may present an impossible handicap. Nevertheless, when one kidney is affected by a lesion the extent of involvement of that kidney must be known. Circumstances such as malignancy may necessitate total nephrectomy. If only part of a kidney is damaged, irrevocable total nephrectomy may be both avoidable and unwise; and so inexorably, the child with only one kindney always presents distinctive problems. Equally it is imperative to know the true status of the contralateral kidney when disease is apparently unilateral. Of course, prognosis may be determined for all time by these considerations.

All these things may appear to be self-evident truths. However, human perception is, on occasion, dominated by intuition and impulse. In infants and children investigation of the kidney and urinary tract should not be such an occasion. From the outset and during surveillance there must always be an objective assessment and analysis to answer the clinical questions.

References

1. Hayek, H. W., Fleishhauer, G., Ecker, G., Kampf, S. C.: Metabolic changes in high dose urography in babies. Ann. Radiol. (Paris) **18**, 325 (1975)
2. Standen, J. M., Nogrady, M. B., Dunbar, J. S., Goldbloom, R. B.: The osmotic effects of methylglucamine diatrizoate (renografin 60) in intravenous urography in infants. Am. J. Roentgenol. **93**, 473 (1965)
3. Tucker, A. S., Izant, R. J.: Inferior venacavography. In: Progress in pediatric radiology. Kaufmann, H. (ed.), Vol. 3, p. 82. Basel, Chicago: Karger, Year Book 1970
4. Saxton, H. M.: Urography. Brit. J. Radiol. **42**, 321 (1969)
5. Cattell, W. R.: Excretory pathways for contrast media. Invest. Radiol. **5**, 485 (1970)
6. O'Connor, J. F., Neuhauser, E. B. D.: Total body opacification on conventional and high dose intravenous urography in infancy. Am. J. Roentgenol. **90**, 63 (1963)
7. Lalli, A. F.: Urographic contrast medium reactions and anxiety. Radiology **112**, 267 (1974)
8. Lalli, A. F.: Urography, shock reaction and repeated urography (Editorial). Am. J. Roentgenol. **125**, 264 (1975)
9. Claus, D.: Systematic use of suprapubic bladder puncture for voiding cysto-urethrography in infants and children. Ann. Radiol. (Paris) **18**, 331 (1975)
10. Hünig, R.: Ultrasonic diagnosis in pediatrics. Pediatr. Radiol. **4**, 108, 175 (1976)
11. Edell, S., Zegel, H.: Ultrasonics evaluation of renal calculi. Am. J. Roentgenol. **130**, 261 (1978)
12. Wilson, D. A., Stacy, T. M., Smith, E. I.: Ultrasound diagnosis of hydrocolpos and hydrometrocolpos. Radiology **128**, 451 (1978)
13. Chervu, L. R., Lee, H. B., Goyal, Q., Blaufox, M. D.: Use of 99 m Tc-Cu-DTPA complex as a renal function agent. J. Nucl. Med. Allied. Sci. **18**, 62 (1977)
14. Wilson, A. J. W., Mistry, R. D., Maisey, M. N.: 99 m Tc DPTA for the measurement of glomerular filtration rate. Br. J. Radiol. **49**, 794 (1976)
15. Enlander, D., Weber, P. M., Remedios, L. V. dos: Renal cortical imaging in 35 patients; superior quality with 99 m Tc DMSA. J. Nucl. Med. Allied. Sci. **15**, 743 (1974)
16. Handmaker, H., Young, B. W., Lowenstein, J. M.: Clinical experience with 99mTc DMSA (dimercaptosuccinic acid). J. Nucl. Med. Allied. Sci. **16**, 28 (1975)
17. Bingham, J. B., Maisey, M. N.: An evaluation of the use of 99 Tcm dimercaptosuccinic acid (DMSA) as a static renal imaging agent. Br. J. Radiol. **51**, 599 (1978)
18. Kereiakes, J. G., Fellner, P. A., Ascoli, F. A., Thomas, S. R., Geltand, M. J., Saenger, E. L.: Pediatric radiopharmaceutical dosimetry. In: Radiopharmaceutical dosimetry symposium, Oak Ridge, Tenn. 1976. HEW Publications (FDA) 76–8044
19. Keriakes, J. G., Wellman, H. M., Simmons, G., Saenger, E. L.: Radiopharmaceutical dosimetry in pediatrics. Semin. Nucl. Med. **2**, 316–327 (1972)
20. Ditzel, J., Vestergard, P., Brinklov, M.: Glomerular filtration rate determined by 51_{Cr}EDTA complex. Scand. J. Urol. Nephrol. **B**, 166–170 (1972)
21. Chantler, C., Barratt, T. M.: Estimation of glomerular filtration rate from plasma clearance of 51 chromium editis acid. Arch. Dis. Child. **47**, 613 (1972)
22. Tamminen, T. E., Riihimäki, E. J., Tahti, E. E.: A gamma camera method for quantiation of split renal function in children for vesico-ureteric reflux. Pediatr. Radiol. **8**, 78–84 (1978)

23. Klopper, J. F., Hauser, W., Atkin, H. L., Eckelman, W. C., Richards, P.: Evaluation of 99 m Tc DTPA for the measurement of glomerular filtration rate. J. Nucl. Med. Allied. Sci. **13,** 107 (1972)

24. Piepsz, A., Dobbeleir, A., Erbsmann, F.: Measurement of separate kidney clearance by means of 99 m Tc DTPA complex and scintillation camera. Eur. J. Nucl. Med. **2,** 173 (1977)

25. Neilsen, S. P., Moller, M. L., Trap-Jensen, J.: 99 m-Tc-DTPA scintillation camera renography: a new method for estimation of single kidney function. J. Nucl. Med. Allied. Sci. **18,** 112 (1977)

26. deleted in production

27. Blaufox, M. D., Grushkin, A., Sandler, P., Goldman, H., Ogwo, J. E., Edelmann, C. M.: Radionucleide scientigraphy for detection of vesico-ureteral reflux in children. J. Pediatr. **79,** 239–246 (1971)

28. Conway, J. J., Belman, A. B., King, L. R.: Direct and indirect radionucleide cystography. Semin. Nucl. Med. **4,** 197–211 (1974)

29. Pollet, J. E., Sharp, P. F., Smith, F. W.: Radionuclide imaging for vesico-renal reflux using intravenous 99 m Tc-DTPA Pediatr. Radiol. to be published (1979)

30. Servadio, C., Nissenkorn, I., Baron, J.: Radioisotope clearance using 99 m Tc sulfur colloid for the detection and study of vesico-ureteral reflux. J. Urol. **111,** 750–754 (1974)

31. Fitzer, P. M.: 99 m Tc-polyphosphate concentration in a neuroblastoma. J. Nucl. Med. Allied. Sci. **15,** 904–906 (1974)

32. Mandel, P., Saxe, B., Spatz, M.: Urologic serendipity in whole body scanning. Urology **3,** 283–287 (1974)

33. Jackmann, S. J., Maher, F. T., Hatterny, R. R.: Detection of renal-cell carcinoma with 99, Tc-polyphosphate imaging of bone. Mayo Clin. Proc. **49,** 297–299 (1974)

34. Sturman, M. F., Moses, D. C., Beierwaltes, W. H., Harrison, T. S., Ice, R. D., Door, R. P.: Radiocholesterol images for the localization of phaeochromocytoma. Surg. Gynecol. Obstet. **138,** 177–180 (1974)

35. Anderson, B. G., Beierwaltes, W. H.: Adrenal imaging with radioiodocholesterol in the diagnosis of adrenal disorders. Adv. Intern. Med. **19,** 327–344 (1974)

36. Beierwaltes, W. H., Sturman, M. F., Ryo, U., Ice, R. D.: Imaging functional nodules of the adrenal glands with 131 I-19-iodocholesterol. J. Nucl. Med. Allied. Sci. **15,** 246–251 (1974)

37. Bergstrom, K., Jorulf, H.: Disposable equipment for percutaneous angiography in infancy and childhood. Pediatr. Radiol. **1,** 241 (1973)

38. Kirks, D. R., Fitz, C. R., Harwood Nash, D. C.: Pediatric abdominal angiography practical guide to catheter selection, flow rates and contrast dosage. Pediatr. Radiol. **5,** 19 (1976)

39. Mortensson, W., Hallbook, T., Lundstrom, N. R.: Percutaneous catheterization of the femoral vessels in children: influence on arterial peak flow and venous emptying rate in the calves. Pediatr. Radiol. **3,** 195 (1975)

40. Mortensson, W., Hallbook, T., Lundstrom, N. R.: Percutaneous catheterization of the femoral vessels in children: thrombotic occlusion of the catheterized artery, frequency and causes. Pediatr. Radiol. **4,** 1 (1975)

41. Cook, W. A.: Techniques and results of urodynamics evaluation of children. J. Urol. **117,** 346 (1977)

42. Whitaker, R. H.: Methods of assessing obstruction in dilated ureters. Br. J. Urol. **45,** 15 (1973)

43. Palm, L.: Micturition cystourethrography combined with simultaneous pressure flow measurements. Ann. Radiol. (Paris) **11,** 451 (1968)

44. Damgaard Pedersen, K., Jensen, J., Hertz, K.: C. T. Whole body scanning in pediatric radiology. Pediatr. Radiol. **6,** 222 (1978)

45. Bolt, D. W., Reilly, B. J.: Computed tomography of abdominal mass lesions in children. Radiology **124,** 371 (1977)

46. Brasch, R. C., Korobkin, M., Gooding, C. A.: Computed body tomography in children: Evaluation of 45 patients. Am. J. Roentgenol. **131,** 21 (1978)

47. Leonides, J. C., Carter, B. L., Leage, L. L., Ramenotsky, M. L., Schwatz, A. M.: Computed tomography in diagnosis of abdominal masses in infancy and childhood: comparison with excretion urography. Arch. Dis. Child. **53,** 120 (1978)

48. Montagne, J. P., Knessel, H. Y., Korobkin, M., Moss, A. A.: Computed tomography of the normal adrenal glands. Am. J. Roentgenol. **130,** 163 (1978)

49. Bueschen, A. J., Evans, B. B., Schlegel, J. U.: Renal scintillation camera studies in children. J. Urol. **111,** 821–824 (1974)

3

Obstruction in the Urinary Tract

3.1 Introduction

Obstruction to urine flow may be complete or incomplete. Since rates of urine flow vary, more so in children than in infants, there may be no effective obstruction at low rates of urine flow, but incomplete obstruction prevents clearance of high volumes of urine.

The evaluation and consequences of acute obstruction are covered in the following way. Acute obstruction of a previously functioning kidney is a rapidly occurring event which prevents flow of urine from the kidney. The causes and sites of obstruction are detailed, the investigation and management are described and late sequelae are noted.

Protracted obstruction to kidney drainage has an impact on the kidney and there is a wide range of causes. In infants and young children these often go under the title of "obstructive uropathy". Whilst there are many causes there are also many effects of protracted obstruction. Many investigatory techniques can and must be used to establish the diagnosis and then monitor progress for a long time. Since repeated investigation is so often required every effort must be made to validate the newer, less invasive modes of examination for these infants and children and also lower radiation dosage.

3.2 Acute Obstruction of the Kidney

3.2.1 The Role of IVU, Ultrasonics and Radioisotope Studies

IVU. When a kidney which was previously normal becomes acutely obstructed its size increases and it slowly becomes heavily opacified at IVU [1]. The increase in size is caused by the increased amount of glomerular filtrate and tubular content. This fluid, increased in volume, gives the kidney its increased density because of the increased number of iodine atoms in the kidney. The nephrogram of acute obstruction is slow to develop (Fig. 3.1) and reaches peak density at perhaps some 2–3 h after injection of the contrast medium. This time sequence reflects the increased absorption of water from the tubular content [2], which is then more concentrated.

Ultrasonics. Echography can be extremely helpful in problems of urinary tract obstruction – sometimes

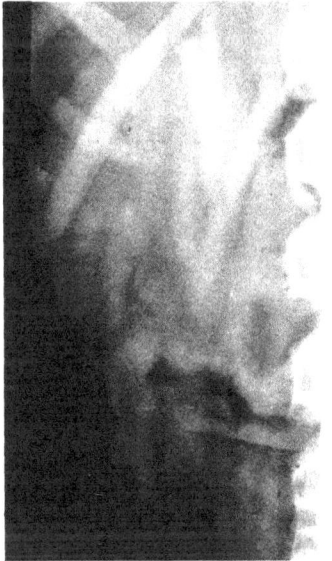

Fig. 3.1. Acute obstruction. IVU radiograph 35 min after injection. The acutely obstructed large kidney shows a late appearance of a nephrogram of progressively increasing density

decisively so. Its advantage over other imaging techniques is that it does not depend on function and therefore the "non-functioning" or "poorly visualizing" kidney ceases to pose such radiological problems as it did in the past.

A further advantage is that preparation is not required and the first study can be performed immediately an obstruction is suspected. Sometimes it may show an unsuspected obstruction, as say in the child with abdominal pain as a result of a PUJ obstruction with acute on protracted obstruction.

At the Hospital for Sick Children ultrasound is often performed during the IVU when a kidney is not opacifying in an expected manner. The benefit that accrues from this facility is a streamlining of the subsequent course of the ongoing IVU which then turns into a confirmatory investigation of the ultrasound findings. Of course this means that many children can leave the X-ray department more speedily with a firm diagnosis, or a better presumptive diagnosis.

Features at Echography. As ultrasound is a relatively new means of investigation it is pertinent at this point to list the information that can be obtained from sonography.

Number of Kidneys: of great importance if the obstructed kidney is solitary.

Size, shape and position of each kidney.

Parenchymal Thickness: valuable with regard to determining chronicity and the possibility of pre-existing protracted obstruction.

Parenchymal irregularity such as cystic change, nephrocalcinosis and scars.

Degree of distension of the pelvi-calyceal system and renal pelvis.

Filling defects in the pelvi-calyceal system and the ability to distinguish calculi by their acoustic shadow (whether or not they are radiolucent) from tumour blood clot and granuloma. The presence of perinephric fluid and the side on on which it lies and urinary ascites, should this be present.

Dilatation of the ureter (at times a normal ureter may be identified).

The level of obstruction of a ureter can be shown as follows:

High – no dilated ureter below the dilated pelvis
Low – dilated ureters visible behind the bladder
Mid-ureteric obstruction by inference (see below)

Bladder size and hypertrophy.

Intraluminal masses including ureteroceles and calculus.

Extraluminal abnormalities such as pelvic tumours or retroperitoneal malignancy.

However, there are limitations and among these are the presence of recent surgical incisions and dress-ings, peritoneal dialysis catheters, and sticky tape used for retaining catheters because they reduce the available potential acoustic windows and make positioning of the child for a satisfactory examination difficult. Furthermore, if the bladder is not filled with urine then examination of the pelvic cavity, including the lower ureters, is not possible.

Intervention. Finally, ultrasound can be used to identify the obstructed kidney for invasive intervention: (a) introducing a needle or catheter for antegrade pyelography, for accurate delineation of the site of obstruction; (b) directing a catheter for continuous drainage (nephrostomy).

Radioisotope Studies: dynamic DTPA radioisotope scan. The acutely obstructed kidney shows a slower build-up of isotope within its substance. As the activity builds up any underlying dilatation of the collecting system is seen as a photon-deficient area which, if late images are obtained, accumulates the isotope. The length of this study is however shorter than the IVU and the level of obstruction is not infrequently determined by $1\frac{1}{2}$–2 h.

IVU and radioisotope studies demonstrate on which side obstruction has occurred. IVU can show, with a precision which radioisotope studies may not have, the site of obstruction and clues as to the cause.

3.2.2 Causes and Sites of Obstruction: Evaluation and Management

Common causes of acute obstruction are calculus and blood clot and both may be associated clinically with colic and pain. An opaque calculus is usually visible on a plain radiograph. Echography has an important role either prior to or during the course of intravenous urography.

At IVU, as contrast medium passes from the kidney into the renal pelvis, transit distally to the level of obstruction takes place. Obstructing calculi, either opaque or non-opaque are localised. Blood clot may be seen as a filling defect in the renal pelvis, ureter and bladder. At IVU as a child changes position from supine to prone to oblique and to the erect position the contrast medium mixes more freely with uncleared urine and this helps to indicate the level of obstruction earlier in an IVU series.

There is a good case for performing an IVU during the acute obstructive episode for it can define the side and the nature of the problem clearly at that time.

As opaque calculi travel down a ureter distally their movement can be recorded on plain radiographs. A repeat IVU can show, after an interval, the relief of acute obstruction and a recovery from acute obstruction. Radioisotope studies using DTPA (a low radiation dose technique) provide quantitative evidence of each kidney's performance, and so recovery or deterioration can be assessed.

3.2.3 Late Consequences of Acute Kidney Obstruction

If a calculus impacts in a ureter or if there has been surgical damage to the ureteric lumen then obstruction continues and *obstructive renal atrophy* develops. This can be shown at IVU when the clubbed calyces are covered by a thinned renal parenchyma. Some renal function may be preserved at IVU but often in a severely reduced form. Radioisotope studies can be used to assess the severity of such renal damage. Even though acute obstruction has been allowed to continue for quite some time, occasionally a remarkable recovery of function can occur if good drainage is achieved.

3.3 Protracted Obstruction

Obstruction often has its origin in the prenatal period. It may be suspected after birth or during childhood because of routine clinical examination, the advent of urinary tract infection, renal failure developing either acutely or over a long period of time, and failure to grow. Pain is especially a feature of pelvi-ureteric junction obstruction. Abnormalities in the act of micturition can also lead to obstruction being suspected. Trauma in a child leads to a clinical examination and obstruction of a kidney which is large may come to light.

In protracted obstruction urine continues to be cleared from the kidney(s) but at a rate of flow which is limited and may be fixed. When urine is cleared at a rate in excess of this limit then there is dilatation proximal to the obstruction. The term "obstructive uropathy" denotes all those changes found in the kidneys and urinary tract as a consequence of protracted obstruction; obstructive uropathy is a term especially applied to the very young with such problems.

The causes of obstruction are numerous and it is useful to summarize these and relate them to the type of investigation which may primarily define them. An IVU is generally capable of localizing precisely sites of obstruction proximal to the bladder. MCU is especially important in showing obstructions to bladder outflow lying in the urethra. Ultrasound studies are very helpful because they can (through inferences drawn from echographic findings) point to the investigatory procedure most likely to produce the decisive information leading to the next step in clinical management. This means that the patient is not subject to unnecessary, unpleasant and costly investigations which have a limited diagnostic yield. The need to take into account these considerations is especially important when investigating infants with acute renal failure, which is often caused by obstructive uropathy (*see* Chapter 2).

Radioisotope studies have a discrete but important role in diagnosis which is indicated subsequently and in the illustrations. Sequential isotope scans are most important in the continuing surveillance of patients.

3.3.1 Summary: The Potential of IVU, Radioisotope Studies, MCU and Ultrasonics in Evaluating Protracted Obstruction

3.3.1.1 Sites and Causes of Obstruction Shown by IVU

Dilatation of the urinary tract proximal to the site of obstruction is a feature of the IVU.

Infundibulum of Major Calyx
Causes: Intrinsic stenosis.
   Vascular compression.
   Tuberculosis.
Effects: Mild obstruction produces partial or localised hydronephrosis.
   Severe obstruction produces a "non-functioning hydrocalicosis" – both are seen most commonly in the upper pole on the right side but may also occur in horseshoe kidney.
Tuberculous disease may produce stenosis and go on to give extensive tuberculous change in the affected segment which becomes a "non-functioning" mass lesion.

High Ureteric and Pelvi–Ureteric Junction Obstruction
Causes: Intrinsic
   Vascular compression.
   Tuberculosis.
   Calculus.
   Intraluminal polyp.
   Malignant disease.
Effects: Dilatation of urinary tract proximal to obstruction – the dilatation may be considerable with loss of parenchymal tissue due to atrophy. If the precise site of the obstruction (e. g. high

ureteric versus pelvi-ureteric) is not defined the operation may be directed to the wrong site.

Mid-Ureteric Obstruction

Causes: Retrocaval ureter has a characteristic course. Neoplastic disease, such as lymphoma, neuroblastoma or ganglioneuroma, metastatic malignancy (Chapter 9) retroperitoneal fibrosis and chronic granulomatous disease.

Effects: Dilatation of urinary tract proximal to site of obstruction – initially the kidney may be large and hydronephrotic but as function deteriorates it may become small and atrophic.

Low Ureteric Obstruction

Causes: Distal ureteral stenosis
Ureterocoele
Paraureteric diverticulum
Intramural lesions as in tuberculosis and bilharzia
Vesical wall thickening in obstructed or neuropathic bladder.
Low ureteric calculus.

Effects: In general as in 3 above.

Intravesical and Bladder Neck Obstruction

Causes: Ectopic ureterocoeles which are large and tense, affect other ureteric orifices and obstruct bladder emptying (Chapter 6).

Vesical calculus impacted in bladder outlet (Chapter 5).

Malignant disease, especially rhabdomyosarcoma of either polypoid or solid type, and neurofibromatosis affecting bladder neck (Chapter 7).

Polyps prolapsing from bladder into urethra (Chapter 7).

Effects: Like low ureteric lesions but with an element of vesical hypertrophy of varying degree.

3.3.1.2 Radioisotope Studies

Dynamic DTPA Radioisotope Scan

Renal failure is always present to a greater or lesser degree in protracted obstruction, and so we tend to be reluctant to give the young infant the high solute load which goes with high dose urography and is necessary to determine the site of obstruction. Further, in the young infants with protracted obstruction and renal failure the intestine tends to dilate and bowel gas patterns mean that either tomography or a renal window view are frequently needed. The dose of contrast medium required for such an IVU is high and the radiation dose tends to be high also.

By comparison, the very small intravenous dose of radioisotope has advantages. It places no extra solute load on the kidneys, the radiation dose is diminutive and bowel gas shadows do not interfere with imaging.

The usual technique is employed and delayed images are obtained between 2 and 4 h. Early on in the examination the isotope accumulates in the renal parenchyma. The dilated collecting system is seen as a "photon-deficient" area. Slowly the isotope accumulates in the dilated collecting system and the level of obstruction can be assessed with some degree of accuracy.

Static DMSA Radioisotope Scan

The indications for this examination are to assess
(i) The amount of renal parenchyma present and
(ii) study split renal function. This examination is especially valuable when the renal function is either poor or very poor.

3.3.1.3 Sites and Causes of Obstruction Shown by MCU

Bladder Base and Proximal Urethra

Tumours such as rhabdomyosarcoma – solid lesions infiltrating bladder base and proximal urethra, and polypoid lesions producing intraluminal obstruction (Chapter 7).

Ectopic ureterocoele – extending across bladder base and involving other ureteric orifices directly, or prolapsing into the urethra (Chapter 6).

Posterior vesical diverticulum extending downwards to compress posterior urethra on micturition.

Post-traumatic stenosis of proximal urethra.

Failure of relaxation in distal part of sphincteric zone in neuropathic bladder.

Stenosis in female urethra.

Junction Posterior and Anterior Urethra in Male

Posterior urethral valves.
Post-traumatic stricture.

Anterior Urethra in Male

Congenital stenosis of urethra – variants are extensive stenosis and stenosis at fossa navicularis.

Post-catheterization stricture at level of suspensory ligament.
Anterior urethral diverticulum.
Meatal stenosis.
Phimosis.

3.3.1.4 Sites and Causes of Obstruction Shown by Ultrasound

Calyceal Infundibulum or Major Infundibulum

Difficult to distinguish from a simple cyst.

*High Ureteric and Pelvi-Ureteric Junction
Obstruction*
- Diagnosed by identifying dilatation of both calyces and renal pelvis, with variable thickness of
renal cortex and absence of a dilated ureter below
the level of the renal pelvis.

Calculi may be identified within the dilated collecting system by virute of their strong proximal echoes
and distal acoustic shadow, and, rarely, a calculus
may be identified at the level of obstruction. A
radiolucent calculus is likely to cast acoustic shadows but the scanning technique is critical. It is
essential to scan at low sensitivities with single
sweeps in order to accentuate possible shadows –
which could be small and lost by virtue of the beam
width effect.

Tuberculosis may be suspected by virute of more
widespread changes of parenchymal destruction in
the kidney with occasional high amplitude echoes
and possible acoustic shadows originating from
areas of calcium deposition (which may not be
visible on radiographs).

Tumours and granulomas (Benign and malignant
tumours) can be distinguished from calculi and also
their extent demarcated; tumours are more likely to
have echogenic properties similar to renal parenchyma, but granulomas in general differ by having
higher echogenicity unless necrosis is a predominant
feature. However, very often these fine distinctions
cannot be made in practice. Obstruction may be a
complication of tumour development with in the
kidney.

Mid-Ureteric Obstruction
The mid-ureteric portion of the ureter is often
frustratingly difficult to visualize echographically
even when it is considerably distended. This is
because this part of the ureter lies in the shadow of
the vertebrae and their transverse processes posteriorly, and gas-filled gut anteriorly and postero-
laterally. And so there is no sonic window allowing
access for the exploring sound beam.

However, if there is a sizeable lesion in the retroperitoneal region, it is likely to displace bowel and
then the ureter is more easily demonstrated. The
combination of a hydronephrosis and a retroperitoneal mass suggests a mid-ureteric obstruction. In
these circumstances the likely causes are lymphomas, metastatic malignancies, tuberculous ade-
nitis, other granulomas and retroperitoneal fibrosis.

*Low Ureteric, Intravesical and Bladder
Neck Obstruction*
When the bladder is at least half-filled or preferably
at maximum capacity echography can show the
presence of a dilated ureter or ureters behind the
bladder. Details of masses outside the bladder, the
state of the bladder wall and intraluminal abnormalities may be detected.

The presence of a dilated ureter behind the bladder
suggests possible obstruction. In the 'megacystis-
megaureter' condition the ureter may be dilated but
not necessarily obstructed. The echographic clue to
the fact that the dilated ureter is not obstructed is
that the calyces are not significantly dilated, and this
feature should be confirmed by study of the kidney.
However the actual cause may elude ultrasonic
evaluation; for instance, distal ureteral stenosis may
not be diagnosed, small tumours and calculi could be
missed, and bladder wall calcification from tuberculosis and bilharzia may not be appreciated if the
acoustic shadows are "lost" in the bowel echo
pattern beyond.

Vesical wall thickening can be effectively demonstrated by ultrasound; the thickness is inversely
related to the degree of bladder filling. If the bladder
is extremely thick walled, shrunken and indistensible
then it may be difficult to demonstrate it at all, and
of course any accompanying ureteral dilatation will
be obscured by bowel gas. The diagnosis of an
intrapelvic obstruction can then be inferred from the
ultrasound examination, but not with confidence. In
echography one can only be confident about positive
findings. Tumours at the bladder base, ureterocoeles
and intravesical tumours, calculi and blood clot can
be seen and demonstrated however.

This summary sets out the scope of various investigatory procedures. Each has a distinctive and
complementary contribution to make in the evaluation of the individual patient's problem. The
purpose of these investigatory procedures is there
fore to define with precision the nature of the
problem so that a rational course of management
can be pursued.

3.3.2 Defining the Site of Obstruction

3.3.2.1 Renal Changes Shown by IVU

(i) The "shell nephrogram". A thin layer of renal
parenchyma surrounds dilated calyces. During
the nephrographic phase the parenchyma is
opacified, but the urine in the calyces retains its
water density. The parenchymal image has a
curvilinear outline on the radiograph (a
"shell"). This phenomenon is seen especially in
young infants and is seldom observed in older
children (Fig. 3.2)

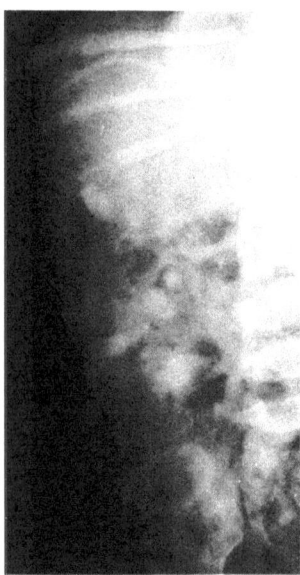

Fig. 3.2. Shell nephrogram. In this infant the contrast medium injected at IVU has faintly opacified the thin layer of renal parenchyma which surrounds the dilated calyces. This nephrographic phase occurs during and after opacification by the contrast medium of all vascular tissues, but non-vascular spaces, such as the dilated calyces, are not opacified. This is the whole body opacification effect enhanced by the nephrogram, which appears as a "shell"

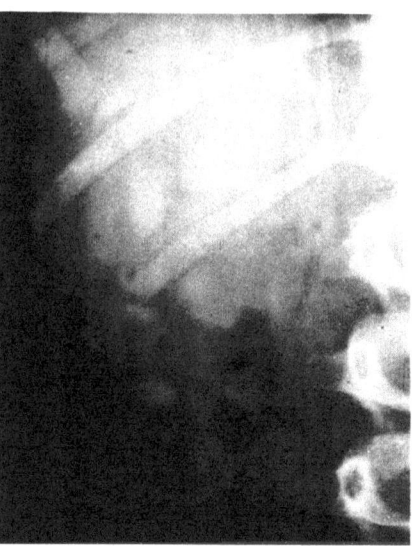

Fig. 3.3. Crescent sign. This young child had obstruction caused by a retrocaval ureter. Dense curvilinear shadows are seen because concentrated contrast medium given at IVU opacifies dilated collecting ducts. On this radiograph only a little contrast medium is seen lying in the posterior, dependent calyces in this supine child

(ii) *The "crescent sign".* [3] The anatomical basis for this feature is dilatation of collecting ducts lying in the medulla. These ducts run tangential to the margin of the papilla which surrounds each dilated minor calyx. As concentrated contrast medium from the tubules enters these ducts they become heavily opacified. Collectively the ducts show as a crescentic image on the radiograph. At a slightly later stage urine in dilated calyces is opacified by contrast medium, but the opacified calyx is separated from the crescentic image by a narrow black line representing the margin of the papilla. The crescent sign is seldom seen in infants. It is a feature observed in the young child especially (Fig. 3.3)

(iii) *Lacunae* in the papillae may be opacified densely during IVU in obstructive uropathy. The precise cause of these lacunae is unknown; they may be a result of long-standing papillary necrosis.

(iv) *Calyx Opacification.* Contrast medium enters dilated calyces from the kidney parenchyma. When there is considerable calyx dilatation the contrast medium may not mix with the urine initially and it collects in a layer in the posterior aspect of each dependent calyx in a supine child.

If a radiograph is then taken with the child erect the heavily opacified urine may form a layer in the lowest parts of dependent calyces. As time passes mixing takes place and the calyces are uniformly opacified: this may take several hours when there is a large pool of undrained urine. When calyx dilatation is not so marked the only distinctive feature in the kidney and calyces may be the early homogeneous opacification of the calyces (Fig. 3.4)

(v) *Changes in Kidney Length and Kidney Size.* The diuretic effect of contrast medium may be sufficient to distend the collecting system and even small changes in kidney length occur normally. In a child with a normal urinary tract very high doses of contrast medium, such as those given at angiocardiography, can produce quite considerable distension; but the free flow of contrast medium is always evident. With the diuresis induced by a high dose of contrast medium in protracted obstruction the dilated parts of the urinary tract may dilate further (Fig. 3.5)

3.3.2.2 Ultrasonics (Fig. 3.6)

The ability of ultrasound to diagnose urinary obstruction rests on recognition of the changed morphology of the kidney, collecting system and ureter.

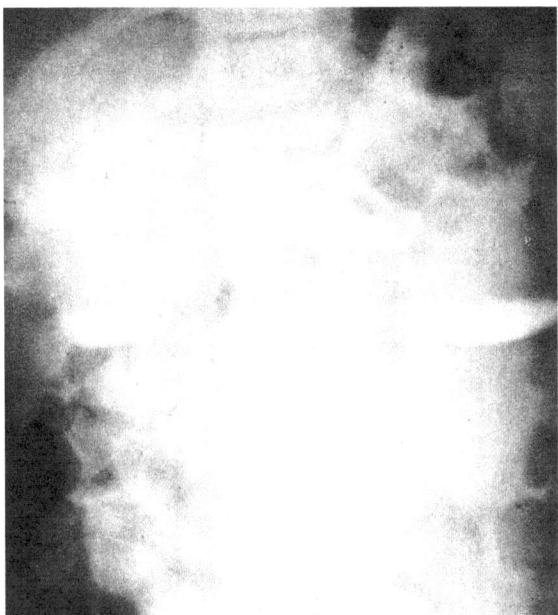

Fig. 3.4. Calyx opacification and layering effect. In this child with large kidneys the contrast medium injected at IVU failed to opacify the calyces when the child was supine. With the child placed erect, the contrast medium is seen as relatively dense layers in the lower parts of the dilated calyces

The Collecting System. The central pelvicalyceal echo cluster often has a small central echolucent area representing the small quantity of urine, in transit, in the renal pelvis. This can be striking in normal cases, but when this echolucent zone is of the same order of thickness as the cortex it probably represents mild dilatation (and by inference obstruction).

If in addition to the central cystic appearance the calyces are also visible as outpouchings, the dilatation is moderate. Marked hydronephrosis is indicated when the renal area is occupied by a virtually cystic mass whose outline resembles a silhouette of "Mickey Mouse." Severe hydronephrosis can be seen when there is almost total effacement of the difference between the renal pelvis and the calyces.

Parenchymal Thickness. Further valuable information is obtained by measuring cortical thickness. The relative thinness of this is related to the severity of the distension, the duration of the obstruction and the resultant degree of atrophy.

The Ureter. Although the normal ureter is rarely visualized a dilated ureter can be demonstrated. Sometimes difficulties may be encountered in establishing the level of ureteric obstruction, a point dealt with previously.

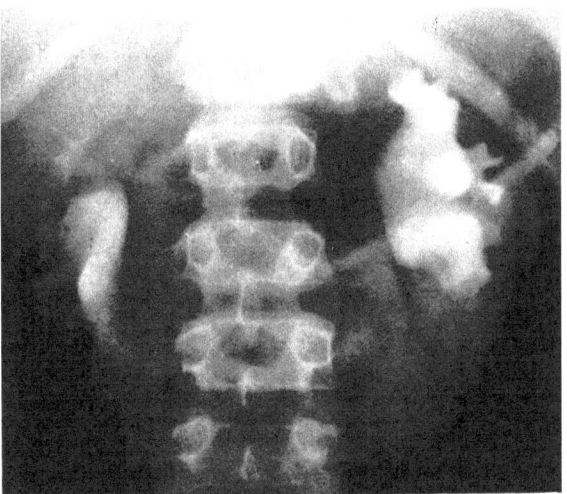

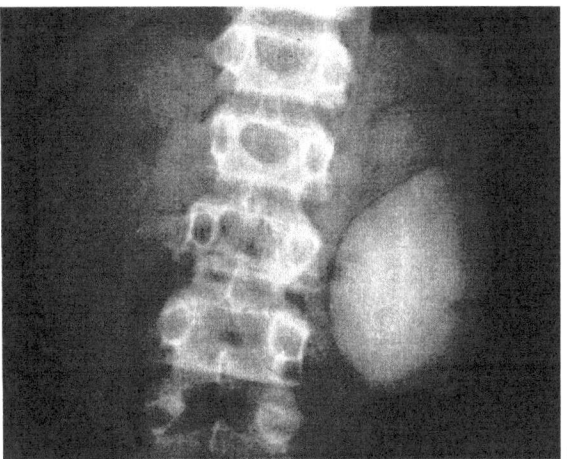

Fig. 3.5 a, b. Obstruction with increase in kidney lenght. **a** This patient with pelvi-ureteric junction obstruction has, in the initial IVU radiograph, well-cupped calyces and a rather box-like renal pelvis in the left kidney. **b** Radiograph taken at 45 min after the child has been put in the erect position shows the right kidney collecting system has emptied its contrast medium distally. On the left side the kidney lenght has increased by 15 mm, the calyces are rather blunted and the renal pelvis is increasingly distended. Similar changes can be observed in children with obstruction more distally in the ureter

Finally it is worth stressing again the advantage of ultrasonic study in the newborn and in older children when one kidney is poorly visualized at IVU or DPTA scan.

3.3.3 Obstruction Proximal to the Bladder

Above the site of obstruction the urinary tract is dilated and below there is no dilatation. Application of this principle in the IVU and in the DPTA scan

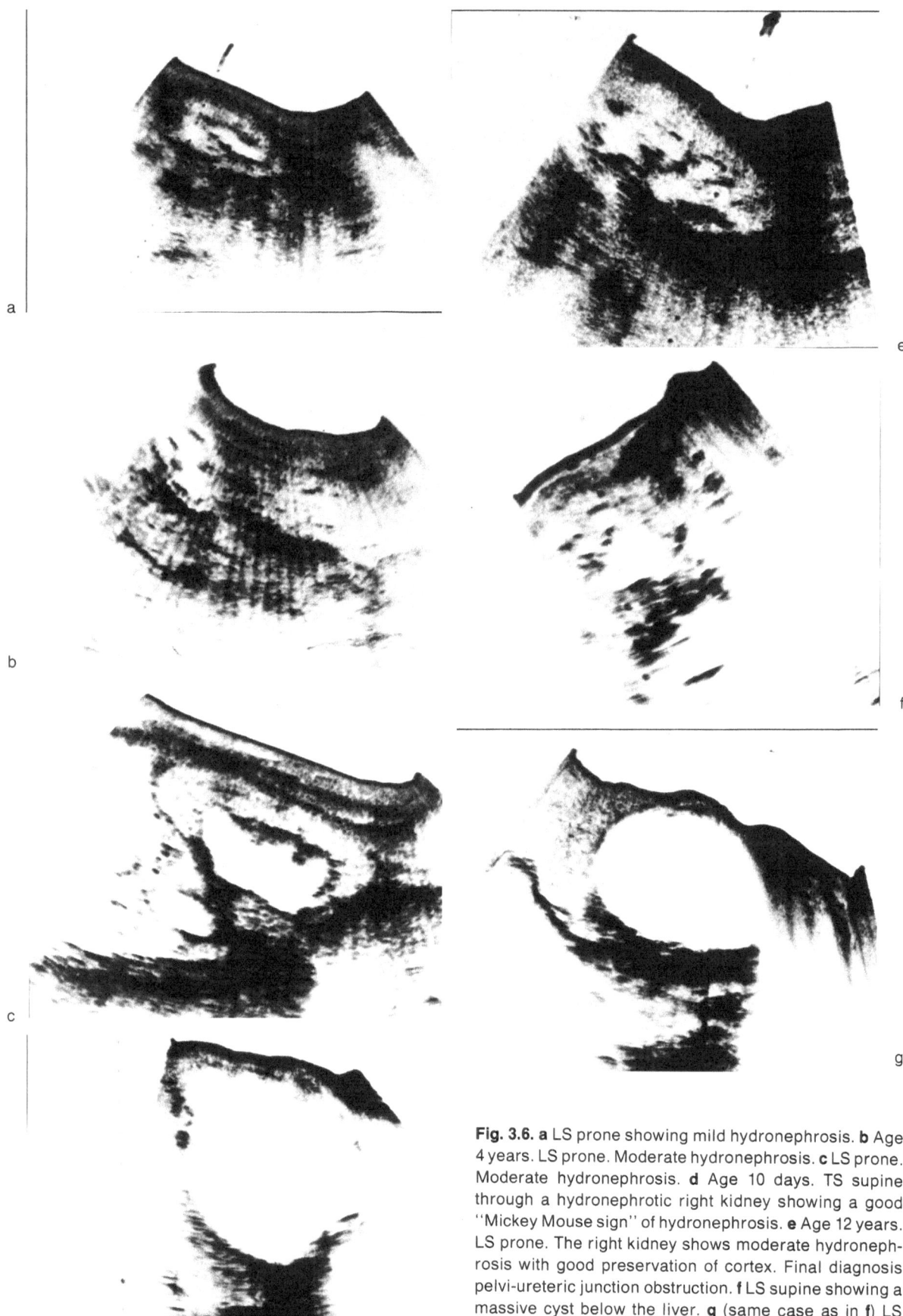

Fig. 3.6. a LS prone showing mild hydronephrosis. **b** Age 4 years. LS prone. Moderate hydronephrosis. **c** LS prone. Moderate hydronephrosis. **d** Age 10 days. TS supine through a hydronephrotic right kidney showing a good "Mickey Mouse sign" of hydronephrosis. **e** Age 12 years. LS prone. The right kidney shows moderate hydronephrosis with good preservation of cortex. Final diagnosis pelvi-ureteric junction obstruction. **f** LS supine showing a massive cyst below the liver. **g** (same case as in **f**) LS prone. A thin rim of cortex posteriorly and virtually effaced calyces show that this is a gross hydronephrosis

gives the site of obstruction and, by inference, the cause of obstruction. The degree of dilatation can be enhanced by high doses of IV contrast medium and by giving in addition a diuretic such as Frusemide. Injection of contrast medium directly either by retrograde catheterization or by antegrade injection pyelography can on occasion be used to highlight this change in calibre in the urinary tract.

3.3.3.1 Characteristic Findings

3.3.3.1.1 Hydrocalycosis and Partial Hydronephrosis
            (synonym: the upper pole syndrome)

The infundibulum of a major calyx may be narrowed either by intrinsic stenosis or by vascular compression. If the minor calyces draining into the infundibulum are grossly dilated and the associated renal parenchyma has poor function then *hydrocalycosis* is present [4]. When calyces are less dilated and they opacify with contrast medium then the term *partial hydronephrosis* [5] is used. Both hydrocalycosis and partial hydronephrosis affect especially the upper pole of the kidney (Figs. 3.7, 3.8, 3.9). Calculi in minor calyces are often associated with calyx dilatation but this is a separate matter dealt with in Chapter 5.

3.3.3.1.2 Pelvi-Ureteric Junction Obstruction
            and High Ureteric Obstruction

(Figs. 3.10, 3.11, 3.12, 3.13, 3.14 and 3.15)

Pelvi-ureteric junction obstruction occurs more commonly on the left side than on the right [6,7]. The narrowing may be caused by either intrinsic stenosis or an extrinsic vascular compression or both of these

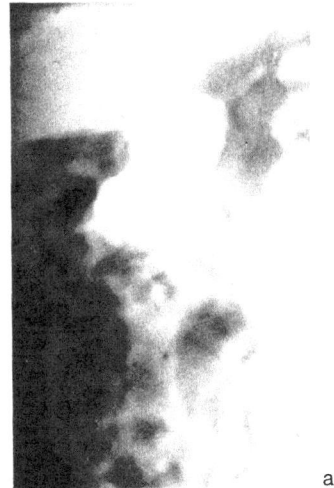
a

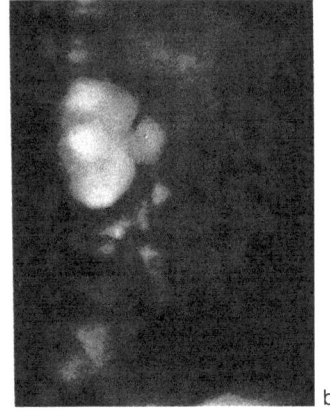
b

Fig. 3.8 a, b. Hydrocalicosis. This IVU shows on a late radiograph of this neonate that the right kidney has a dense cavity containing contrast medium at its upper pole (**a**). There is downward displacement of the normal calyces in the remainder of the kidney, well shown on the lateral projection (**b**)

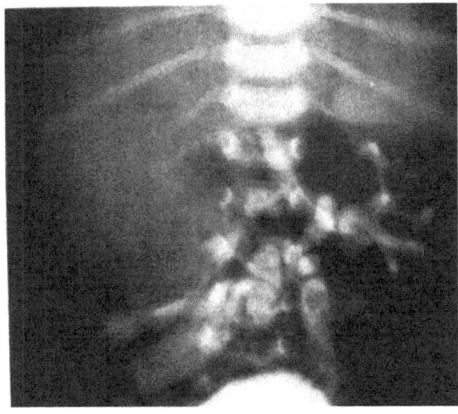

Fig. 3.7. Hydrocalicosis. At IVU this infant with posterior urethral valves shows distension of the normally located left kidney calyces. On the right side the calyces are displaced downward by gross dilatation of the uppermost right renal calyx – hydrocalicosis – and there is non-function in this cyst-like lesion

together. Rarely, polyps [8] in the ureteric lumen produce high obstruction, as may calculi. Typically the minor calyces and the renal pelvis are dilated and the kidney parenchymal thickness may be reduced. In sequential radiographs during an IVU series the dilatation may increase as the diuresis develops and the kidney length may also increase. The lumen at the site of obstruction may not be opacified on the radiograph when it is severely narrowed but the ureter below is undilated.

In doubtful cases a radiograph with the child erect will show contrast medium retained in the upper tract above the site of obstruction. It is imperative to define whether the obstruction lies in the pelvi-ureteric junction or in the uppermost part of the ureter. When operative correction is carried out the site of obstruction may not be so clear because there is no diuresis at the time. Obviously an operative

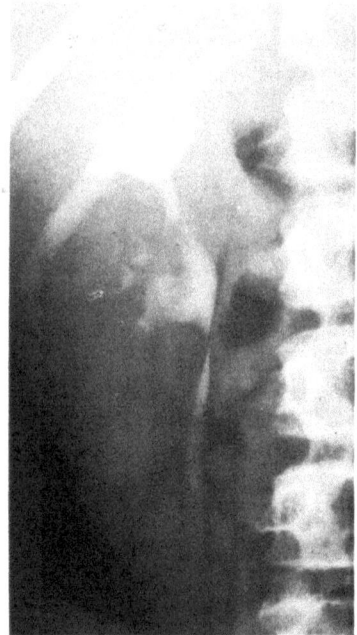

Fig. 3.9. Partial hydronephrosis. The upper pole calyces are dilated and there is loss of cupping of the minor calyces. The adjacent parenchyma is thinned. Across the upper pole infundibulum a vascular impression is visible

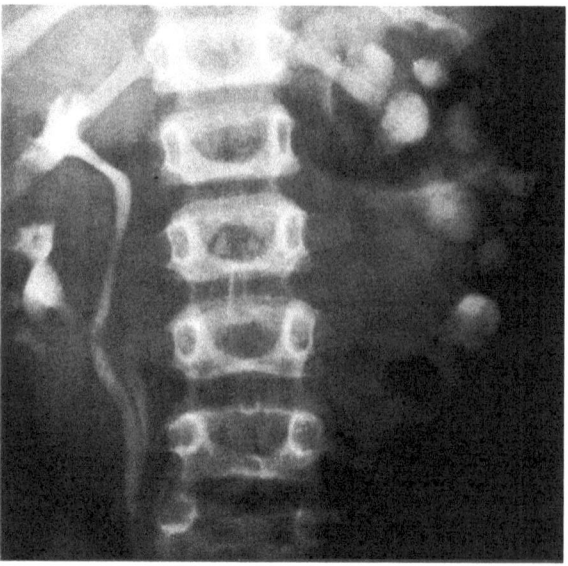

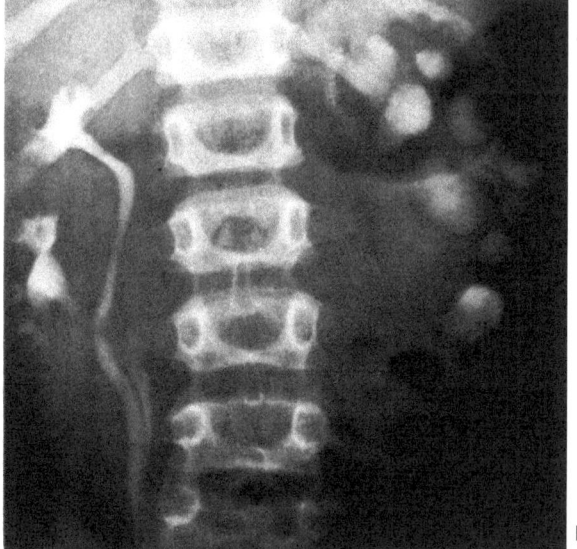

a

b

▷

Fig. 3.10 a, b. Pelvi-ureteric junction obstruction. **a** At IVU the right kidney is a simple duplex kidney, but the left has dilated calyces on the initial radiograph. **b** After injecting the diuretic Frusemide, the right kidney calyces clear contrast medium but the obstructed left kidney does not

procedure carried out on the pelvis and pelvi-ureteric junction is misdirected when the lesion is a high ureteric one.

3.3.3.1.3 Obstruction in the Middle Third of the Ureter

Obstruction in the middle part of the ureter is produced by relatively few lesions. Some of these are distinctly uncommon and they may be part of a more generalised disease process.

1. *Retrocaval Ureter.* The ureter becomes retrocaval [9] during those complex events involving the development of the inferior vena cava. At IVU the dilated ureter descends from the right kidney then sweeps upward and medially to a point where it passes behind the cava and is obstructed. Beyond this point the ureter is narrow as it descends down towards the bladder (Fig. 3.16).

2. *Retroperitoneal fibrosis and chronic granulomatous disease* with continuing inflammatory change and fibrosis narrow the ureter [10]. Dilatation proximal to the obstruction is present [11].

3. *Malignant disease* in the retroperitoneal region, especially Hodgkin's disease, leukaemia, lymphosarcoma (including ileocaecal lymphosarcoma) and sarcoma can also produce ureteric narrowing, displacement and obstruction.

3.3.3.1.4 Distal Ureteric Obstruction

There is dilatation of the calyces of the kidney which may also show atrophic changes. The ureter is dilated down to the point of obstruction. Among the causes of obstruction at this level, as a specifically urological problem, is distal ureteral stenosis [12, 13, 14] (Figs. 3.17, 3.18, 3.19, 3.20). Continuing dilatation of a ureter after reimplantation in the bladder

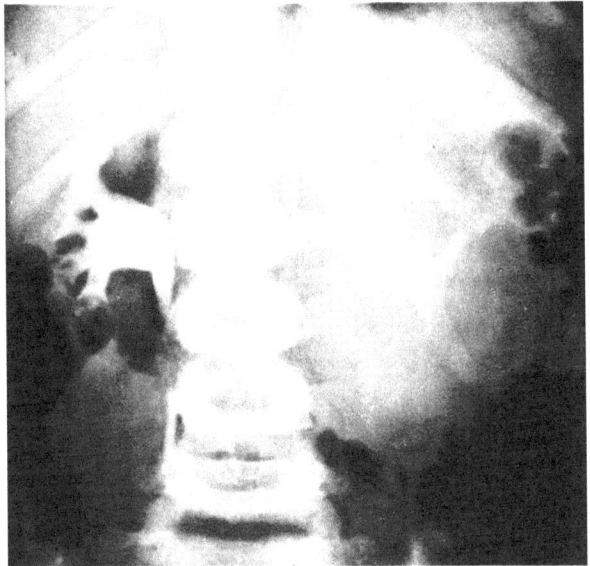 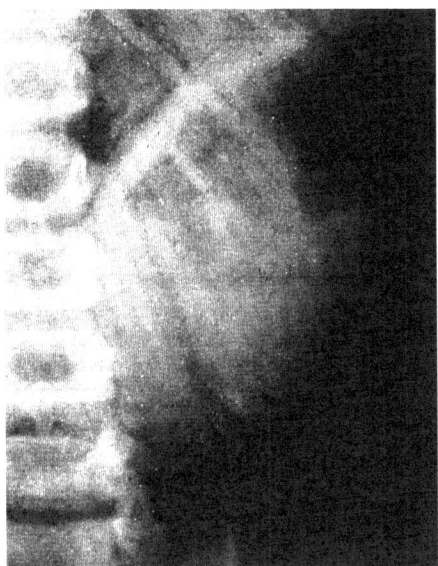

a, b

Fig. 3.11 a, b. Pelvi-ureteric junction obstruction. **a** High-dose IVU in this boy with periodic pain in the left flank shows on the radiograph at 40 min a dense left nephrogram containing non-opacified circular zones occupied by dilated calyces. The kidney is rotated with its lower pole lying laterally. **b** Late radiograph at 17 h shows the faint opacification of the dilated renal pelvis

does not necessarily indicate persisting obstruction (Fig. 3.21). Occasionally the nature of the obstruction is immediately evident and clear-cut, as in ureterocoele (Fig. 3.22). Para-ureteric vesical diverticulum (Fig. 3.23) may be an isolated finding or may occur in conjunction with severe vesical wall hypertrophy due to either neuropathic bladder or vesical outflow obstruction. Changes in the wall of the bladder and ureter either in tuberculosis or in bilharzia may be associated with mural calcification and produce distal ureteral obstruction. Disorders, both local and general, may cause ureteric obstruction in the pelvis. Such lesions include continuing pelvic inflammation (e. g. appendix abscess in the infant or toddler, or post-operatively following "pull through" procedures for Hirschsprung's disease or anorectal anomaly), malignant disease, neurofibromatosis and genital tract lesions, such as haematometrocolpos and ovarian masses.

With a lower urinary tract obstruction and even with a high dose IVU the study may need to be continued for a long time before radiographs diagnostic of the site of obstruction are obtained. This delay reflects diminished renal clearance of contrast medium which then has to reach a high enough level to give an image of the residue of urine trapped above the obstruction. Ultrasound study is indicated as it may be able to define the presence, site and nature of a pelvic mass.

When bilateral dilatation of the collecting system and ureters is present a possible obstruction to bladder emptying must always be considered. A vesical outlet obstruction may be excluded by MCU in all cases except those where the cause, as in large extrinsic masses, is clearly evident. The combination of lower tract obstruction with vesico-ureteric reflux, so often associated with an obstruction to bladder emptying, is especially deleterious to kidney function; in obstructive uropathy it commonly causes non-function at IVU.

3.3.4 Causes of Obstruction to Bladder Emptying

Clinical examination may indicate the bladder is large and does not empty, the urine stream may be seen to be poor and there may be incontinence. These findings have led, in common practice, first to an IVU and ultrasound study and then to an MCU. This gives a definitive answer to the question of obstruction of vesical emptying.

Retrograde urethral catheterization or suprapubic puncture are commonly employed techniques for introducing contrast medium into the bladder. Less commonly and usually in older children, bladder emptying can be assessed late in an IVU study. Injection of viscous medium into the male urethra is used principally to define distal urethral obstruction. A description of the causes and findings in lower urinary tract obstruction follows. Some of the lesions are found in both sexes, but some such as posterior urethral valves are found only in males.

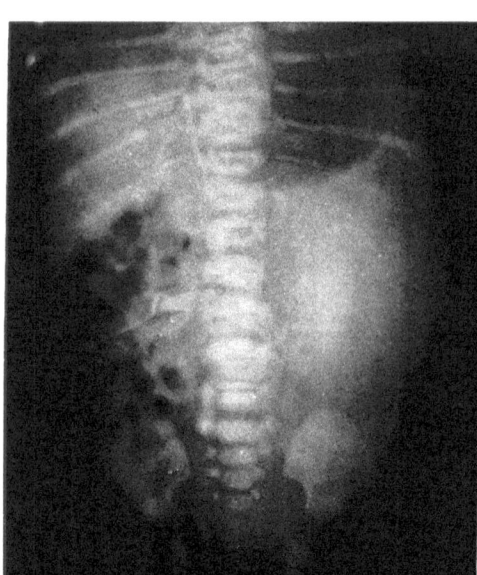
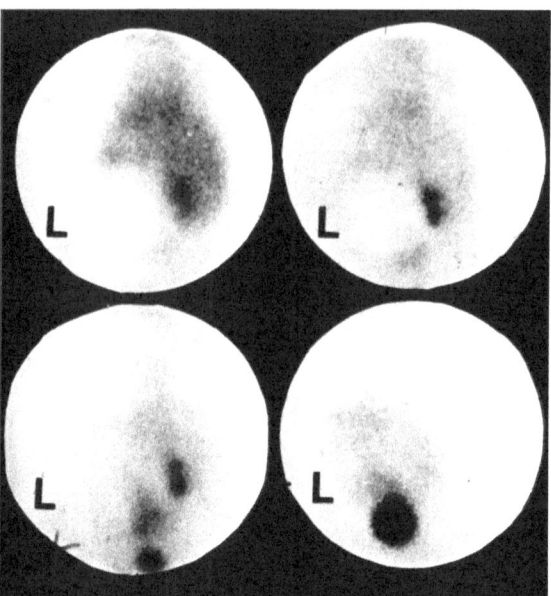

a, b

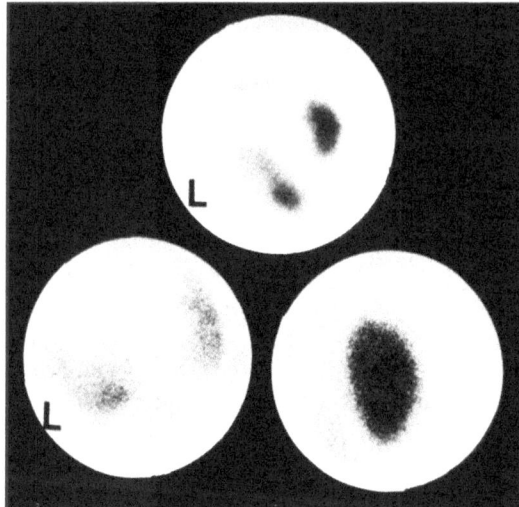

c

Fig. 3.12 a–c. Pelvi-ureteric junction obstruction. **a** This neonate had an abdominal mass diagnosed on antenatal ultrasound examination. IVU within 24 h of delivery showed the left-sided mass with a little contrast medium along its supero-lateral margin. No sign of any right kidney was seen in the urogram series. **b** DTPA study shows a normal right kidney. The left kidney has an early "Photon negative" zone centrally (*top left*) and 3 h (*bottom right*) this central zone has accumulated isotope within the previously negative area. **c** DMSA scan shows on the upper image using the converging/diverging collimator the two kidneys and, the two lower images present views of the left and right kidneys respectively. *Comment.* This series shows (i) how misleading an IVU in the first 24 h of life can be, (ii) the value of the DTPA scan in assessing function and (iii) how the DMSA scan in this case establishes that renal tissue is present and normal on the right side – prognosis being determined by the status of the contralateral kidney

The conditions are listed according to location, the most proximal appearing first.

3.3.4.1 Vesical Diverticulum

A large posteriorly located diverticulum lying behind the bladder base distends as the bladder contracts. The most inferior part of the diverticulum, as it distends, compresses the bladder neck and the most proximal part of the urethra. Incomplete urethral obstruction results. The detrusor relaxes after micturition ceases and the bladder refills from the distended diverticulum. This condition is seen in males (Fig. 3.24). Young boys can have quite serious associated upper tract problems which are characterized as obstructive uropathy, but there may be a considerably amount of ureteric reflux also present.

3.3.4.2 Bladder Neck Obstruction

In former times and long ago this diagnosis was not uncommon and applied mistakenly to male infants who had posterior urethral valves (Fig. 3.25). The reason for this mistake was simply that the bladder neck was undoubtedly narrow relative to the posterior urethra, but in itself the bladder neck was not absolutely narrowed. Obstruction at the bladder neck does occur but as a part of other problems. These include ectopic ureterocoele (Fig. 3.26), rhabdomyosarcoma and polyp (Fig. 3.27).

3.3.4.3 Posterior Urethral Valves

Bladder emptying is obstructed by a membrane of tissue arising from the anterior aspect of the urethra.

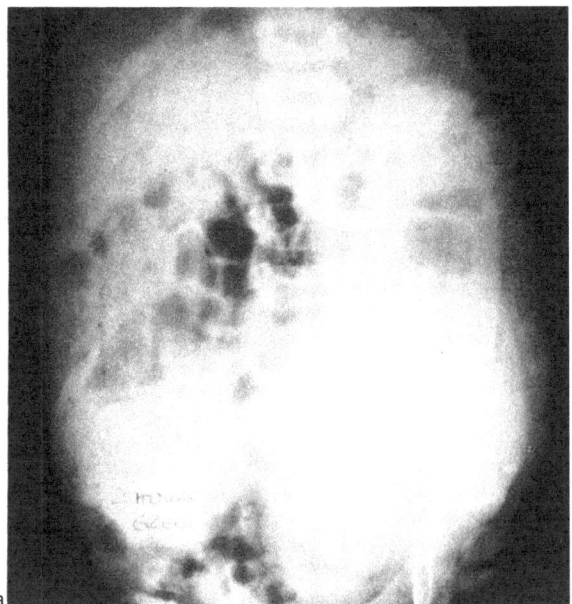

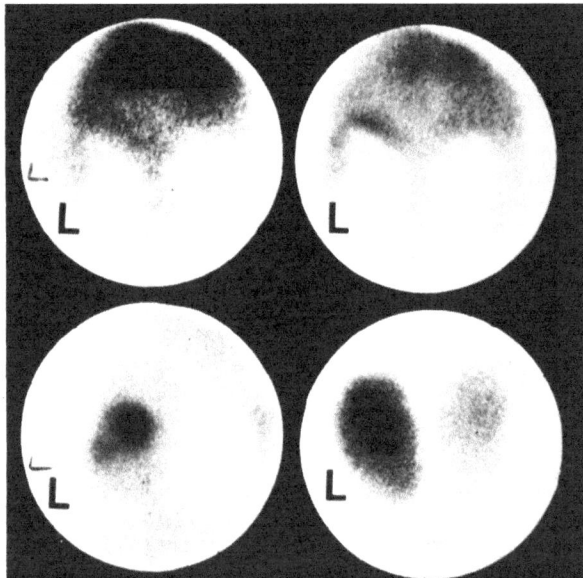

Fig. 3.13 a–c. Bilateral pelvi-ureteric junction obstruction. **a** IVU in this 2-year-old with abdominal distension, polyuria and polydipsia shows no function in the right kidney and at 2 h in the erect position a grossly dilated faintly opacified lesion of the left kidney. **b** DTPA scan shows at 2 h (*bottom right*) the accumulation of isotope in the dilated renal pelves (much more being in the left renal pelvis), a sequence indicating obstruction. **c** Bilateral retrograde pyelograms show gross distension of the renal pelves with malrotation of the left kidney. *Comment.* This series shows how the IVU may be of very limited help in children with severe chronic obstruction and verging on renal failure. The renogram shows that the level of obstruction is high in the urinary tract and indicates that the next (and decisive) investigation should be a retrograde study

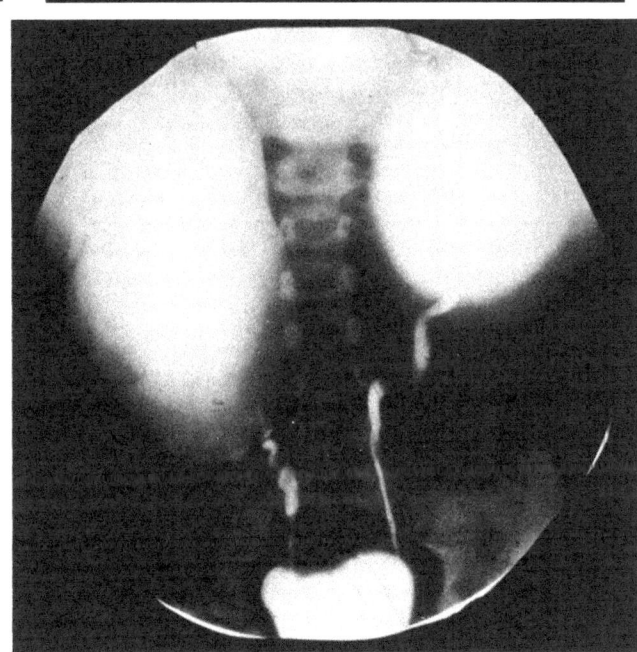

c

As the urethra fills from the bladder the membrane distends, and, valve-like, occludes the lumen of the urethra [15, 16, 17, 18]. Distal to the valves the urethral lumen is narrow; proximal to the valves the posterior urethra is dilated and elongated. The membrane of the valve tissue can be seen on high-quality radiographs at the point of transition in urethral calibre (Fig. 3.28). To demonstrate urethral valves adequately it is essential to have a good detrusor contraction for only then will the posterior urethral dilatation, the valves and the anterior urethra be shown. The junction between the bladder lumen and the urethra, although narrower than the dilated urethra below, is not absolutely narrowed.

In practice posterior urethral valves when adequately defined do not have a differential diagnosis. However, prolapsing ectopic ureterocoele can sometimes mimic these appearances.

Posterior urethral valves in a male is one of the common causes of obstruction. The obstruction itself is relatively easily treated by diathermy. The problems lie elsewhere and proximally (Figs. 3.29, 3.30, 3.31). A minor problem is prostatic duct reflux which, if infection is present, may hinder its eradication. Detrusor hypertrophy occurs and the bladder may have many saccules along its contour. This bladder wall hypertrophy may be associated with no undue increase in bladder capacity but it can in

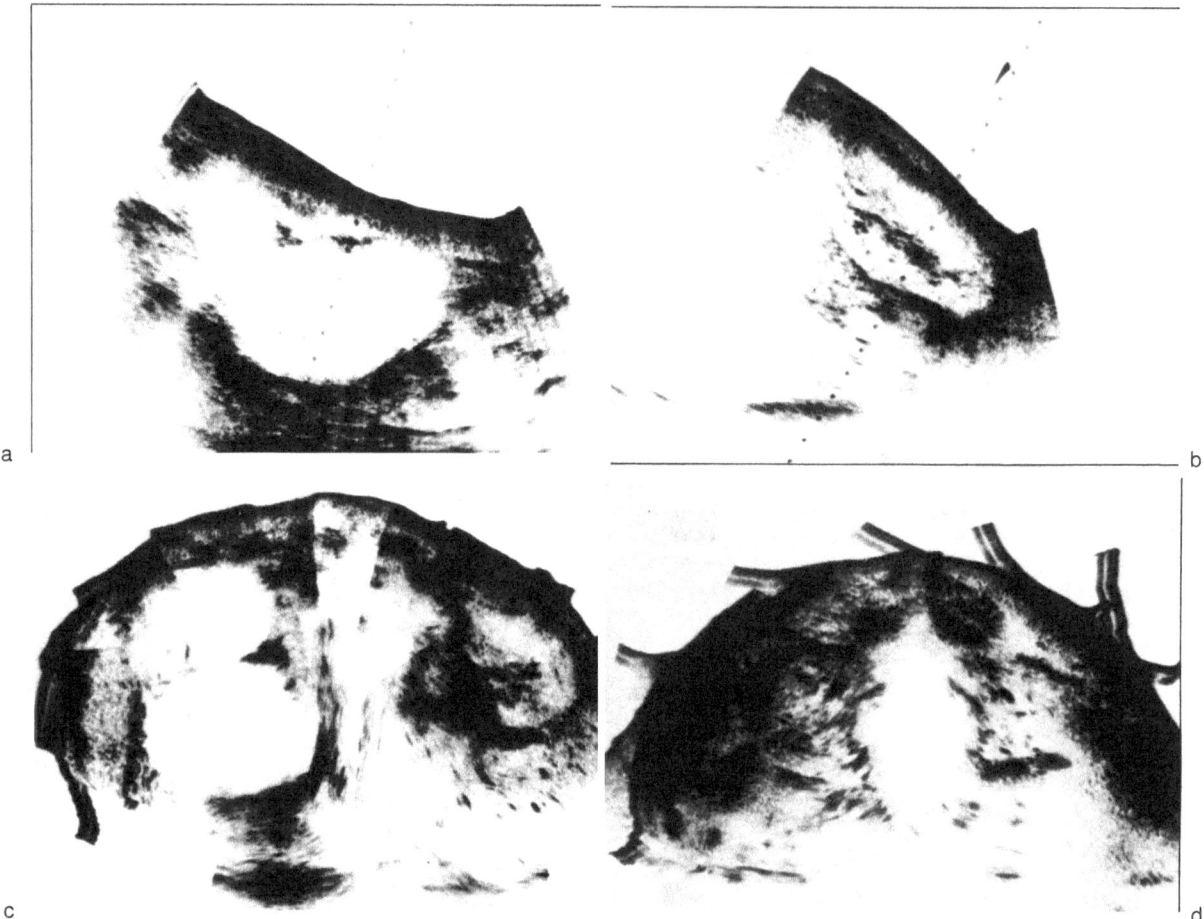

Fig. 3.14. a Age 9. LS prone. Gross hydronephrosis of the left kidney in a boy who presented with abdominal pain and a mass on the left. b (same case as in a) LS prone showing a normal right kidney. c (same case as in a) TS prone demonstrating again the large hydronephrosis with a massive dilated renal pelvis anteriorly. d (same case as in a) TS prone beneath the level of the kidneys, no evidence of a dilated ureter on the left, suggesting a high ureteric obstruction most probably at the pelvi-ureteric junction

terfere with the opening of the intramural section of the ureter; thus, serious bladder wall hypertrophy can lead to ureterovesical junction obstruction and this persists even when the valves have been ablated. Vesico-ureteric reflux may occur and the combination of distal obstruction with reflux into the upper tract usually produces a sharp reduction in the performance of the kidney subject to reflux. In both obstruction alone and reflux with obstruction there is often serious widening and increased tortuosity of the ureter.

As will be discussed later, cystic disease is often associated with obstruction. Infants with posterior urethral valves are no exception and such cystic changes add to the problems they have. Furthermore, since there is a large undrained urinary residue urinary infection may occur and lead to pyelonephritic scarring. Add to these the elements of either obstructive renal atrophy or compromised renal

development and there is a concatenation of damaging influences which can compromise renal function and jeopardise long-term survival. The prognosis in posterior urethral valves is determined by factors other than the primary obstruction – and this applies to other obstructing lesions such as ectopic ureterocoele.

Even so, there are many young infants who have a rapid recovery and a good potential for the future after the urethral obstruction has been removed. Careful follow-up studies are always needed.

3.3.4.3.1 Tactics and Strategy in Investigating Patients With Posterior Urethral Valves

The newer modes of investigation and their role are exemplified by the changed pattern of investigation of the young male suspected of having obstructive uropathy and posterior urethral valves. Usually, the clinical evaluation leads to a high level of suspicion

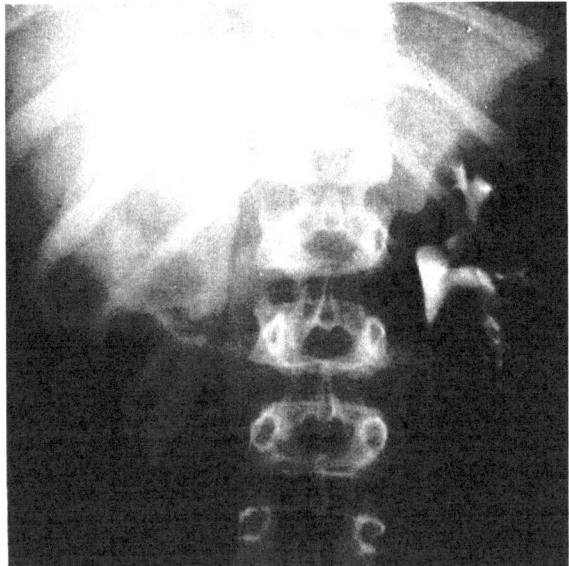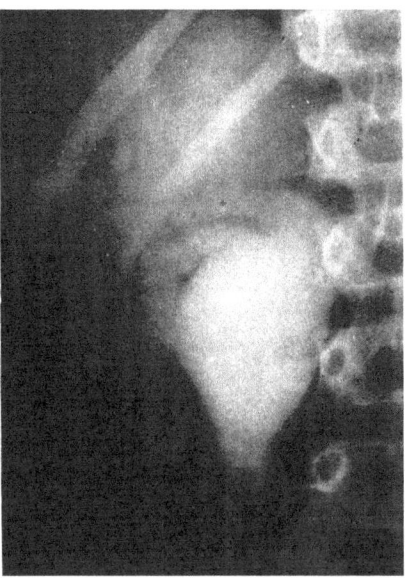

Fig. 3.15 a, b. High ureteral polyp. **a** Initially the IVU shows the right kidney is much larger than the normal left kidney. The right nephrogram at 2 h is dense because the kidney is acutely obstructed. The circular zones of increased transradiancy are due to non-opacified urine in dilated calyces – a sequel to protracted obstruction as an underlying feature. **b** A later radiograph in the prone position shows contrast medium passing into the upper part of the ureter which is obstructed apparently completely by the intraluminal polyp. *Comment.* It is important to define accurately the level of obstruction in the upper tract (e.g. high ureteric versus pelvi-ureteric) so that surgery takes place at the correct level

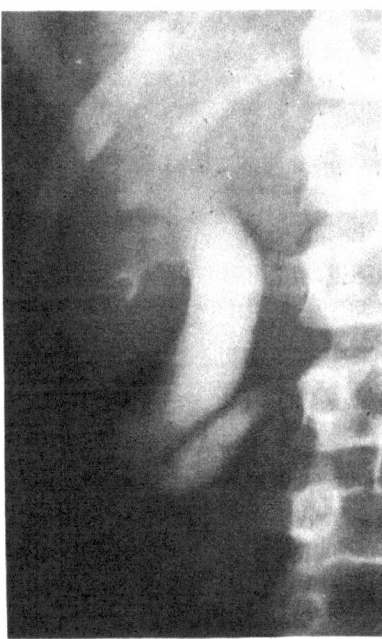

Fig. 3.16. Retrocaval ureter. This right-sided lesion may have serious obstructive effects (see Fig. 3.2). At IVU the course of the dilated ureter is diagnostic; it passes downward to its middle third, then sweeps upward to the point of obstruction, where it passes behind a component of the cava, on this radiograph with the child prone. It is not necessary to carry out contrast medium studies of the caval system, just as it is unnecessary to undertake vascular studies in obstructed retroiliac ureters

of the diagnosis because the kidneys are palpable, the bladder is large, the urine stream on voiding is poor and there may be an accompanying urinary tract infection.

In such circumstances and without upset to the young infant ultrasonics can be expected to yield the following information. It will confirm the dilatation of the pelvicalyceal system in the kidneys and show the parenchymal thickness. Perinephric collections of urine caused by leakage from the upper tract will be defined, as will any possible urinary ascites. When the bladder is examined its overall capacity can be assessed, at least in a semi-quantitative way, and the vesical wall thickening, sacculation and diverticula can be shown. Dilated ureters entering the posterior aspect of the bladder will be demonstrated unless they have particularly hyperdynamic peristalsis and when, by coincidence, a ureteric contraction occurs at the moment when the sound beam sweeps across the area. Real time ultrasound study should avoid this combination of events producing diagnostic problems. Thus, echography confirms the clinical impression and indicates there is a lower urinary tract obstruction.

MCU is the logical next investigatory step. It demonstrates the cause of obstruction, confirming the diagnosis of urethral valves and the vesical wall hypertrophy. If reflux into a ureter is present, then the upper tract on the side subject to reflux is shown.

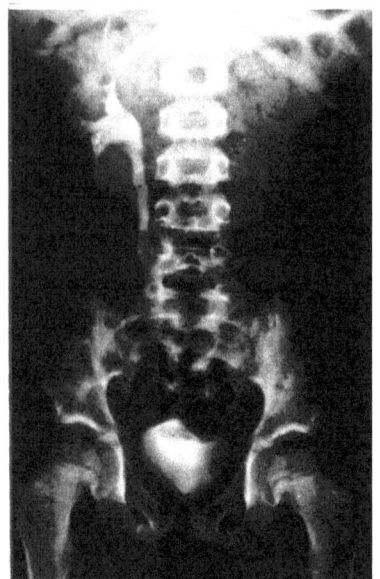

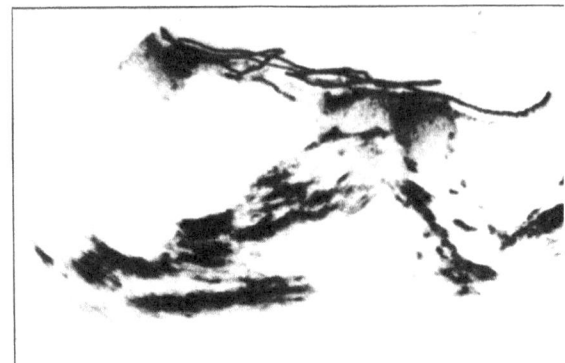

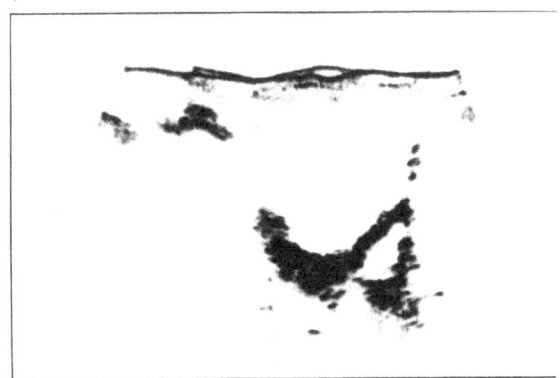

Fig. 3.17 a–c. Ureterovesical junction obstruction. Age 11. **a** At IVU there was no evidence of function in the left kidney 5 min after injection of contrast medium. Patient was therefore studied by echography. Full-lenght post-echographic radiograph is shown. **b** LS supine, left of midline, shows a massive hydronephrosis, tortuous dilated ureter and normal full bladder. **c** TS supine view of bladder showing the dilated left ureter. As a result of this examination a late post-voiding radiograph was taken to show that there was no evidence of reflux. Diagnosis: ureterovesical junction obstruction on the left

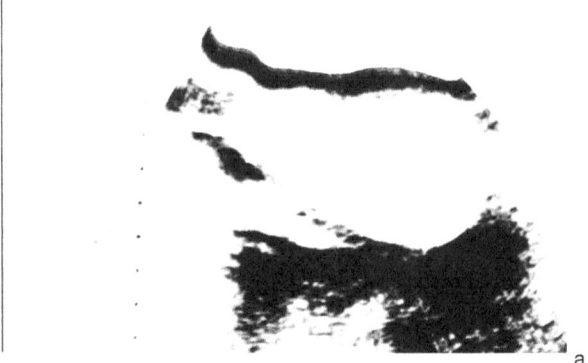

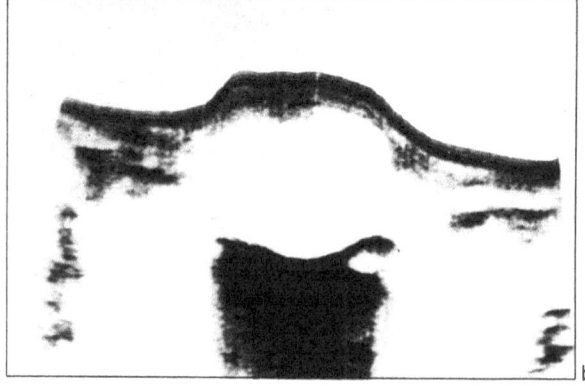

Fig. 3.18. a Age 3. LS supine view of the bladder. The dilated ureter is seen tapering behind this. Unilateral ureterovesical obstruction. **b** (same case as in **a**) TS supine view of the bladder showing a single dilated ureter on the left. The normal right ureter was not demonstrated

Once the valves have been defined they can, at the elective moment, be ablated by diathermy. Even when there is no reflux sufficient information will generally have already come from echography about the status of the upper tract to make any additional study of its status superfluous at this stage.

The next phase is concerned with evaluating the upper tract and bladder once the valve ablation has been carried out or other drainage procedures, such as nephrostomy, performed. Echography can confirm at any time that there are no upper tract complications such as perinephric collections which may have become infected. Upper tract dilatation often rapidly improves after urethral obstruction has been relieved. The bladder capacity falls sharply following valve ablation although residual thickening of the wall can be expected to persist for some time.

Surveillance of the patient over the long term must be contemplated and the baseline investigations for this carried out. There is also great need to recognise that complications can develop sooner rather than later. Isotope scans are used to estimate the contribution of each kidney to overall renal function and

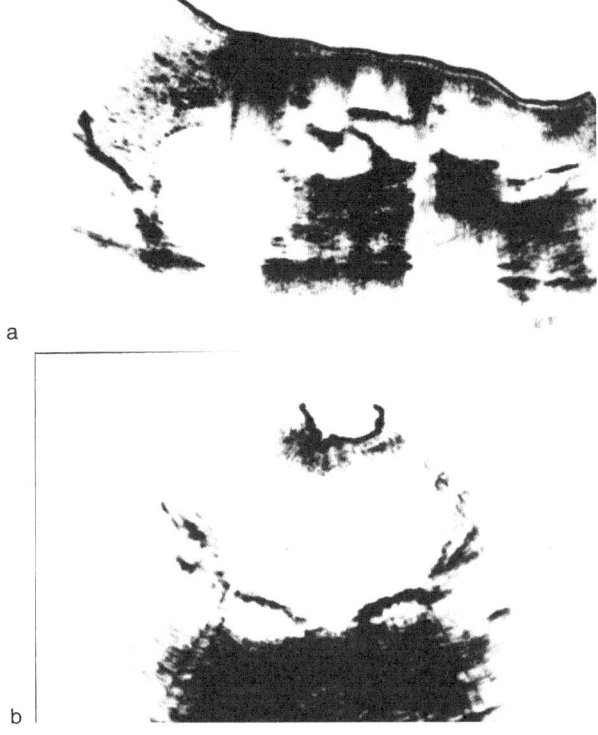

a

b

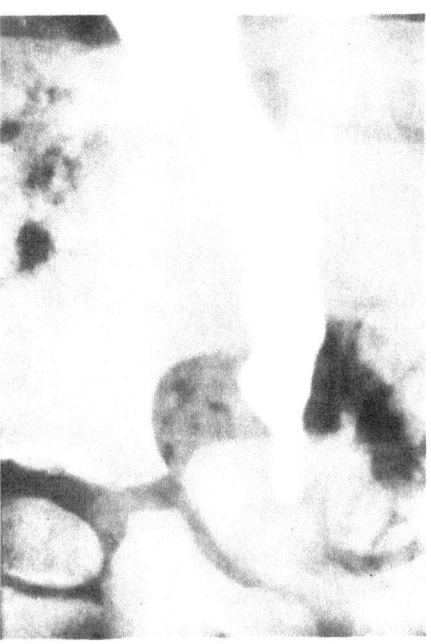

Fig. 3.20. Distal ureteral stenosis. Previous serve upper tract dilatation detected on the right side with no evidence of vesico-ureteric reflux at MCU. Nephrostomy drainage instituted. Contrast medium injected through the nephrostomy tube passes down the dilated ureter, but only a small volume enters the normal bladder. Such drainage procedures enable an obstructed kidney function to be studied directly on clearance studies and by split function renography. If function is exceptionally poor and the condition is unilateral, nephroureterectomy may be the next step. Should it be decided to retain the kidney and carry out ureteric reimplantation, then fluoroscopic studies of ureteric function can be useful

Fig. 3.19. a LS supine. There is a large hydronephrotic sac under the liver, beneath this a serpignous dilated ureter. There was a similiar appearance on the left. **b** (same case as in **a**) TS supine view of the bladder. Dilated ureters can be seen behind the bladder indicating possible bilateral ureterovesical obstruction

assess the significance of any continuing upper tract dilatation (Fig. 3.32). IVU demonstrates the anatomy of the upper tract and the vesical volume once the primary obstruction has been relieved. MCU confirms satisfactory urethral flow and indicates whether reflux is persisting. This is one upper tract problem which may well demand a further surgical intervention. Reflux may be associated with exceptionally poor and declining function in the kidney; nephroureterectomy may be appropriate if the contralateral kidney takes over urine clearance but, more hopefully, ureteric reimplantation will be possible when the kidney continues to function. The second upper tract problem is persisting or increasing dilatation without vesico-ureteric reflux. This eventuality most often results from vesical wall hypertrophy although a para-ureteric diverticulum or saccule may contribute to the problem. When the bladder volume is sharply reduced (either because of catheter drainage or valve ablation) the already hypertrophied wall becomes exceptionally thick and narrows the intramural course of the ureter. Furthermore, incompetent ureteric peristalsis in a di-

lated ureter is yet an additional factor in the upper tract dilatation. If reimplantation of a dilated ureter into a grossly hypertrophied bladder is to be satisfactory great skill is needed. The objective of surveillance is to enable those appropriate steps to be taken which ensure good renal function and a good potential for kidney growth.

Although the topic of posterior urethral valves has been singled out for detailed analysis among the causes of obstructive uropathy similar principles of investigation and evaluation are applicable in varying degrees to other lesions causing lower urinary tract obstruction.

3.3.4.4 Anterior Urethral Diverticulum

This condition [19] is sometimes called "anterior urethral valve". As contrast medium is voided along the male urethra the calibre is seen to be increased proximal to the site of the diverticulum. The diverticulum itself is located inferiorly and as voiding occurs it distends. The distal mucosal lip of the

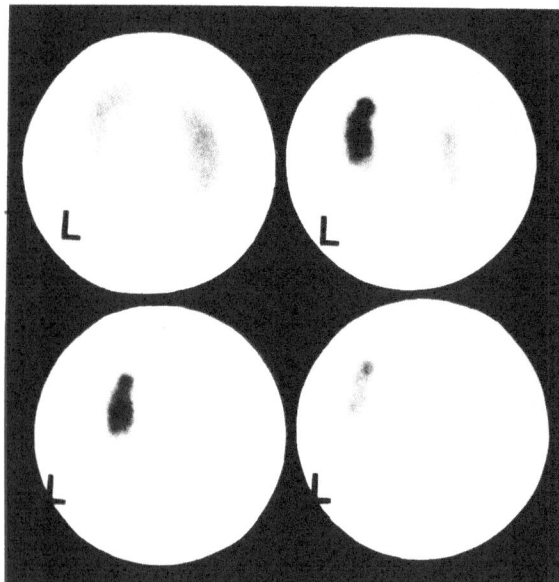

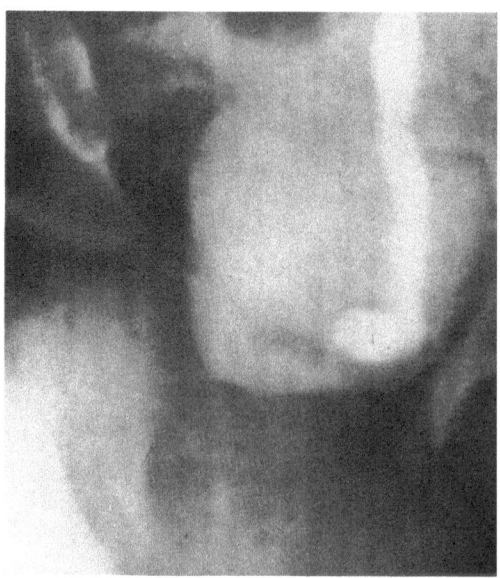

Fig. 3.21. DTPA scan following reimplantation of the left ureter for reflux shows no post-operative obstruction. At 5 min, isotope has accumulated in the renal substance of both kidneys (*top left*). There is subsequent filling of a dilated left pelvicalyceal system. After the intravenous injection of the diuretic Frusemide, there has been good clearance of isotope from the left side (*bottom right*). This indicates that the left system is dilated but not obstructed. Isotope studies of this sort are particularly valuable in the post-operative follow-up of a child with poorly functioning and dilated systems on IVU

Fig. 3.22. Orthotopic ureterocoele. On this descending study, following nephrostomy drainage for non-function on IVU, the dilated submucosal segment of ureter, proximal to the ureteric meatal stenosis, is densely opacified by contrast with the less dense urine in the bladder. The thin transradiant rim of the wall of the ureterocoele is clearly seen

diverticulum obstructs flow into the urethra beyond and so the urethra distal to the diverticulum is of narrow calibre (Fig. 3.33).

3.3.4.5 Distal Urethral Obstruction

This may be caused by phimosis (Fig. 3.34), meatal stenosis [20] (Fig. 3.35) or urethral stenosis (Figs. 3.36 and 3.37) just proximal to the meatus. The first two of these conditions may be suspected clinically. All give distinctive appearances on voiding cystograms. Phimosis with infection can give severe obstruction.

3.3.4.6 Calculus Obstruction

A calculus may pass into the urethra, impact, and cause obstruction. The calculus may lodge in the bladder neck, in the posterior urethra above the membranous urethra, and in the fossa navicularis distally.

3.3.4.7 Urethral Duplication

Most urethral duplications are complete and non-obstructive. Rarely they are incomplete [21, 22] and

produce obstruction at the junction of the two urethral lumina. The single distal urethral lumen is not dilated.

3.3.4.8 Urethral Stricture

Obstruction by stricture may follow accidental trauma (usually to the perineum) and is followed by urethral scarring and narrowing. Urethral operations for repair of hypospadias and exstrophy can sometimes result in stricture formation. Protracted periurethral inflammatory changes may produce a stricture, sometimes over quite a long distance.
Fortunately, the incidence of strictures in the vicinity of the suspensory ligament and following catheter drainage of the bladder is now virtually an event in past history.

3.3.5 Effect of Obstruction on the Bladder

Generally, when the bladder's outflow is seriously obstructed it fails to empty completely. This can be observed clinically, on post-micturition films at IVU and at MCU. However, it is quite common, because of the circumstances of the procedure, for the

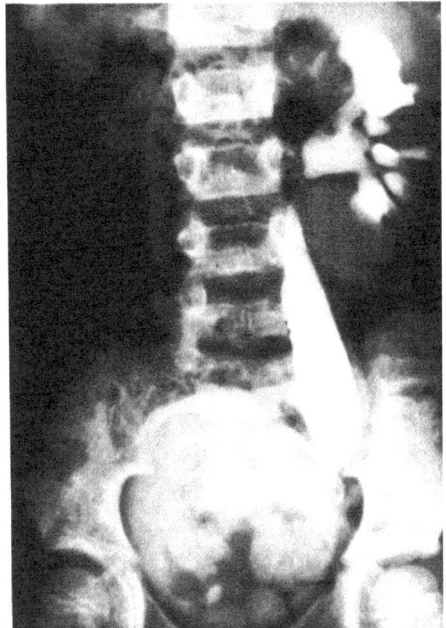
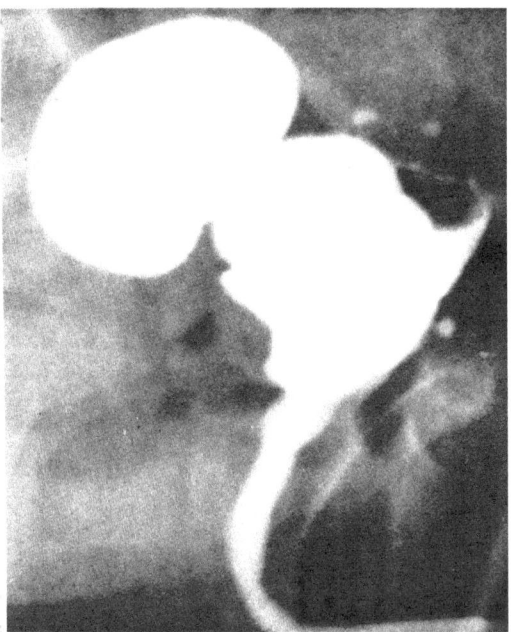

a, b

Fig. 3.23 a, b. Para-ureteric diverticulum. **a** IVU shows the dilated collecting system and ureter draining the left kidney. Dilatation extends down to the vicinity of the bladder. **b** MCU demonstrates the para-ureteric diverticulum, which obstructs the lower end of the ureter. Such a finding and the difficulty of distinguishing severe primary reflux at IVU from obstruction in the very young underline the need for MCU in cases of suspected lower ureteric obstruction

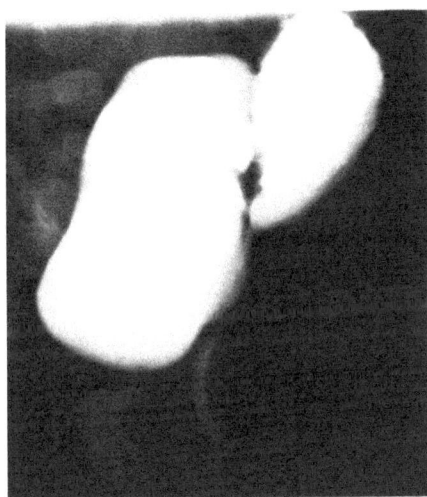

Fig. 3.24. Vesical diverticulum obstructing urethra. MCU shows, as the bladder contracts, a large posterior diverticulum extending downward to obstruct the urethra

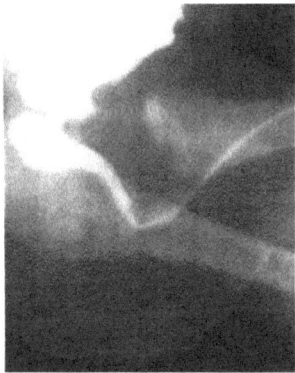

Fig. 3.25. Posterior urethral valves. Infant aged 3 months who voided slowly and who had posterior urethral valves. The distal part of the urethra is narrow. At the valve site there is additional narrowing and slight dilatation immediately proximal to the valves. The vesico-urethral junction is narrower than the diameter of the bladder above and the urethra below, but it is not absolutely narrow. Such findings are a feature of rather poor detrusor contraction at the time of MCU, combined with vesico-ureteric reflux, which was also present

bladder not to be emptied completely at MCU, even when there is no obstruction. The post-micturition vesical residue can be studied in more natural circumstances by ultrasonics.

Acute obstruction to vesical emptying results in painful retention. Such retention can sometimes occur in young males whose micturition is inhibited by local problems, such as painful meatal ulcer.

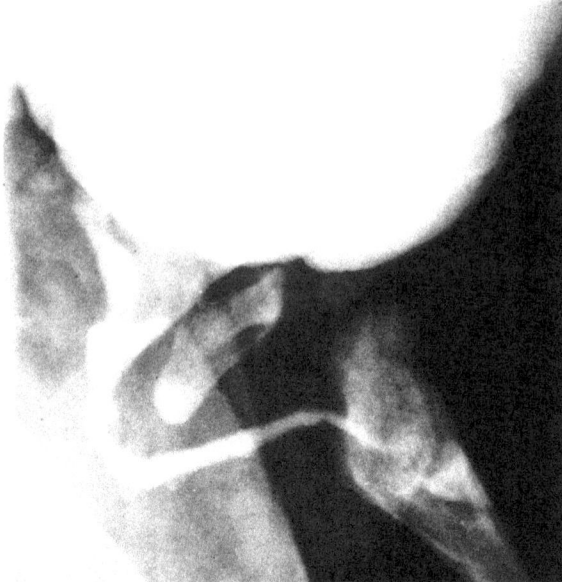

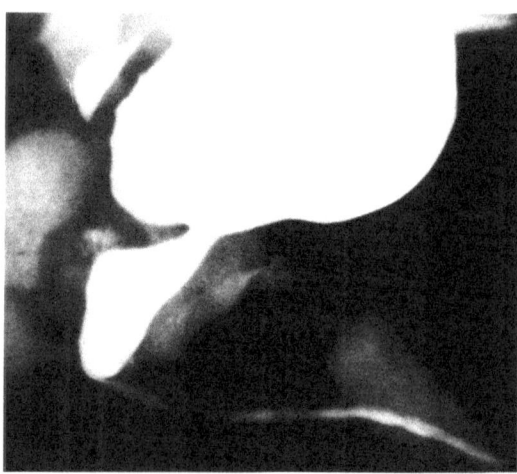

Fig. 3.26. Prolapsing ectopic ureterocoele in a male. At MCU in a boy, if the ureterocoele prolapses into the urethra while the bladder neck is widely open on voiding, the proximal part of the urethra has the appearance of an inverted cone and the filling defect of the non-opaque ureterocoele is shown. This appearance must be distinguished from that of posterior urethral valves, and very careful study of the upper tract features is essential

Fig. 3.28. Posterior urethral valves. The delicate membranous folds of the valve tissue present no obstruction to transit of the catheter into the bladder, but when voiding at MCU occurs the valves severely occlude the lumen. In this young infant the valve membrane can be seen below the dilated proximal urethra and at the point where the lumen is abruptly narrowed. A little reflux into the prostatic ducts, which is seen in this example, is quite common. Some reflux into an ureter is also shown

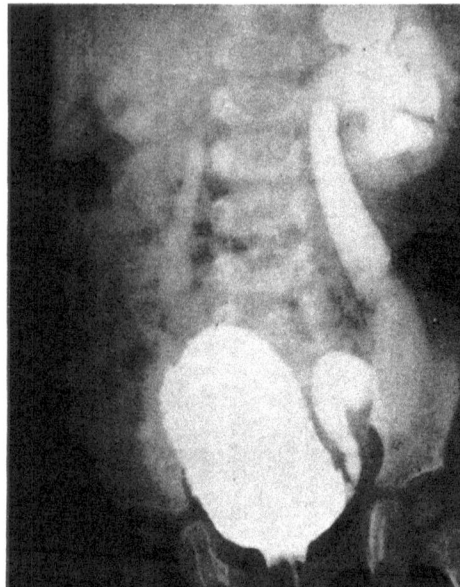

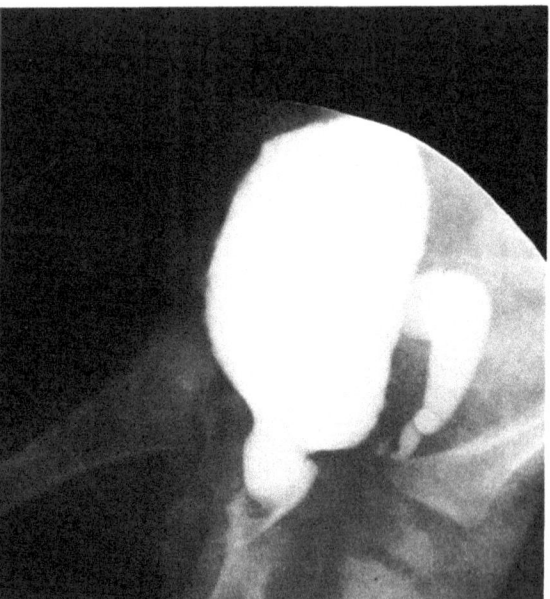

Fig. 3.27 a, b. Simple polyp at the vesico-urethral junction. Retention, haematuria, and urinary infection are presenting clinical features of varying prominence. a At MCU during the vesical filling phase the polyp lies in the vesico-urethral junction. There is bilateral vesico-ureteral reflux, with parenchymal opacification of the left kidney caused by intrarenal reflux. There is persistent undrained urine in the upper tract which dilutes the contrast medium as it enters the ureter (see right side). b During voiding the polyp descends through the wide bladder neck into the urethra. The proximal part of the urethra in which the polyp lies is dilated, but distally the urethra is narrow

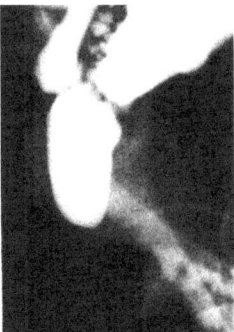

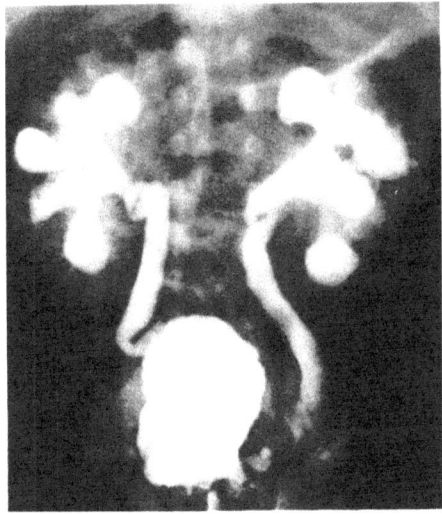

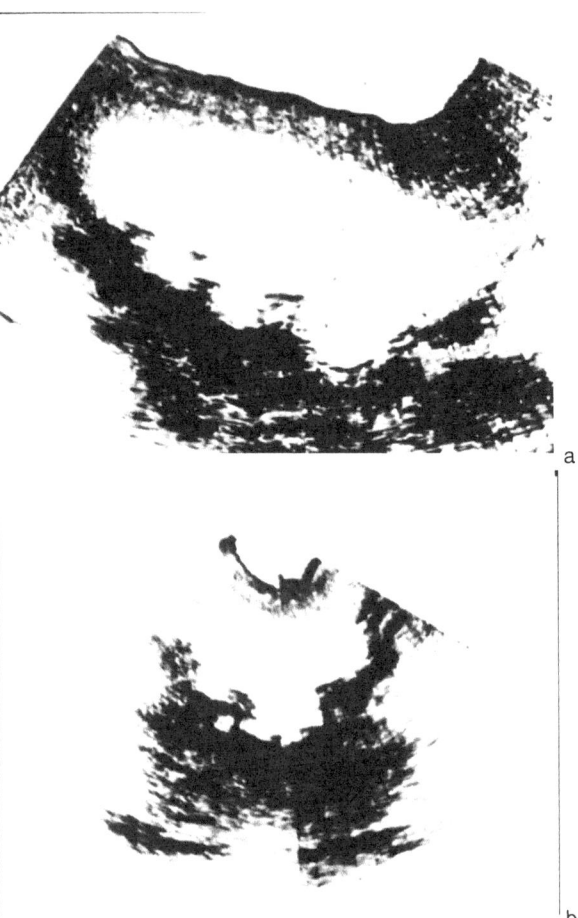

Fig. 3.29 a, b. Posterior urethral valves. **a** A male neonate aged 3 weeks in renal failure with urinary infection. MCU shows the smooth, elongated and dilated posterior urethra. At the valve site the urethra changes calibre very sharply and is narrow beyond the valve site. The bladder above the dilated posterior urethra has many saccules on its posterior aspect. At this stage of the cystogram reflux of contrast medium into an ureter (*right*) is seen. **b** MCU: The infant has failed to empty the bladder which is trabeculated as well as sacculated. Bilateral reflux into dilated, rather tortuous ureters is shown. All the calyces of the kidneys are dilated and there is opacification of the renal parenchyma; in part this is intrarenal reflux with diffuse opacification, but there are also some small spots of contrast medium indicating cystic change in the kidneys. In this infant the combination of urethral valve obstruction, a powerful detrusor action and bilateral vesico-ureteric reflux has dilated the upper tract. However, there is in this young infant a good renal parenchymal thickness present. After medical treatment and a short period of catheter drainage, the valves were cauterized by diathermy

Fig. 3.30. a LS supine view of bladder. The bladder wall is thickened with saccule-like trabeculation. **b** (same case as in **a**) TS supine scan shows the irregular bladder contour with dilated ureters posteriorly. Both kidneys were hydronephrotic. These scans indicated that the obstruction was at the urethral level

Protracted obstruction to bladder emptying can develop in utero or later in life. Detrusor hypertrophy, saccule formation and diverticula are all consequences of obstruction. Such alterations in bladder structure need to be differentiated from those of neuropathic origin. Not all obstructed bladders are large, indeed, marked detrusor hypertrophy may be sufficient to overcome the urethral obstruction and bladder capacity may remain normal. All these features can be shown by MCU, but sonography can be a decisive non-invasive technique yielding similar information.

If vesico-ureteric reflux is present in addition to obstruction to bladder emptying, then as the detrusor contracts, upper tract distension of considerable degree often develops.

Obstruction, caused by for example urethral valves in a male infant, can be relieved and the previous considerable upper tract dilatation may rapidly ameliorate.

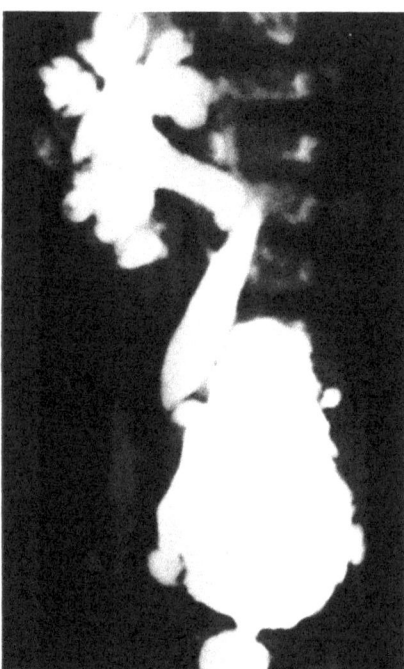

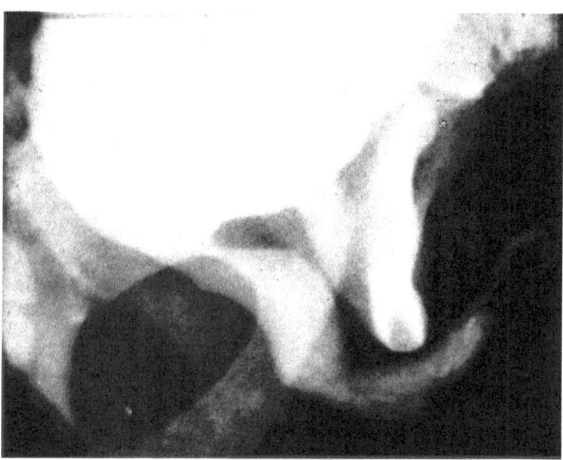

Fig. 3.33. Anterior urethral diverticulum. At MCU the voided contrast medium enters the diverticulum; this may have been perceived by the astute clinician on his examination. On voiding, contrast medium enters the diverticulum freely, but egress is impeded by a mucosal flap which partially closes the lumen and so the urethra distal to the diverticulum is much narrower then the lumen proximal to the diverticulum

Fig. 3.31. Posterior urethral valves. MCU in a child with posterior urethral valves shows some filling of proximal part of the urethra with prostatic duct filling. The bladder is cone-shaped with multiple saccules and a grossly thickened wall. Reflux into the dilated, rather tortuous ureter opacifies the calyces and the tips of the papillae by intrarenal reflux. It is important to differentiate this type of apperance from that due to a neuropathic bladder

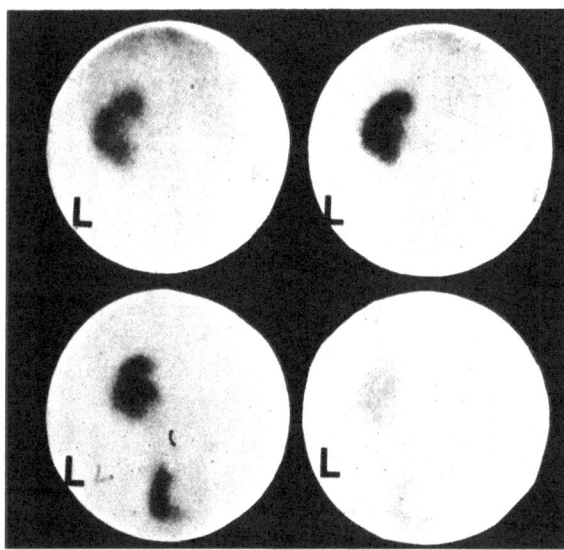

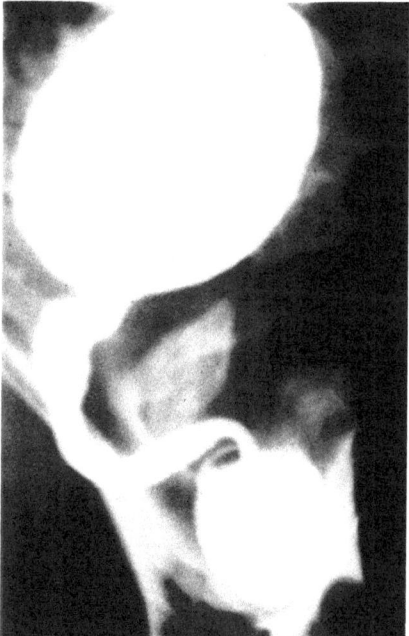

Fig. 3.32. DTPA scan in a child with a solitary left kidney and a persistently dilated system following resection of posterior urethral valves. At 5 min (*top left*) there is good perfusion of the solitary left kidney. After the intravenous injection of Frusemide there has been good clearance of isotope (*bottom right*) indicating that there is no continuing obstruction in the dilated system

Fig. 3.34. Phimosis. As in meatal stenosis, a narrow-gauge catheter must be used for injection into the bladder per urethram. On the voiding phase of MCU the urethra is not unduly wide, but the preputial sac distends with contrast medium. Unless urinary infection supervenes (when the young boy may become seriously ill) the lesion is easily treated

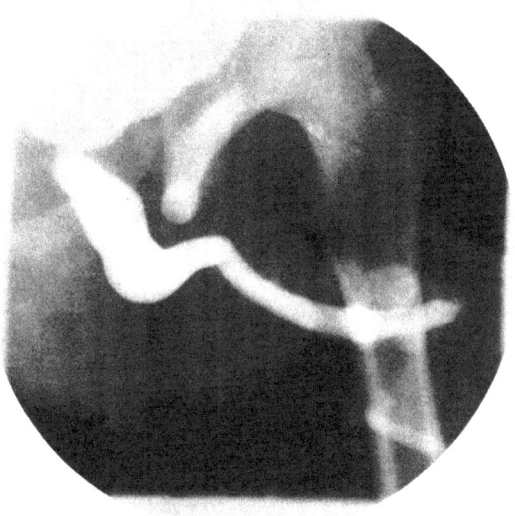

Fig. 3.35. Meatal stenosis. In meatal stenosis the urethra must be catheterised by a narrow-calibre catheter of 4FG or 6FG size. This example, in a boy aged 9 years, shows dilatation of the urethra proximally and a narrow jet of contrast medium voided past the stenosis. The impact of such obstruction is usually slight by comparison with proximal urethral obstruction caused by posterior urethral valves and upper tract dilatation is usually slight even when it is present

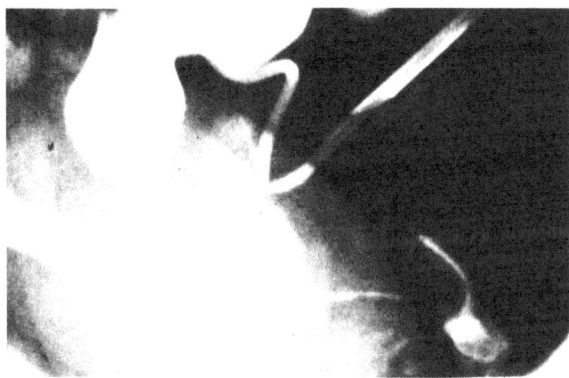

Fig. 3.36. Urethral stenosis. Congenital urethral stenosis may be an exceptionally serious condition when the anterior male urethra is narrowed over much of its length. It is impossible to catheterise the urethra, so contrast medium must be introduced into the dilated bladder by the suprapubic route. Bilateral and serious renal maldevelopment results in "non-function" at IVU and severe bilateral vesico-ureteric reflux can be the only way to opacify the upper tract via the dilated tortuous ureters at cystography. The male anterior urethra has a narrow lumen if an erection occurs, but simple observation should mean no diagnostic problems arise. Urethral stenosis in girls is exceptionally rare and a sense of the obstruction can usually be perceived at catheterisation per urethram

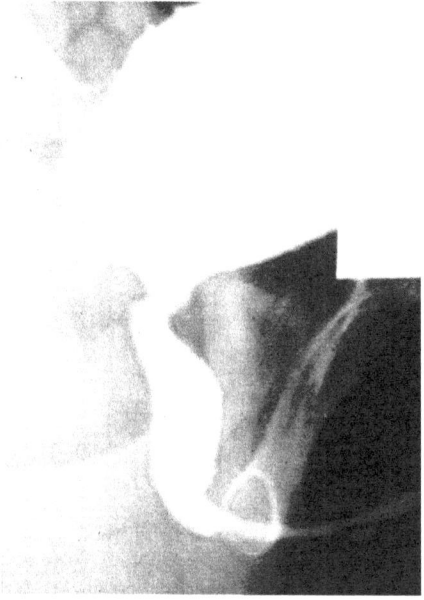

Fig. 3.37. Acquired urethral stenosis. This is a rare event in infants and children. In this boy peri-urethral inflammatory changes with small abscess cavities opacified by the voided contrast medium have together narrowed the urethral lumen. Although proximal urethral dilatation is present, no dilatation of the upper urinary tract had occured. Periodic painful retention was the presenting symptom and the boy was a diabetic.

Stricture due to trauma used to be a not uncommon event in boys who had rubber indwelling catheters in situ; fortunately such strictures localized to the vicinity of the suspensory ligament are now very rarely seen with modern catheters and modern drainage techniques. Post-operative stenosis of the reconstructed urethral lumen following plastic procedures still occurs from time to time

3.3.6 Urinary Ascites and Perinephric Urinoma
(Figs. 3.38, 3.39 and 3.40)

Although extravasation of urine can occur at any age, neonates are especially vulnerable to this event. The combination of prenatal obstruction and the trauma of delivery probably account for this. The urinary leak can be confined to the perinephric tissues and produces a "urinoma"; this may be palpable clinically as an ill-defined loin mass. When urine leaks into the peritoneal cavity urinary ascites develops [23, 24, 25]. In both types of leakage complex serum electrolyte disturbances ensue as part of the renal failure.

The precise site of extravasation from the urinary tract may not be demonstrated by IVU or at surgical exploration. When vesico-ureteric reflux is present the MCU can show the site of leakage which is often

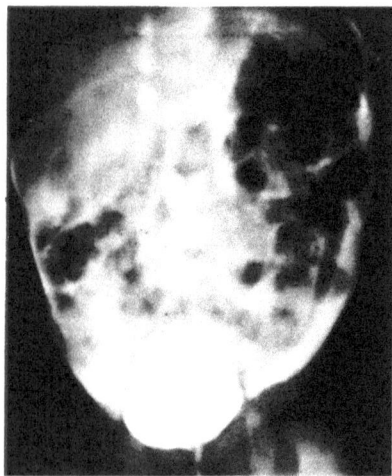

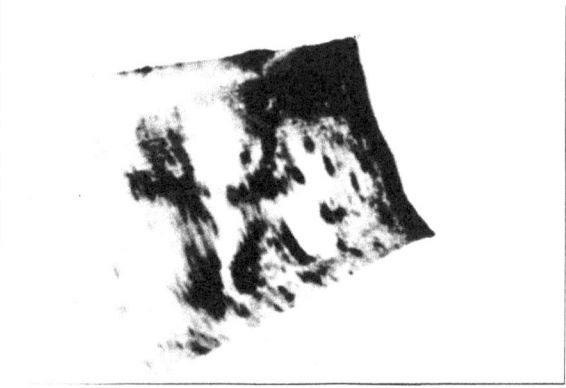

Fig. 3.40. Age 10 days. TS supine view of the left kidney. Moderate hydronephrosis is seen with an appreciable renal cortex. Between the kidney and the spine is another echolucent area: a perinephric leak of urine secondary to a lower urinary tract obstruction. There was a similar appearance on the right side, but neither were seen during the prone examination

Fig. 3.38. Urinary ascites. This neonate, whose spinal problem is shown, had a distended abdomen. The distension was caused by leakage of urine from the neuropathic bladder, with quite free spillage of contrast medium into the peritoneal cavity at cystography

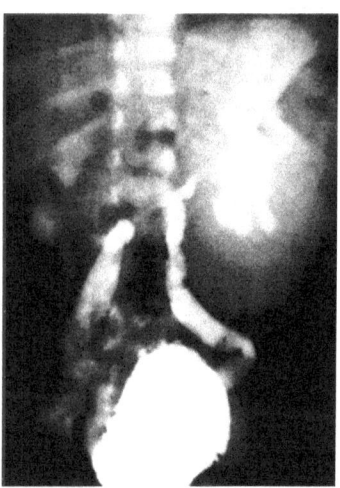

Fig. 3.39. Urinoma in infant with posterior urethral valves. At MCU, reflux up the ureter has opacified the collecting system of the left kidney. Leakage through the renal parenchyma into the space around the left kidney (the urinoma) is shown

through the fornix of a calyx or from a bladder saccule. Common causes of urinary leakage are, primarily, urethral valves [27] and neuropathic bladder. Much rarer causes include pelvic tumours (such as neuroblastoma), urethral atresia associated with imperforate anus, urethral stenosis, ectopic ureterocoele, and pelvi-ureteric junction obstruction [26].

When leakage is from the kidney the perinephric collection can be difficult to identify at IVU al-

though sometimes a vague perinephric haziness develops late in the IVU series. The non-opacified perinephric collection may be seen as a radiolucent area around the kidney and posterior abdominal wall. Ultrasonics studies can be decisive in showing such perinephric collections (Fig. 3.40).

Urinary ascites, as with any other form of severe ascites, characteristically shows on a plain radiograph; features in the supine film are the central location of gas-containing loops of gut within the abdomen, the overall abdominal distension, and the inability to define the margins of the liver, spleen or posterior abdominal wall structures. Urinary ascites is seldom a minor clinical feature and ultrasonics studies are rarely needed to confirm its presence. Nevertheless sonography is a decisive investigatory technique in assessing abdominal distension because it will differentiate in clear-cut fashion intraperitoneal fluid collections from all other causes of abdominal distension and if the cause is urinary ascites due to renal leakage it will identify the side. One important and interesting fact is that, when perinephric leakage has occurred, the kidney often has a very good potential for function and growth. Effective clinical management realises this potential and such infants can have an excellent long-term prospect.

In older children with hydronephrosis, minor trauma can lead to either haematuria or perinephric leakage of urine. Such kidneys may be severely hydronephrotic and their function at IVU much diminished. Ultrasonic studies can usually show the nature of the kidney problem and the perinephric urine collection. Injury at the pelvi-ureteric junction may lead to encapsulation (and a parapelvic cyst) or downward extension alongside the ureter at the acute stage of damage.

3.3.7 "Non-Functioning" Kidney

In the concept of the "non-functioning" kidney it is presupposed that an IVU had led to this finding. The contralateral kidney must be studied carefully. Considerable compensatory hypertrophy in the contralateral kidney suggests the condition of nonfunction has been present for a long time. Since very young patients grow quickly compensatory hypertrophy can develop in a period of months, which in the life span of a young infant is along time. Bilateral disease patterns in kidney conditions are well recognised and include obstruction, calculi, Wilms' tumour and atrophic scarred kidneys. Finally, prognosis for a child is very often determined by the status of the contralateral kidney when nonfunction is present on the one side.

There are two broad groups of non-function – a kidney mass may or may not be *palpable* on the side of non-function.

A. When there is a mass present clinically the following more common diagnostic possibilities are present:
1. Hydronephrosis – due to obstruction or obstruction and vesico-ureteric reflux.
2. Wilms' tumour.
3. Pyonephrosis – often with an opaque calculus being visible on plain radiograph.
4. Multicystic kidney – with possible contralateral dysplasia or obstruction.
5. Adult-type polycystic disease with predominant involvement of one kidney.
6. Renal venous thrombosis in young infants.
7. Compensatory hypertrophy with severe damage in the contralateral kidney.

B. When there is no mass clinically detectable the following diagnostic possibilities are present:
1. Unilateral renal aplasia, severe hypoplasia, severe dysplasia (maybe in an ectopic kidney), small multicystic kidney.
2. Obstructive atrophy from any cause.
3. Severe chronic atrophic pyelonephritic scarred kidney.
4. End-stage renal venous thrombosis.

In Group A ultrasonics is especially helpful in distinguishing between Wilms' tumour and obstruction to a kidney. Pyonephrosis may give the clinical impression of being solid because of inflammatory change and so it is easily differentiated from Wilm's tumour because of its echo pattern.

Sonography is useful in Group B because it can be expected to show if any kidney-like structure is present at all. Furthermore, radioisotope studies, especially the DMSA scan, can help in locating small amounts of kidney tissue or ectopic kidneys which are apparently non-functioning at IVU.

3.4 Tactics in Investigation of Patients with Suspected Obstruction

3.4.1 Investigation to Establish Diagnosis of Obstruction

Sonography can establish, by non-invasive means, whether there is dilatation in the upper urinary tract, the lower ureter and bladder. An IVU, in conjunction with these findings and the clinical features, will generally dictate the subsequent course of management if obstruction appears to be high in the upper tract at ultrasound examination. This is because an IVU can establish the diagnosis of obstruction when there is either singly or in combination:
   calyx dilatation;
   dilatation of calyces and pelvis;
and dilatation of calyces, pelvis and upper ureter.
Supplementary retrograde or antegrade injection studies can usefully highlight the nature of the problem in a very few selected cases.

If a kidney is non-functioning at IVU, ultrasonics studies can usually elucidate the nature of the problem, but a DMSA scan will also be helpful on occasion. Both DMSA scan and DTPA scan can be used to quantify each kidney's function and the findings may influence decisions about management, such as whether it is worth conserving a kidney whose function is very severely compromised when the contralateral kidney functions well and has a favourable morphology.

3.4.2 Evaluating the Upper Tract Problem in Lower Ureteric Obstruction

Obstruction high in the upper tract, above the middle third of the ureter, can be defined with certainty as to site and cause by IVU in the majority of patients. However, when the ureter is dilated down to its lower reaches fluoroscopic study either at IVU, or after direct antegrade injection at urodynamic studies or after ureterostomy diversion can help in assessing obstruction. Normally peristaltic waves start high in the ureter and descend towards the bladder. At the level of peristaltic contraction the lumen of the ureter is occluded and a small amount of contrast medium in the urine is propelled towards the bladder by the peristaltic wave. In distal ureteral obstruction the peristaltic wave passes down the ureter but the whole of the ureteric content in front of the wave does not. As the wave approaches the point of obstruction some of the ureteric content passes backward through the advancing peristaltic wave which does not occlude the ureteric lumen. Thus, the ureteric peristaltic wave is incompetent and the severity of obstruction can be related to (i) the degree of occlusion of the ureteric lumen by the peristaltic wave, (ii) the volume of urine entering the bladder with each wave, and (iii) the amount of urine passing proximally through the advancing peristaltic wave.

Although these are subjective assessments they can be very helpful, for if reimplantation of the ureter into the bladder is being contemplated it is encouraging to know the ureter contracts well. On the other hand, when the ureter does not contract well and it is exceptionally dilated and kidney function is deteriorating, then urinary diversion may be preferred. Such a diversion may be the one way of relieving obstruction with certainty and arresting the progress of obstructive renal atrophy.

3.4.3 Role of Cystography

MCU is a logical further step when there is dilatation extending down to the lower part of the ureter shown by either echography or radioisotope scan. An IVU is a debatable early investigation of choice in patients who may have a lower ureteric obstruction. The reason is simply that so often a lower ureteric obstruction is secondary to a vesical problem or a urethral obstruction. Obviously there are exceptions such as mass lesions in the pelvis which cause obstruction, or intramural lesions such as bilharzia and then an IVU may be the preferred examination.

Not all patients who have dilatation in the urinary tract have got obstruction. The child with the absent abdominal muscles syndrome is but one example. Free primary vesico-ureteric reflux in an infant or young child is a rather more subtle problem but it is quite common and this simply underlines the value of MCU when suspected obstruction is not clearly high in the upper tract.

3.5 Monitoring Progress

After any intervention to relieve obstruction studies are needed to demonstrate its efficacy. Such studies are directed towards establishing that (i) obstruction has been relieved and previous proximal dilatation has receded, (ii) kidney function is improving and (iii) satisfactory kidney parenchymal growth is occurring. Classic radiological studies, sonography and radioisotope examinations each have a role. Many examples of obstruction are encountered early in life and follow-up studies are needed to ensure satisfactory continuing management over the childhood years. In such studies radiation dose must be kept to a minimum.

After surgical intervention to relieve obstruction a range of investigations is carried out (sooner rather than later in, for example, infants who have posterior urethral valves) to establish a baseline against which subsequent follow-up studies can be assessed. In the follow-up of patients, radioisotope studies attain particular significance because they yield information about the way in which each kidney's function is developing. IVU indicates what trends, either favorable or unfavorable, are unfolding as time passes. MCU is especially important because (i) it demonstrates the efficacy of measures taken to relieve urethral obstruction and any complication, such as urethral stricture, which may have supervened, and (ii) it will show the development or continuation of vesico-ureteric reflux, this being of distinctive importance in the follow-up of patients with posterior urethral valves, obstructing ectopic ureterocoele, and patients in whom reimplantation of the ureter has been carried out. Echography demonstrates morphology in the upper tract including renal parenchymal growth and it may be used to assess residual urine volumes after micturition.

Initial post-operative studies may be very encouraging. For example, after posterior urethral valves or an ectopic ureterocoele have been dealt with there may be a dramatic reduction in the distension in the upper tract; the amount of renal parenchyma may clearly then be sufficient to ensure a good prognosis.

One of the chief problems arises when upper tract dilatation continues. Such a feature predicates one of the two questions – is the dilatation a consequence of continuing obstruction or is it a consequence of long standing anatomical changes produced by obstruction? Help in getting the right answer can be obtained by careful study of sequential films in an IVU series as diuresis due to the contrast medium injection begins, reaches a peak and recedes. Urodynamic studies with perfusion through the site of possible obstruction can be decisive in selected cases; by adding some contrast medium to the perfusion fluid it is possible to assess the potential of ureteric peristalsis to propel urine distally. Sequential radio-isotope studies, with a timely injection of a diuretic, is another way in which the answer to these questions may be sought.

In all this endeavour there is the need to prevent progressive obstructive atrophy [28] and secure the potential for renal growth. This is but one of the differences between the infant or young child with obstruction and the adult patient. The differences are substantial and many in number.

References

1. Fry, I. K., Cattell, W. R.: The nephrographic pattern during excretion urography. Br. Med. Bull. **28**, 227 (1972)

2. Barratt, T. M., Chantler, C.: Obstructive uropathy in infants. Proc. R. Soc. Med. **63**, 1248 (1970)

3. Dunbar, J. S., Nogrady, N. B.: The calyceal crescent – a roentgen sign of obstructive hydronephrosis. Am. J. Roentgenol. **110**, 520 (1970)

4. Williams, D. I., Mininberg, D. T.: Hydrocalicosis; report of 3 cases. Br. J. Urol. **40**, 541 (1968)

5. Benz, G., Willich, E.: Upper calyx reno-vascular obstruction in children; Fraley's syndrome. Pediatr. Radiol. **5**, 213 (1977)

6. Johnston, J. H.: Pathogenenis of hydronephrosis in children. Br. J. Urol. **41**, 724 (1969)

7. Nixon, H. H.: Hydronephrosis in children. Br. J. Surg. **40**, 601 (1953)

8. Williams, D. I., Neiderhausen, W. V.: Les polypes de l'uretère. J. Urol. Nephrol. (Paris) **69**, 145 (1963)

9. Considine, J.: Retrocaval ureter. Br. J. Urol. **38**, 412 (1966)

10. Forbes, G. S.: Genitourinary involvement in chronic granulomatous disease of childhood. Am. J. Roentgenol. **127**, 683 (1976)

11. Sutcliffe, J., Chrispin, A. R.: Chronic granulomatous disease. Br. J. Radiol. **43**, 110 (1970)

12. Rudhe, U., Ericsson, O.: Lower urinary tract obstruction in infancy and childhood. Ann. Radiol. (Paris) **10**, 247 (1967)

13. Pagano, P., Passerini, G.: Primary obstructed megaureter. Br. J. Urol. **41**, 469 (1977)

14. Reid Pitts, W., Muecke, E.: Congenital megaloureter: a review of 80 patients. J. Urol. **111**, 468 (1974)

15. Eklof, O., Ringertz, H.: Pre- and post-operative urographic findings in posterior urethral valves. Pediatr. Radiol. **4**, 43 (1975)

16. Cass, A. S., Stephens, F. D.: Posterior urethral valves; diagnosis and management. J. Urol. **112**, 519 (1974)

17. Johnston, J. H., Kulatilake, A. E.: The sequelae of posterior urethral valves. Br. J. Urol. **43**, 743 (1971)

18. Williams, D. I., Whitaker, R. H., Barratt, T. M., Keaton, J.: Urethral valves. Br. J. Urol. **45**, 175 (1973)

19. Rudhe, U., Eringsson, O.: Congenital urethral diverticula. Ann. Radiol. (Paris) **13**, 287 (1970)

20. Mowad, J. J., Michaels, M. M.: Meatal stenosis associated with reflux in boys; management of 25 cases. J. Urol. **111**, 100 (1974)

21. Fellows, G. J., Johnston, J. H.: Incomplete urethral duplication and urinary retention. Br. J. Urol. **46**, 449 (1974)

22. Selvaggi, F. P., Goodwin, W. E.: Incomplete duplication of the male urethra. Br. J. Urol. **44**, 495 (1972)

23. Wynne, J. M., Cywes, S., Retief, P. J., Louw, J. H.: Ascites in the newborn. S. Afr. Med. J. **42**, 919 (1968)

24. Mann, C. M., Leape, L. L., Holder, T. M.: Neonatal urinary ascites: report of 2 cases and review of literature. J. Urol. **111**, 124 (1974)

25. Leonides, J. C., Letter, E., Gribetz, D.: Congenital urinary tract obstruction presenting with ascites at birht. Radiology **96**, 111 (1970)

26. Friedland, G. W., Tune, B., Mears, E. M.: Ascites due to rupture of the renal pelvis in an 11 month old infant with uretero-pelvic junction obstruction. Pediatr. Radiol. **2**, 263 (1974)

27. Morgan, C. L., Grossman, H.: Posterior urethral valves as a cause of neonatal uriniferous perirenal pseudocyst. Pediatr. Radiol. **7**, 29 (1978)

28. Hodson, C. J.: Post-obstructive renal atrophy. Br. Med. Bull. **28**, 237 (1972)

4   Urinary Infection and Vesico-Ureteral Reflux

4.1 Introduction

Urinary infection is a complex subject and so it is fraught with controversy. Reflux of urine from the bladder provides a path by which bacteria may enter the kidney and cause pyelonephritis. Renal damage in the form of local scarring or renal growth failure may ensue. Investigatory protocols are needed to cover the requirements of current concepts of management of the individual child's problem. Reflux from the bladder into the ureter may be a feature which runs in families and so the implications of this problem must be discussed. Not all urinary infection is symptomatic and screening of schoolgirls has shown a high incidence of covert bacteria; the relevance of this finding to infants and children in general is analysed.

Although most organisms infecting urine are inhabitants of the intestinal tract there is a group of miscellaneous infections producing, for example, tuberculous disease, bilharzia and moniliasis, and these may occur in rather special circumstances. Nevertheless, it is the commoner type of urinary infection which is the primary subject of this section. Urine is an excellent culture medium for bacteria [1]. Infection in the urinary tract is common but it is not normal, and so the question arises – what ordinarily prevents urinary infection in the normal infant or child? [2] There must be many factors at work; salient among these is the continuing flow of urine into the calyces and down the ureter so that there is no undrained residue of urine in the upper tract. In the bladder normal voiding occurs periodically and the bladder is emptied completely [3]. Uro-epithelium

has the capacity to prevent bacterial growth on its surface [4]. It may be that the urethral mucosa with these characteristics prevents entry of bacteria into the bladder. However, during voiding the urethral lumen opens widely, allowing urine to pass through the sphincteric zone. When voiding ceases the urethral lumen is closed by the sphincter and the mucosa folds in a longitudinal way to occlude the lumen. If the urine is colonized by bacteria then the normal urinary tract has, in theory, the capacity to eliminate such bacteria.

In infancy and childhood urinary tract infection is common. The infecting organism is very often *E. coli* or some other bacterial inhabitant of the gut. When infection is present it is rational to think of those possible changes in function in the urinary tract which predispose to colonization by bacteria. Of course any congenital abnormality which results in an undrained urine residue can predispose to infection; this is why any obstruction in the urinary tract can first present with a urinary tract infection. A urinary calculus gives both a nidus for infection (and reinfection), and very often there is also an element of obstruction. Even when all such examples are excluded there remains a very large group of infants and children who have urinary tract infection but without any of these distinctive underlying problems.

4.2 Infection and the Bladder

Altered patterns of bladder emptying may be present. Amongst school children, especially girls, infection is common and it may be because unusual voiding habits develop. Fluid intake may be low and vesical emptying may be infrequent, say twice a day, and this very effectively gives the urinary residue which predisposes to infection. Fluid intake may be normal but voiding may occur very infrequently; in these circumstances the capacity of the bladder may be very large although complete emptying occurs at micturition cystourethrography (Fig. 4.1). Both the diurnal pattern of voiding urine and the fluid intake may be apparently normal and yet at MCU the bladder capacity is found to be increased; when asked to void the child will pass only a part of the vesical content, leaving an unvoided vesical residue.

Any infection, such as an upper respiratory tract infection with fever or gastro-intestinal upsets with vomiting and diarrhoea, leads to diminished fluid intake, increased fluid loss, an element of dehydration and a diminished volume of fluid being cleared by the kidneys. Such clinical features are often present in infants and young children who develop urinary infection.

When urinary tract infection is discovered an urgent MCU is not indicated, provided that no serious lesion needing immediate surgical intervention is suspected. Occasionally the intravenous urography

Fig. 4.1. Infrequent bladder emptying. This 8-year-old girl had recurrent urinary infection. IVU was normal and there was no vesico-ureteric reflux at MCU. However, she voided 550 ml contrast medium in a normal way after vesical filling was terminated. At this vesical volume she had no especial urge to void. In daily life she voided once or twice each day

(IVU) will show the features of acute cystitis; the bladder is small and its contour irregular because of the inflammatory change in the mucosa. If the circumstances are appropriate it is best do delay cystography until clinical symptoms are controlled. Rarely in patients who have protracted infection the bladder mucosa undergoes a cystic change – cystitis cystica. The cysts lying within the bladder mucosa indent the vesical contour and this can be seen at either MCU or IVU. The larger of these cysts should be identifiable by sonography, but this has yet to be reported. A rather similar cystic change may occur rarely in the ureter or pelvis – ureteritis cystica and pyelitis cystica, respectively.

4.3 Ureterovesical Junction: Functional Characteristics

If MCU can reasonably be delayed for an interval after discovering infection and after the acute episode has been controlled, it is more likely that circumstances predisposing to infection can be realistically assessed. The bladder function and capacity can be studied along the lines previously indicated. However, the function of the uretero-vesical junction is of crucial importance; this assessment of function must not be influenced by acute inflammatory changes in the vicinity.

The normal uretero-vesical junction permits urine flow from the ureter into the bladder and there is never retrograde flow from the bladder into the ureter. Except when flow from the ureter into the bladder is occurring, the uretero-vesical junction remains closed. As in other parts of the body, closure of the lumen is achieved by the mucosal folds and muscular action. During micturition there is no retrograde flow from the bladder into the ureter and the uretero-vesical junction remains competent.

The abnormal event at the uretero-vesical junction is reflux of urine from the bladder and into the ureter [3]. Inevitably urine enters the upper tract and there is a residue in the urinary tract which would otherwise have been voided – this residue predisposes to infection.

At MCU reflux may occur as the bladder is filled and during the early stages of filling; as the bladder distends no further reflux may occur. In other patients reflux may occur only towards the end of vesical filling, and in yet another group reflux may occur throughout the filling procedure. Reflux in this last group may be a continuing feature rather than an intermittent phenomenon and reflux may continue during the act of micturition. Finally, there are those patients in whom reflux occurs only when the bladder contracts.

In some patients undergoing an IVU or MCU appearance of contrast medium in the ureter and collecting system may be a late event. When a kidney is slow to clear contrast medium at IVU the sudden appearance of increased concentration of medium late in the IVU series may be a consequence of reflux. This type of sequence is well demonstrated by isotope cystography following clearance studies.

4.4 Significant Factors in Vesico-Ureteral Reflux

Two considerations about reflux now follow: one is concerned with the volume of urine entering the upper urinary tract and the other is related to the moment at which reflux occurs. When the amount of urine passing into the upper urinary system is small then at the end of micturition the unvoided residue is small. If large amounts pass upward as a result of reflux, then at the end of micturition the bladder refills and the volume entering the bladder may be sufficient for the child to void again (Fig. 4.2). Even though reflux may be considerable at MCU the IVU

can be surprisingly normal in appearance. This is because the bladder does not contract and empty during the procedure. Sometimes at IVU and MCU a clue about the undue distensibility of the upper tract may be detected if longitudinal striation in the pelvis or ureter is seen (Fig. 4.3). On other occasions

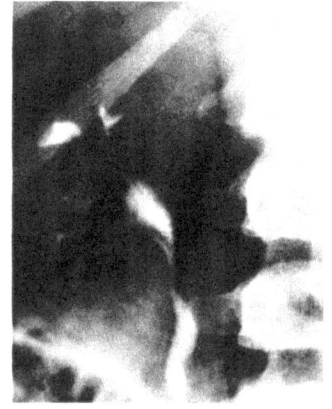

Fig. 4.3. Striation of the renal pelvis. At IVU this girl, who had vesico-ureteric reflux, shows striation of the renal pelvis on the right side. Such striation may also be seen in the ureter at IVU. The cystogram demonstrated that the upper tract is distended at times to a greater degree than is present at IVU. The striation simply represents the longitudinal folds of the uro-epithelium and may be found in patients who have reflux or obstruction

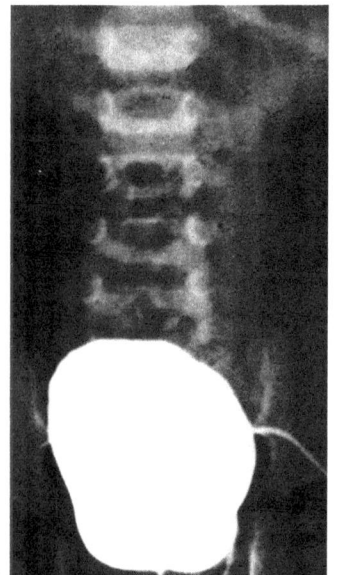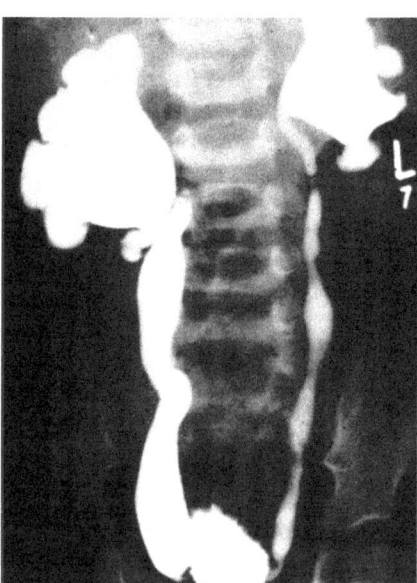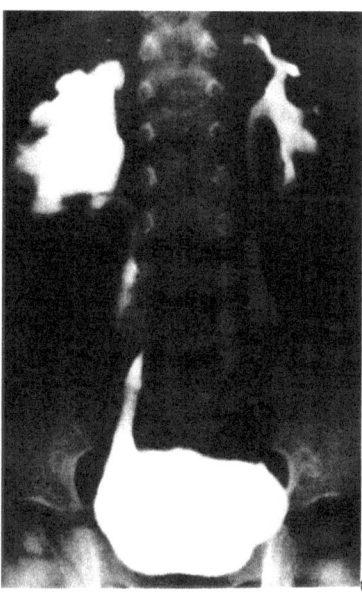

a, b   c

Fig. 4.2 a, b–c. Vesico-ureteric reflux. This boy had recurrent urinary infections. His MCU shows there is no reflux on vesical filling (**a**), but on voiding there is gross reflux into both ureters at the end of micturition (**b**). Although at the end of micturition the bladder was empty, rapid emptying of the ureters occurs because of quite efficient ureteric peristalsis (**c**). As the distension of the upper tract diminishes and the upper tract empties, the bladder refills with contrast medium. After a short interval he was able to void again. Note the continuing distension of the right renal pelvis

upper tract distension may be gross (Fig. 4.4). When the upper tract is distended considerably the papillae of the kidney are subjected to the transmitted force of the detrusor contraction of the bladder. It becomes clear that patients with substantial volumes of reflux can be considered for reflux-preventing surgery at an early stage.

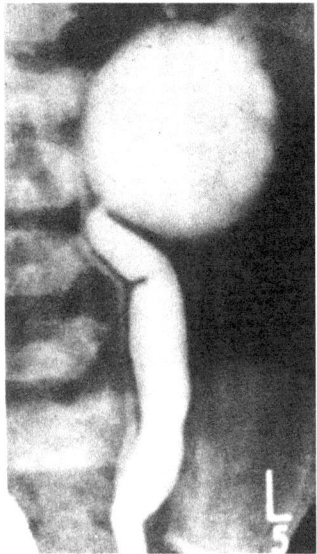

Fig. 4.4. Gross distension of the upper tract at MCU. This boy had pain in the left loin on voiding. He has a duplication on the left side. The upper renal element has a narrow ureter and undistended calyces. The lower renal element has a grossly dilated ureter through which contrast medium passes to enter and distend the left renal pelvis. At the pelvi-ureteric junction there is a narrowing which permits the forcible entry of urine during voiding, but traps the urine in the distended pelvis after voiding ceases. See also Fig. 4.2

The normal ureter enters the bladder through its intramural pathway which lies tangential to the convexity of the full bladder (Fig. 4.5) [5]. In some

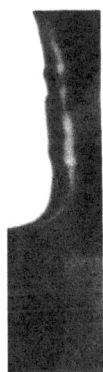

Fig. 4.5. Uretero-vesical junction. In this male infant who had a urinary infection, the MCU shows the ureter has a normal angle of entry into the bladder. Some 18 months later, repeat MCU showed the reflux had disappeared. IVU was normal

patients with reflux, especially those with severe reflux, the intramural ureter lies at right angles to the normal expected tangent (Fig. 4.6). Only carefully positioned oblique projections obtained by fluoroscopy will yield this type of information about the intramural course of the ureter. An assessment of the ureteric orifice can also be made at endoscopy; when the normal ureteric orifice is closed a small mound is formed by the mucosa, but when there is a severe degree of reflux the ureteric orifice can be seen as a "golf hole". If the intramural course of the ureter is at right angles to the convexity of the bladder and if there is a golf hole type of ureteric orifice seen at endoscopy the prospect for a spontaneous recovery of competence at the uretero-vesical junction must be very poor [5, 6].

Surgical treatment for reflux can be necessary in other patients at an early stage. When a diverticulum

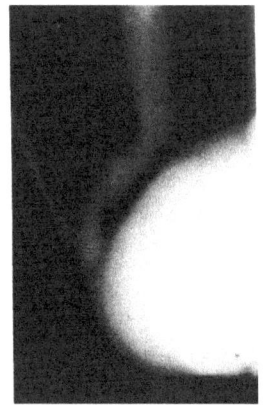

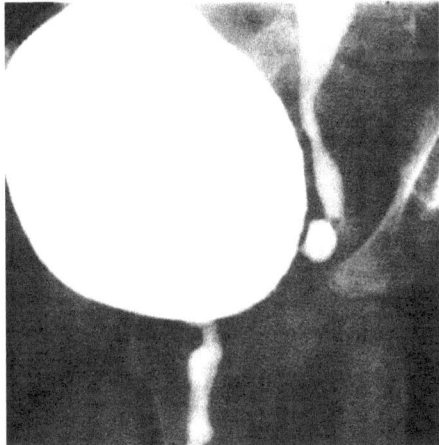

Fig. 4.6 a, b. Uretero-vesical junction. **a** In this boy with recurrent infections, the right ureter enters the bladder through a narrow intramural course which lies along a radius of the bladder contour. MCU shows there is also considerable reflux into the dilated ureter. **b** At the left uretero-vesical junction there is a small diverticulum which fills as voiding occurs and reflux into the left ureter begins

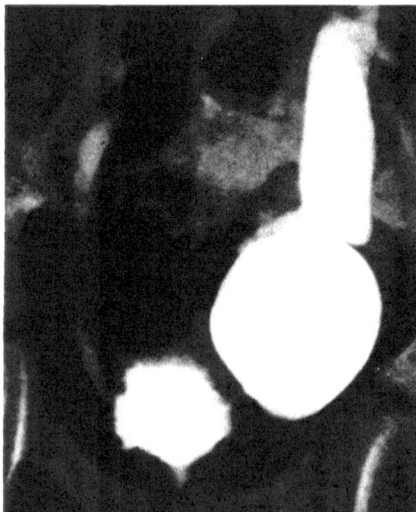

Fig. 4.7. Bilateral reflux with para-ureteric diverticulum at MCU. MCU shows some reflux on the right side, but gross reflux on the left side associated with a diverticulum which distends considerably as micturition comes to an end

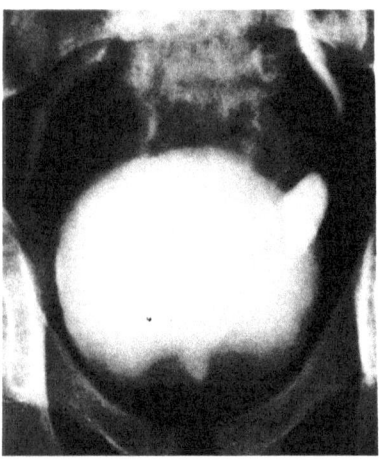

Fig. 4.8. Paraureteric diverticulum at IVU. The urogram shows the ureter sweeping alongside the undistended but heavily opacified diverticulum. This ureter drained a heavily scarred small kidney

is present at the uretero-vesical junction (Fig. 4.6) the ureter may pass alongside the para-ureteric diverticulum (Figs. 4.7 and 4.8) or it may enter the diverticulum itself (Fig. 4.9). With such anatomical abnormalities there is no prospect of reflux stopping spontaneously. Such diverticula may only be seen towards the end of micturition at MCU.

Other structural abnormalities rule out any likelihood of spontaneous recovery from reflux. Such abnormalities include all those ectopic points of entry of the ureter into the lower urinary tract, and

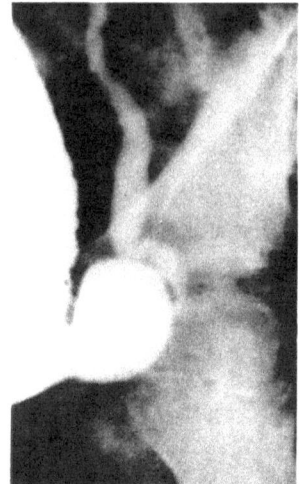

Fig. 4.9. Ureter entering a diverticulum. The MCU shows reflux into a diverticulum and thence into the ureter, which enters the diverticulum directly

these are especially associated with the variants of duplication.

There are many children in whom such clear-cut features are not present and at the first examination there is no distinctive evidence to indicate surgery is required sooner rather than later. Satisfactory control of urinary infection can be achieved with chemotherapy. In about two-thirds of such children reflux will disappear spontaneously during a 2-year interval (Fig. 4.5) [7, 8]. This time factor is important. For children who have otherwise had a satisfactory development in the kidneys and urinary tract and in those approaching the age of maturity the prospects are good. The problem lies among those infants and young children who need good kidney growth and a satisfactory outcome at the end of the many years which lie ahead before maturity is reached. During these years there is the possibility of breakthrough infection during periods of chemotherapy or the recurrence of infection after a period of chemotherapy, and there are the rare untoward side-effects of chemotherapy itself. For these children and for many others with lesions in the lower urinary tract concern centres on the development of the kidney itself.

4.5 Acute Kidney Infection and the Advent of the Pyelonephritic Scar

In infants and children who have clinical features suggesting an acute pyelonephritis the kidneys are often large and tender to palpation. Systemically effective chemotherapy controls the kidney infection and the clinical features abate rapidly.

Infants undergoing intravenous urography during the acute episode may show delay in clearance of contrast medium by the enlarged kidneys even when the calyces are not increased in size, as in infants who have obstructive uropathy. There is very occasionally an increase in density of the nephrogram in association with acute pyelonephritis. The pathology of acute pyelonephritis is one of acute interstitial renal inflammatory changes with inflammatory changes also present in the renal pelvis. In children with acute pyelonephritis in whom the kidneys have not been damaged by some antecedent lesion the IVU shows renal enlargement with compression of the calyx system and an apparent increase in parenchymal thickness [9]. If appropriate clinical measures are taken to combat acute infection, the previously undamaged kidney may recover fully. In children who have had successful treatment of urinary infection and pyelonephritis there may be a retardation in the rate of accumulation of isotope in the scintigram of the kidneys for a period even though by other methods of assessment the urinary tract and kidneys appear normal. The association between reflux and pyelonephritic scarring has long been recognised [10]. Recently it has become fashionable to describe such scars as reflux nephropathy; [11] this simply reflects current thinking which holds as one of its tenets that such lesions are a consequence of reflux of urine from the lower tract up to the kidney [12]. With reflux, infected urine carries bacteria through the minor calyces into the parenchyma of the renal medulla through papillae whose tips are susceptible to such intrarenal reflux [13, 14]. There is no doubt that intrarenal reflux of contrast medium can be demonstrated at MCU and the more carefully it is sought the more often it is seen (Fig. 4.10) [15].

Since the human kidney has many minor calyces and associated pyramids such intrarenal reflux and infection of the kidney can lead to the development of new pyelonephritic scars. In any carefully controlled group of children who have urinary infection the transition from a normal status to a scarred kidney is rarely seen; [16, 17] this simply reflects the skill and efficacy of clinical management and it does not represent a study of the natural progress of disease. The pyelonephritic scar in the infant or child is acquired and it develops rapidly in a period of a few months (Fig. 4.11), may be in a very few months [18]. It appears to be a special feature of the infant and young child since adults who have acute pyelonephritis seem not to acquire localised scarring.

The radiological hallmark of the pyelonephritic scar is clubbing of a minor calyx or dilatation of a minor

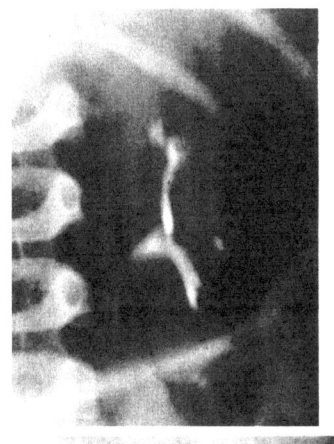

a

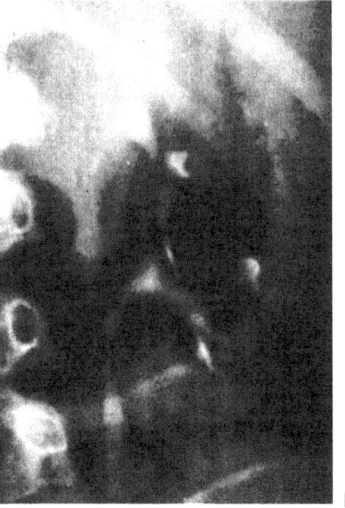

b

Fig. 4.11 a, b. Acquired renal scarring. This boy has exstrophy of the bladder and his urogram showed no renal abnormality initially (**a**). Fifteen months later the repeat urogram (**b**) demonstrates pyelonephritic scarring with calyx clubbing and parenchymal thinning. It is exceptional to see such a sequence

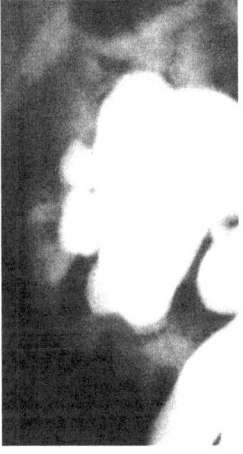

Fig. 4.10. Intrarenal reflux. This infant has severe reflux into a dilated tortuous ureter, which then enters the dilated renal pelvis. The calyces are dilated and many papillae permit the transit of contrast medium through the papillary tips into the parenchyma

calyx with destruction of the renal pyramid (19). There is indentation of the margin of the renal parenchyma adjacent to the affected calyx and this reflects the damage to the parenchyma at the site of the scar (Fig. 4.12). Such a solitary scar may seem a minor phenomenon but this is not the case as a DMSA scan can show the zone of diminished uptake (Fig. 4.13). Furthermore, at IVU the margin of the scar may not be profiled by IVU and yet echography can then demonstrate such lesions clearly (Fig. 4.14)

because of the reduced parenchymal thickness and possible increase in echogenicity where sound is reflected from the scar. Most often the scars lie at one or both poles of the kidney. As a result at IVU the kidney alignment in relationship to the fixed structures of the posterior abdominal wall changes (20). When the upper pole is scarred the clubbed

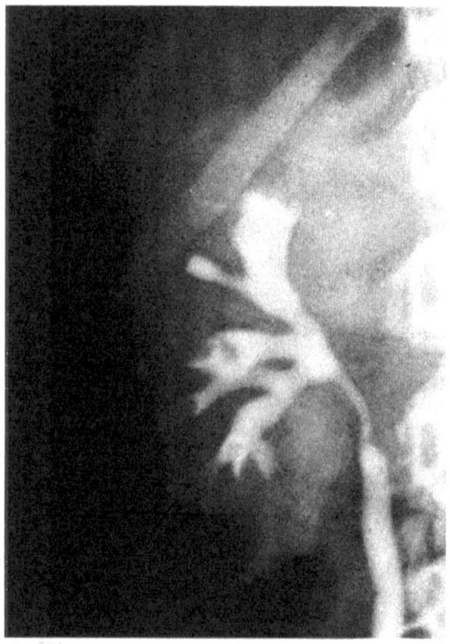

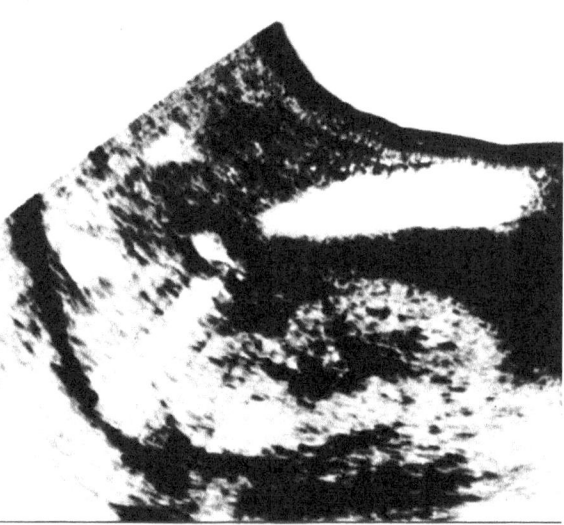

Fig. 4.14. Age 10 years. LS supine showing liver, gall-bladder and right kidney. The indentation of the upper pole is a scar. This child has scarring, but the IVU appeared to be normal

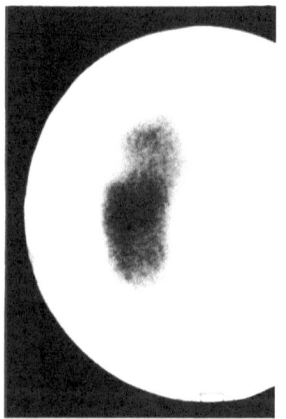

Fig. 4.12. The pyelonephritic scar. This young girl had vesico-ureteric reflux on the side of the scarred kidney. One calyx shows clubbing and there is contiguous thinning of the renal parenchyma. There appears to be a minor structural change, but the IVU gives a limited knowledge of the reality

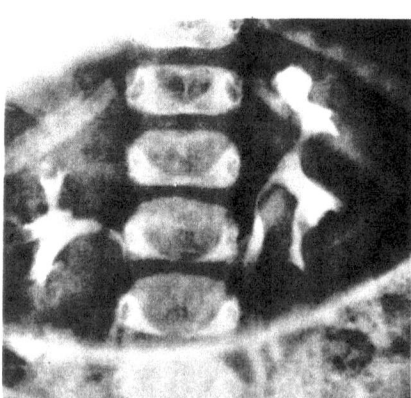

Fig. 4.15. Changes in calyx relationships with scarring and atrophy. In this young child one kidney is unaffected, but the damaged kidney shows scarring at both the poles, bringing the upper calyx in closer proximity to the spine and the lower calyx nearer the ureter. This change is a consequence of reduction in parenchymal thickness at the sites of scarring. If the renal contours are not clearly visible such changed relationships can be of diagnostic value. In addition, note the bulge in the contour at the site of hypertrophy in the undamaged middle part of the kidney

Fig. 4.13. DMSA scan in a kidney with a pyelonephritic scar. In the damaged zone there is no uptake of isotope and this feature indicates more truly the loss of functioning renal tissue in the kidney

calyces come to lie unduly close to the spine as the parenchymal loss occurs. Lower pole scarring brings the clubbed calyces in closer proximity to the ureter (Fig. 4.15). Oblique views at IVU can sometimes enhance the prospect of seeing scars on the ventral and dorsal aspects of the kidney. The renal window view and tomography can also be useful radiological projections. However, scars not revealed at IVU may be effectively demonstrated by sonography.

4.6 Sequels to Renal Scarring and Reflux [21, 22]

Once a scar has developed it represents a loss of parenchyma which is irreversible and also a loss of growth potential in the scarred area. If one kidney is heavily scarred and the other is relatively unscarred the less damaged or undamaged kidney undergoes compensatory hypertrophy (Fig. 4.16). In fact compensatory hypertrophy can occur in any undamaged area and when scarring is bilateral such local hypertrophy can further distort the renal outline. This means that simple measurements of kidney length are not a very good method of assessing

kidney development in all patients who have pyelonephritic scarring. This has been known for a long time and it led to defining kidney contours by line drawing so that contours from one urogram can be compared with those from another [8].

Even quite heavily scarred kidneys can produce good opacification of the clubbed calyces at IVU. The reason is that the undamaged hypertrophied part of the kidney still functions well. In a child this appearance of kidney performance is deceptive. The potential for kidney growth can be outstripped by the continuing growth of the child. With failing reserves of kidney function the capacity to concentrate contrast, medium falls until there may be virtually no pyelogram at IVU and the kidneys may not be visible. Hypertension occurs with increasing frequency as the individual with pyelonephritic scarring grows older and hypertensive nephropathy further diminishes kidney function. When the kidneys are not visible at IVU, sonography can identify anatomical features and if reflux has persistend MCU may make it possible to demonstrate the calyx deformity (Fig. 4.17). However, it is also important to monitor renal function; split renal function studies using the radioisotope DTPA enable the contribution of each kidney to the total glomerular clearance to be assessed.

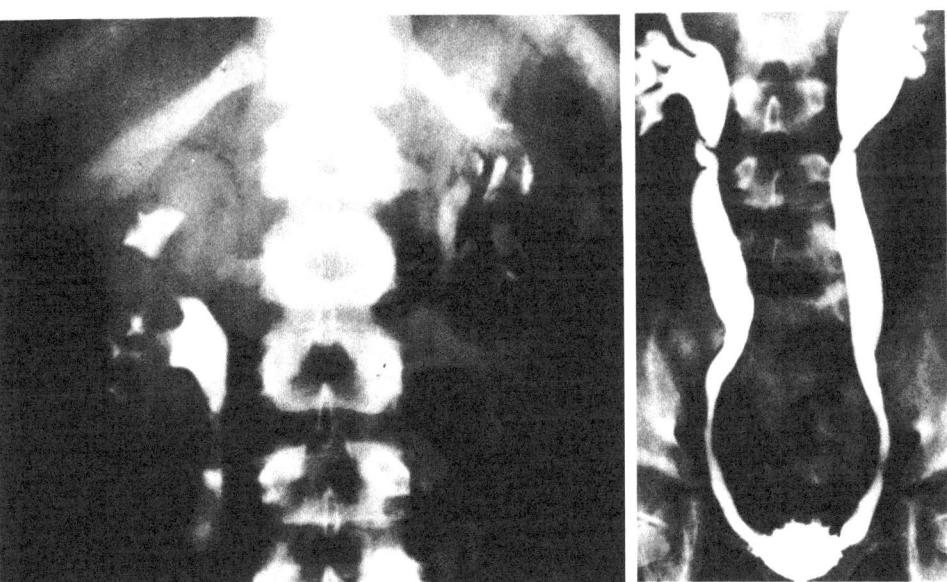

a, b

Fig. 4.16 a, b. Contralateral compensatory hypertrophy and renal scarring. **a** At IVU one kidney is very heavily scarred and atrophic – the clubbed calyces are crowded together in a very small kidney which still appears to concentrate well. The other kidney has a normal structure and is large owing to compensatory hypertrophy. The ureter on this side is dilated and shows striations. **b** MCU in this girl with recurrent urinary infection shows severe bilateral vesico-ureteric reflux, apparently equally severe on the two sides. It might be inferred that the papillae in the undamaged kidney had not been susceptible to intrarenal reflux whereas on the damaged kidney they had been. Intrarenal reflux does not seem to occur into a scarred zone

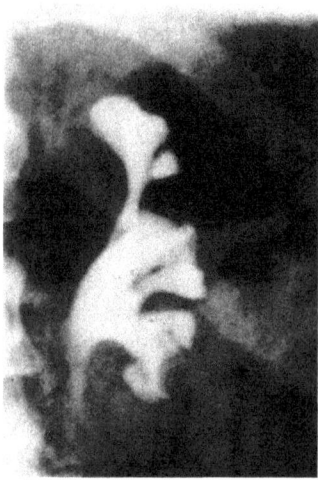

Fig. 4.17. Renal failure and hypertension. In this girl with end-stage disease, neither kidney functioned at IVU. Nevertheless at MCU there was bilateral vesico-ureteric reflux sufficient to show the clubbed calyces crowded together in the small heavily scarred kidney on one side

4.6.1 Differential Diagnosis of the Small Kidney

Differential diagnosis of reflux nephropathy is not an easy subject to discuss. Theoretically *segmental hypoplasia*, which has distinctive pathological characteristics, has radiological features at IVU identical to those of pyelonephritis. Some authors report segmental hypoplasia as being a less than rare phenomenon. However, this has not been the experience in many institutions where it is considered to be an exceptionally rare lesion as compared to the very common pyelonephritic scar. Not all patients who have pyelonephritic scarring have reflux which can be demonstrated; in these circumstances it has to be presumed that scarring develops in the context of a urinary tract infection in which reflux was transiently present with renal papilla susceptible to intrarenal reflux. Reflux without renal scarring but with infection is found and it must be presumed that the renal papillae are not susceptible to intra-renal reflux and parenchymal infection and damage (Fig. 4.16) or that medical management has been effective in preventing scar formation. Urinary tract infection is such a common phenomenon that one can never be certain that infection has not been present at some time in any one individual.

The other main group of renal lesions which must be considered in differentiation are *renal dysplasia* and *hypoplasia*. However, this group of disorders is found in rather special circumstances (*see* Chapter 6).

The late stage of *medullary (papillary) necrosis,* acquired in infancy, can present a differential diagnostic problem. When medullary necrosis is complete the calyx has a clubbed appearance but the indentation of the renal contour seen in the pyelonephritic scar is not present on the IVU. As in pyelonephritis, medullary necrosis does not result in uniform damage to all papillae. Illnesses, such as gastroenteritis, a common precipitating feature of the shock state that can lead to medullary necrosis, is also often found as a background feature in the infant with urinary infection. If adrenal calcification, which is a sequel to adrenal haemorrhage, is present, then a concomitant renal lesion is likely to be medullary necrosis or late stage renal venous thrombosis.

In children who have both a history of infection and reflux, the kidney may fail to grow in size without developing scars [8]. This is an event which has some parallels with that seen in adults who have acute pyelonephritis; in the adult who has an acute renal infection a reduction in kidney size may follow, but without local scarring. When the kidney fails to grow in a young child the long-term outcome is compromised. Simple measurements of kidney length can elucidate such growth failure but the use of contour diagrams can be much more helpful. When pyelonephritic scarring is also present contour diagrams are even more helpful. Echography can be used to measure the kidney; measurements of length, antero-posterior and coronal diameters can all be made, and from these measurements a knowledge of kidney volume can be derived.

4.7 Investigation and Implications for Management in Urinary Infection

4.7.1 Indications for Surgical Treatment

The foregoing is a statment of facts and deductions as well as a synthesis on which a rational strategy for management can be based. Surgical intervention and reimplantation of the ureter into the bladder is considered in the following circumstances:

1. Severe degrees of reflux where there is a sizeable volume of urine in the upper tract at the end of micturition.
2. Structural abnormalities which make it unlikely that reflux will abate and such abnormalities include:
   Para-ureteric diverticulum (when large)
   Unfavourable intramural ureteric course, maybe with unfavourable findings at endoscopy

Variants of duplication in which reflux is a continuing feature

3. Reflux with renal parenchymal opacification, for this indicates parenchymal vulnerability of a high order.

4. Reflux persisting over a period of time in a young child in whom medical measures have failed to control infection; there is in these circumstances a long period of growth ahead for the child and this must not be compromised by damage to the kidney.

There are now two caveats to be made. The first is that reimplantation surgery in the young infant presents exceptional technical difficulties and should be avoided whenever reasonable. The second is that parenchymal scarring seems unlikely to develop after about 6 years of age and so there is little point in reimplantation for older children who have reflux and who have scarred kidneys – such a possible tactic is unwise because it is too late.

Nevertheless most patients who undergo reimplantation surgery will lie within the categories 1–4 above and they will be under 6 years of age. Protracted reflux without kidney damage (where there is, despite medical management, a repeated tendency to recurrent infection) may constitute an indication for reimplantation in a tiny minority of children.

Before undertaking reimplantation surgery obstruction to bladder emptying and neuropathic bladder must be excluded. Ureteric performance must be assessed and the presence and efficiency of ureteric peristalsis noted at fluorosocopy, as in certain types of ureteric obstruction. There is a very small number of children who have (generally in late childhood) two grossly dilated non-peristaltic ureters; for these a diversion procedure may constitute the best prospect for preserving heavily compromised function in both kidneys. If such a very gross degree of dilatation is present on one side only, nephroureterectomy may be the best course of action; isotope studies can show the low contribution to total renal function of a kidney draining into such a ureter.

4.7.2 Indications for Medical Management

Careful medical management will have every prospect of ensuring good kidney growth and abatement of reflux in infants and children who fortunately do not have the type of problem for which surgery is clearly required.

4.7.3 Timing of Investigation

Current evidence suggests that the first clear-cut clinical infection is sufficient to warrant investigation. In children over 6 years who are found to have a normal intravenous urogram (this includes cases of simple duplication) no further radiological investigation appears to be warranted. Younger patients are more vulnerable and so MCU generally follows the IVU once infection is clearly under control and inflammatory changes have subsided. Urinary tract surgery necessitates follow-up studies and repeat IVU and MCU after an interval of some 3–6 months will be the correct procedure. With skilled surgical teams it is very rare that an earlier study to evaluate a possible complication needs to be undertaken.

Subsequently all patients will require further follow-up studies at increasingly longer intervals throughout childhood if the urinary tract is not normal. Initially, a study at 1 year and then 2-yearly intervals will suffice. All these studies are not pleasant for the child, and modern techniques are beginning to make it possible to envisage a less burdensome line of follow-up and initial study.

Sonography can estimate kidney size at the time of the first baseline radiological study. Afterwards kidney growth may be assessed by ultrasound study alone. Likewise isotope studies carried out concurrently with the first radiological studies will give an estimate of the contribution of each kidney to overall renal function. If DTPA is used and late examination shows the kidneys to be clear of isotope, the presence of significant degrees of reflux can be demonstrated by voiding the isotope which has accumulated in the bladder. It can be expected that such a strategy for investigation will be increasingly important since it both reduces radiation dosage and is virtually non-invasive by comparison with classic radiological studies. Nevertheless before this style of long-term follow-up can be established each department must be confident that its skills in these fields have been validated. But the MCU still gives a range of information not quite matched by other methods.

4.8 Collateral Considerations

4.8.1 Covert Urinary Tract Infection

Up to this point attention has been focused on the infant or child whose urinary infection produces symptoms and investigation is then directed towards finding any functional or structural problem in the kidney and urinary tract. However, not all urinary infection is symptomatic – the covert urinary infection; and reflux may occur in brothers or sisters of an affected child.

About 1 girl in 20 may be expected to have a clinically asymptomatic "covert" urinary infection in her years at school: epidemiological studies show this to be so [23, 24, 25, 26]. If such girls have normal kidneys at the moment of discovery of infection it would appear they will continue to have undamaged kidneys irrespective of whether they are treated or not. Should the kidney be already scarred there is the possibility that scarring may progress.

However, it is surely true to say that these epidemiological studies have in part been carried out in this particular age group because schoolgirls constitute a population which is easy to assess. The findings, among other things, underline that scarring is acquired at an earlier age. It has been emphasized here and many times previously, that the vulnerable kidney is especially that of the child below school age. Perhaps energies should be directed more to epidemiological studies of the pre-school child and infant [27, 28, 29].

Prevention of kidney scarring is of the essence because of the increasing risk of hypertension as years pass [30], quite apart from the gross degrees of scarring which lead to renal failure sooner rather than later.

4.8.2 Reflux in Families

For years it has been recognised that symptomatic infection and reflux may occur in more than one child in a family. Recent studies of apparently well brothers and sisters of a sympomatic child have shown that they too may be affected by reflux [31, 32].

This is an interesting finding but its implications are considerable. It is questionable whether the invasive and unpleasant procedures of IVU and MCU are appropriate for investigating asymptomatic siblings. Sonography and perhaps radioisotope studies with a late voiding scintigram are better methods of study if investigation in this area is deemed necessary and worthwhile.

4.9 Miscellaneous Urinary Infections

In infants and children the infecting organisms are commonly those which may be found in the large intestine. Strains of *E. coli* are by far the commonest infecting organisms, but others such as *Pseudomonas* and *Klebsiella* do occur. Infection by *Proteus* must always lead to the suspicion of calculus disease in the urinary tract.

Fortunately in developed countries tuberculosis of the urinary tract is rare. The renal damage may simulate chronic pyelonephritic scarring with damage to the renal medulla leading to caliectasis. Stenoses at the infundibulum of a calyx, pelvi-ureteric junction and uretero-vesical junction may produce obstruction. Tuberculous disease of the bladder wall leads to a contraction of the bladder's capacity and increased frequency. Clearly routes of infection in the urinary tract other than the intraluminal one may be implicated in tuberculosis; the onset of the infection may be haematogenous and the spread may be via the lymphatic channels as well as directly through the tissues.

Rarer opportunistic infections may be found in children with immunodeficiency states, such as those infections encountered in chronic granulomatous disease and in children under treatment for leukaemia and malignant disease.

References

1. Asscher, A. W., Sussman, M., Waters, W. E., Davies, R. H., Chick, S.: Urine as a culture medium for bacterial growth. Lancet *1966 II*, 1037
2. Cox, C. E., Hinman, F.: Experiments with induced bacteriuria, vesical emptying and bacterial growth. J. Urol. **86,** 739 (1961)
3. O'Grady, F., Cattell, W. R.: Kinetics of urinary tract infection I. Upper urinary tract. II. The bladder. Br. J. Urol. **38,** 149 (1966)
4. Norden, C. W., Green, G. M., Kass, E. H.: Antibacterial mechanisms of the urinary bladder. J. Clin. Invest. **47,** 2689 (1968)
5. Fendel, H., Devens, K.: The radiographic and endoscopic appearance of the uretero-vesical junction in vesico-ureteric reflux. Ann. Radiol. (Paris) **17,** 403 (1974)
6. Fendel, H.: The radiology of the vesico-ureteric junction. In: Current diagnostic pediatrics. Vol. 1: Current Concepts in pediatric radiology. Eklöf, O. (ed.), p. 94. Berlin, Heidelberg, New York: Springer (1977)
7. Heikel, P. E., Parkkulainen, K. V.: Vesico-ureteric reflux in children. Ann. Radiol. (Paris) **2,** 37 (1966)
8. Edwards, D., Normand, I. C. S., Prescod, N., Smellie, J. M.: Disappearance of vesicoureteric reflux during long-term prophylaxis of urinary infection in children. Br. Med. J. **3,** *1977 III*, 285
9. Hugosson, C. O., Chrispin, A. R., Wolverson, M. K.: The advent of the pyelonephritic scar. Ann. Radiol. (Paris) **19,** 1 (1976)

10. Hodson, C. J., Wilson, S.: Natural history of chronic pyelonephritic scarring. Br. Med. J. **2**, *1965 II,* 191

11. Hodson, J., Maling, M. J., McManomon, P. J., Lewis, M. G.: Reflux nephropathy. Kidney Int. **8,** S-50-S-58 (1975)

12. Smellie, J., Edwards, D., Hunter, N., Normand, I. C. S., Prescod, N.: Vesico-ureteric reflux and renal scarring. Kidney Int. **8**, S-65-S-72 (1975)

13. Rolleston, G. L., Shannon, F. T., Utley, W. L. F.: Relationship of infantile vesicoureteric reflux to renal damage. Br. Med. J. *1970 I,* 460

14. Rolleston, G. L., Maling, T. M. J., Hodson, C. J.: Intrarenal reflux and the scarred kidney. Arch. Dis. Child. **49,** 531 (1974)

15. Ransley, P. G.: Opacification of the renal parenchyma in obstruction and reflux. Pediatr. Radiol. **4,** 226 (1976)

16. Blank, E.: Caliectasis and renal scars in children. J. Urol. **10,** 255 (1973)

17. Shah, K. J., Robins, D. G., White, R. H. R.: Renal scarring and vesicoureteric reflux. Arch. Dis. Child. **53,** 210 (1978)

18. Hugosson, C. O., Chrispin, A. R., Wolverson, M. K.: The advent of the pyelonephritic scar. Ann. Radiol. (Paris) **19,** 1 (1976)

19. Filly, R., Friedland, G. W., Govan, D. E., Fair, W. R.: Development and progression of clubbing and scarring in children with recurrent urinary tract infections. Radiology **113,** 145 (1974)

20. Friedland, G. W., Filly, R., Brown, B. W.: Distance of upper pole calyx to spine and lower pole calyx to ureter as indications of parenchymal loss in children. Pediatr. Radiol. **2,** 29 (1974)

21. Kaas Ibsen, K.: The growth of the kidneys in children with vesicoureteric reflux. Acta Paediatr. Scand. **66,** 741 (1977)

22. Aperia, A., Broberger, O., Ekengren, K., Erisson, N. O., Wikstad, I.: Correlation between kidney parenchymal area and renal function in vesicoureteral reflux of different degrees. Ann. Radiol. (Paris) **20,** 141 (1977)

23. Kunin, C. M., Zacha, E., Paquin, A. J.: Urinary tract infections in school children: Prevalence of bacteriuria and associated urological findings. N. Engl. J. Med. **266,** 1287 (1962)

24. Meadow, S. R., White, R. H. R., Johnston, N. M.: Prevalence of symptomless urinary tract disease in Birmingham school children. Br. Med. J. *1969 III,* 81

25. Edwards, B., White, R. H. R., Maxted, H., Deverill, I., White, P. I.: Screening methods for covert bacteriuria in schoolgirls. Br. Med. J. *1975 II,* 463

26. Cleasson, I., Lindberg, H.: Asymptomatic bacteriuria in schoolgirls. Radiology **124,** 179 (1977)

27. Davies, J. M., Gibson, G. L., Littlewood, J. M., Meadow, S. R.: Prevalence of bacteriuria in infants and pre-school children. Lancet *1974 II,* 7

28. Boothman, R., Laidlaw, M., Richards, I. D. G.: Prevalence of urinary tract infection in children of pre-school age. Arch. Dis. Child. **49,** 917 (1974)

29. Kunin, C. M., Groot, J. E. De, Uehling, D., Ramgopal, V.: Detection of urinary infection in 3 to 5 year old girls by mothers using a nitrite indicator strip. Pediatrics **57,** 829 (1976)

30. Heale, W.: Chronic pyelonephritis in the adult. Aust. N. Z. J. Med. **1,** 283 (1971)

31. Reflux in families (editorial). Br. Med. J. *1975 IV,* 726

32. Redman, J. F.: Vesico-ureteral reflux in identical twins. J. Urol. **116,** 792 (1976)

5 Nephrocalcinosis – Nephrolithiasis – Urolithiasis

5.1 Introduction

Calcium deposits in the kidney and urinary tract always predicate a problem. They can be difficult to identify by radiography because in the young child gas and other gut content obscures the kidney area, the ureteric pathway, and, to a lesser extent, the bladder. Although calcium is radio-opaque there may be so little calcium in any one place that it is hard to produce an image of it and this can be an almost insuperable problem on X-ray examination. Urinary calculus is a stone against which every radiologist, paediatrician and urological surgeon has stubbed his toe at one time or another; for the child and his doctor the pain and cost of this event is perceived sooner or later. Fortunately for everyone many calcium deposits in the kidney and urinary tract are easy to identify on radiological and ultrasonics examination.

5.2 Causes of Nephrocalcinosis, Nephrolithiasis, and Urolithiasis

5.2.1 Nephrocalcinosis

In overall terms nephrocalcinosis is a rare feature of paediatric renal disease, but the causes are clear cut [1, 2]. Calcium may be deposited in the kidney in the following conditions and in those identified by* stone formation may also occur:

Renal tubular acidosis* (Figs. 5.1, 5.2 and 5.7)
Hypercalciuria

Post-parenchymal necrosis and cortical necrosis
Calcium deposits in malignancies, notably Wilms' tumour
Xanthogranulomatous pyelonephritis*

Nephrocalcinosis may be a reflection of more general metabolic problems such as:
Hyperparathyroidism* (Fig. 5.3)
Cushing's syndrome in infancy*
Hypophosphatasia with severe bone disease (Fig. 5.4)
Metaphyseal dysostosis (mistaken for rickets) and treated with high Vitamin D doses*
Vitamin D intoxication resulting from a variety of reasons Idiopathic hypercalcaemia (Figs. 5.5 and 5.6) Immobilization*

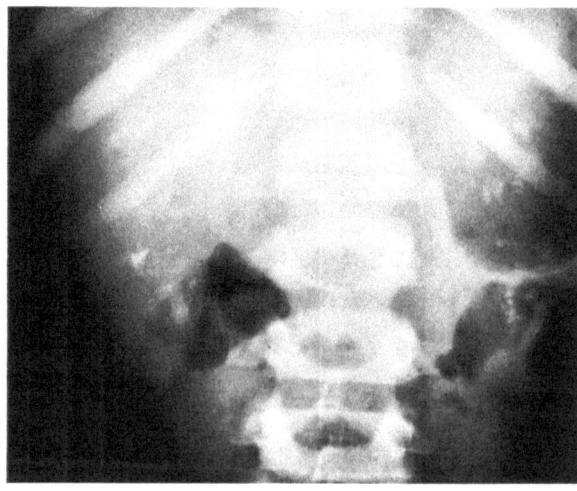

Fig. 5.1. Nephrocalcinosis and nephrolithiasis in renal tubular acidosis. Plain radiograph shows deposits of calcium in the medullary zones of both kidneys

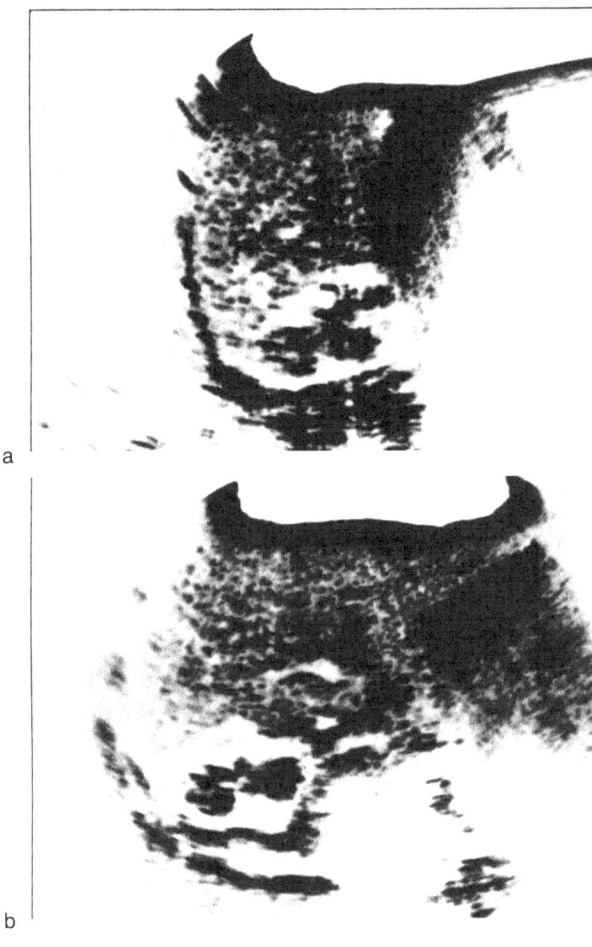

a

b

Fig. 5.2 a, b. **Fig. 5.2 a, b.** Age 1 year. **a** LS supine, through the right kidney and liver. The usual collecting cluster is replaced by a more stellate appearance of very high echoes. **b** TS supine. This appearance is caused by collections of small medullary calculi: in this child they are a result of renal tubular acidosis

◁

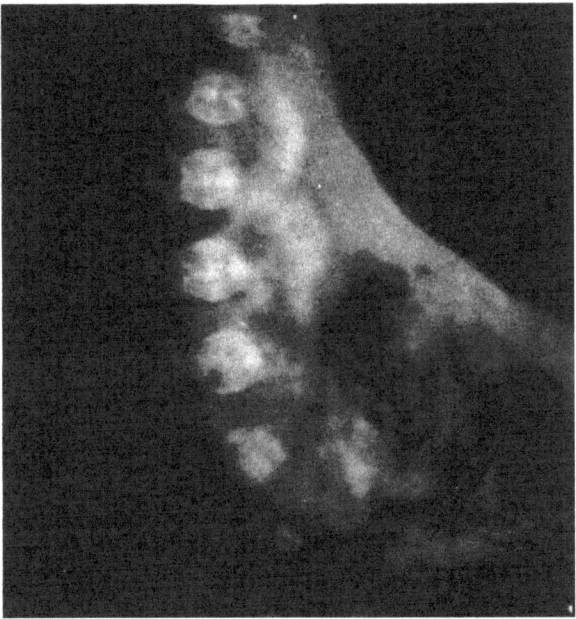

Fig. 5.4. Nephrocalcinosis in hypophosphatasia. On the skeletal survey of this infant with severe bone lesions the lateral radiograph of the spine showed the extensive calcification in the kidneys

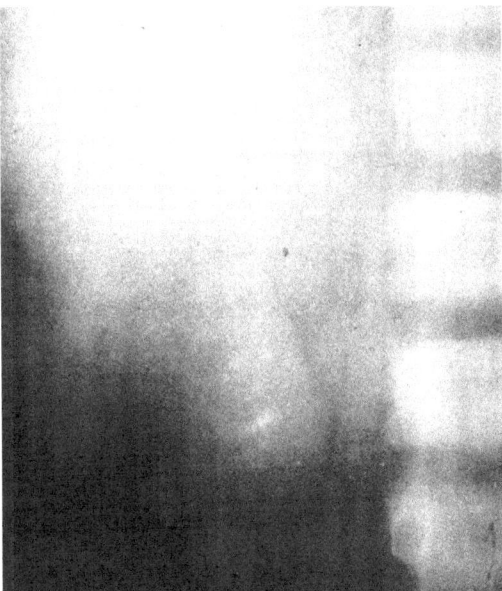

Fig. 5.3. Nephrolithiasis in primary hyperparathyroidism. Nephrotomogram showing two small calcific densities in the kidney. These were the only radiological lesions (apart from the hyperparathyroid lesion) seen in this patient

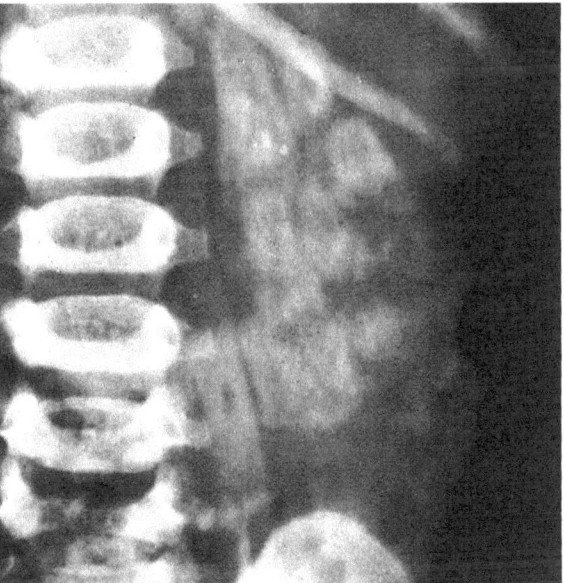

Fig. 5.5. Nephrocalcinosis in idiopathic hypercalcaemia. Extensive calcific deposits in the kidney are shown, as well as the increased bone density. Contrast the bone lesion with that in Fig. 5.3

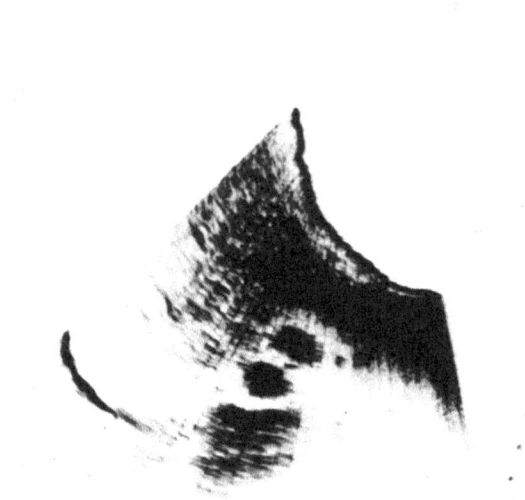

Fig. 5.6. Age 3y. LS supine. Only the upper pole of the right kidney can be seen, but there is striking echogenicity of the medullary portion of the kidney, suggesting the presence of calcium deposition. This child has idiopathic hypercalciuria. The plain abdominal film is unremarkable

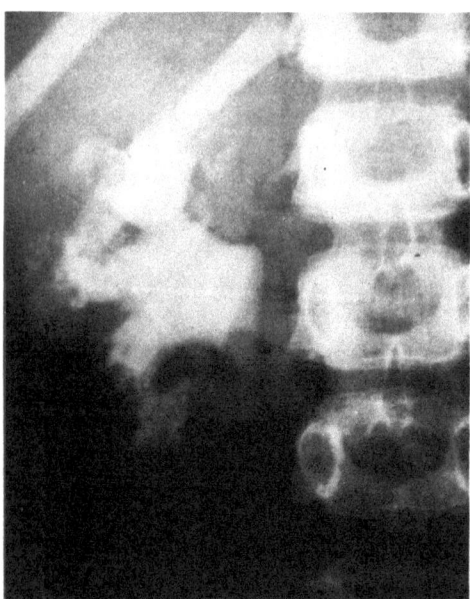

Fig. 5.7. Renal tubular acidosis at IVU. The urogram shows the normally cupped calyces in relationship to the centrally located calcium deposits in the kidney

The rarity of some of these lesions in conjunction with nephrocalcinosis is such that very often only one example has been encountered during the last 15 years at the Hospital for Sick Children.

5.2.2 Nephrolithiasis

Calculus formation within the kidney, is described as nephrolithiasis [1, 2]. Radiologically such calculi tend to be localised to the renal pyramid; this is unlike the calcium deposition of nephrocalcinosis which is more widespread throughout the parenchyma and may be localised discretely, as in cortical necrosis, to the cortico-medullary junction.

Many of the conditions listed above (those indicated by*) may also be associated with stone formation in the kidney. To these may be added the following conditions, namely, medullary sponge kidney and a variety of metabolic disorders such as cystinuria, xanthinuria and hyperoxaluria.

5.2.3 Urolithiasis

The presence of calculi in the collecting system of the kidneys and maybe also in the urinary tract distally is denoted as urolithiasis. Stones formed within the kidney may pass into the urinary tract where they may then increase in size by accretion. If they pass down the ureter there may be an acute onset of ureteric colic or if they remain proximally they may cause protracted pain. The downward transit of ureteric calculi can be arrested at the pelvi-ureteric junction or the uretero-vesical junction. Urinary calculus at any level can cause haematuria.

Urinary infection by *Proteus* is often the first clue to the presence of urinary calculus. The causes of urinary calculus are as follows:

All causes of nephrolithiasis
Urinary infection, especially *Proteus* infection and infection by *E. coli*
Any congenital anomaly associated with urinary tract stasis or obstruction
Endemic calculus disease varies in incidence throughout the world, the reasons for this being uncertain [3, 4].

5.3 Investigation

Many of the circumstances which lead to the investigation for calcium deposition and calculus disease are implicit in the causes of these events. Symptoms and features which directly suggest there may be urolithiasis are pain in the loin, colicky pain, mass lesions in the loin, haematuria and infection.

5.3.1 Techniques

Not all patients who have a renal deposit of calcium have enough calcium present to show on even the best quality radiographs. In fortunate circumstances the gut shadows overlying the renal areas and urinary tract may allow calcium to be seen. The likelihood of seeing calcium increases when the X-ray beam is kept below 70 KV (often well below 70 KV). When the kidney areas are not clearly seen the renal window view (Chapter 2) will help project the kidney areas against the images of the liver, heart and stomach. Modern high-performance image intensifiers give a good prospect of seeing even small deposits of calcium and the manual selection of a low KV helps; fluoroscopy times must however be kept to a minimum to contain the radiation dosage. Calcium deposits, radio-opaque and radiolucent stones can be shown by sonography because of their high echogenicity and acoustic shadows. As with plain radiological techniques, there are times when ultrasound examination fails; the course of the ureter is difficult to follow throughout its length in infants and children by ultrasound study.

Doubt sometimes still exists after all the above procedures and then tomography of the renal areas may provide the answer. Opaque calculi are likely to be either oxalic acid stones, xanthine stones or triple phosphate stones (Fig. 5.8). The density of the calculus on the abdominal radiograph is no indicator of its chemical composition.

At IVU the density of contrast medium in the urinary tract may be so great that calculi (especially soft matrix calculi containing not much calcium) can

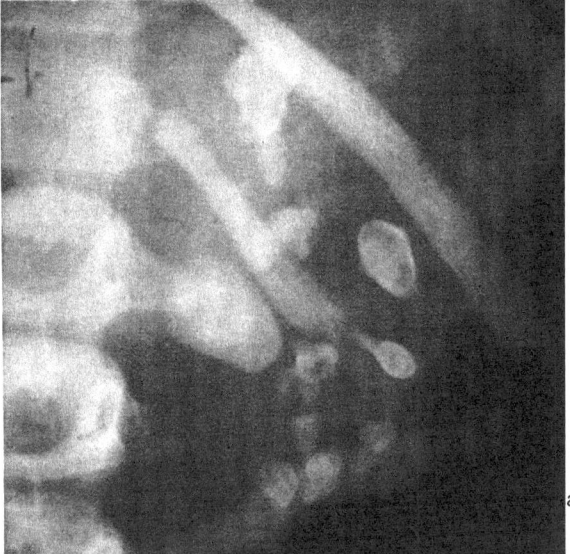

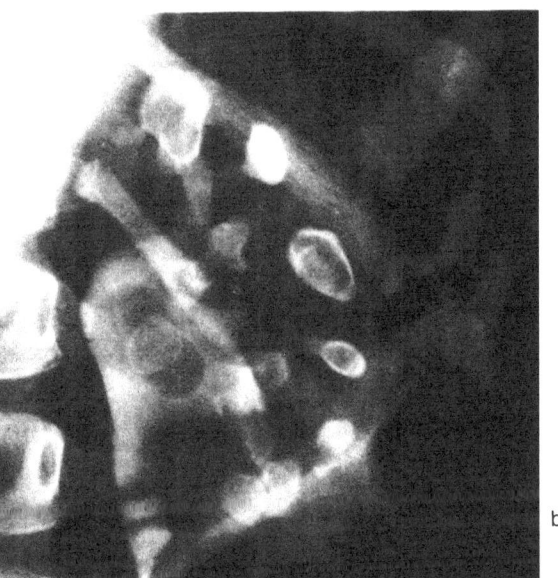

Fig. 5.8 a, b. Urinary calculus disease. **a** Many opaque calculi are present in the calyces and renal pelvis. **b** IVU shows dense contrast medium in the calyces within which the calculi appear as filling defects, as in the pelvis

be obscured. Non-opaque urinary calculi, however, are highlighted as filling defects within the contrast medium (Fig. 5.9). Clearly some calculi are easy to demonstrate but others are not (Figs. 5.10 and 5.11). Echography can confirm that the defect is a calculus and not a granuloma or tumour. One objective of the investigation is to determine the location of a calculus. It is generally wise to carry out radiography of the abdomen and pelvis in children immedi-

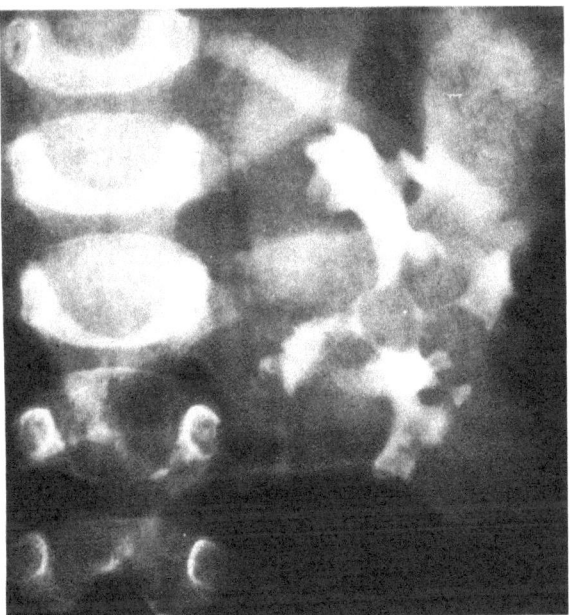

◁
Fig. 5.9. Non-opaque urinary calculus. IVU showing non-opaque calculus lying in the renal pelvis

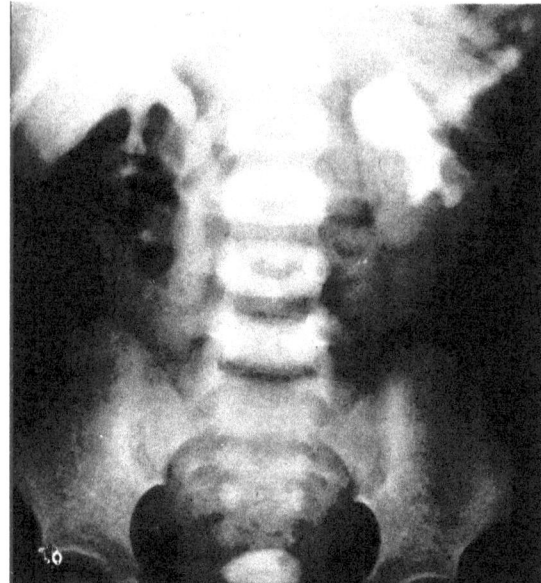

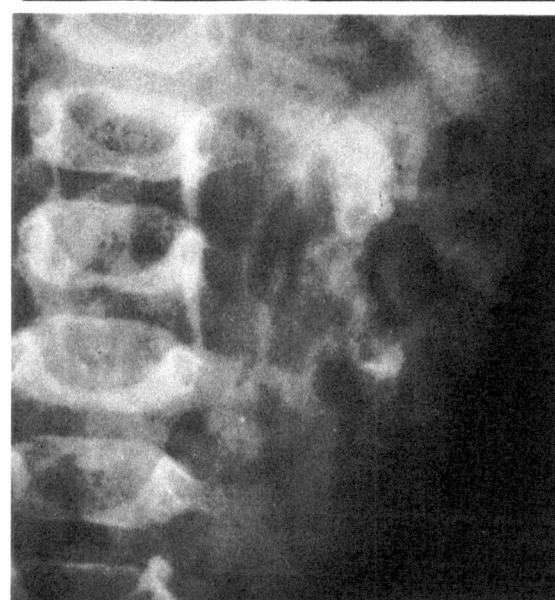

a

b

able and may become anuric but "calculus anuria" in children with two kidneys is a very rare event. Following the passage of a ureteric calculus into the bladder the ureter may appear relatively adynamic and indeed in a state of ileus and subject to vesico-ureteric reflux.

5.4.2 Obstruction and Atrophy of the Kidney

Patients who have had calculi in the upper urinary tract for some time very often have kidneys which are rather small [5]. The atrophic parenchymal thinning may be localised if only a part of a kidney is partially obstructed by calculus related to the group of calyces. More generalised atrophy is seen when calculi have lain in the renal pelvis for a protracted period (Fig. 5.12). Clearance of contrast medium through such kidneys is often good and a common unexplained finding is slight ureteric dilatation distally even though there is no distal obstruction – this feature disappears after the calculi have been removed. If atrophy is unilateral, the unaffected kidney undergoes compensatory hypertrophy as the child grows (Fig. 5.13).

Practically no child with a congenital anomaly of a kidney and the urinary tract is immune to developing a calculus. Sometimes the anomaly itself may be associated with renal growth failure (Fig. 5.14) and calculus formation may lead, in addition, to renal atrophy. It is surprising but calculi may develop even in the presence of vesico-ureteric reflux which ordinarily might be expected to inhibit calculus disease on theoretical grounds.

There is no doubt about the deleterious effect of calculi on renal function (Fig. 5.15). Dynamic DTPA isotope studies can show the serious depression of a kidney's performance when its pelvis contains calculi. Not all calculi which enter a ureter cause renal colic and clinically apparent haematuria. Some ureteric calculi are encountered in which there is already severe obstructive renal damage without an apparently dramatic episode in the preceding period.

ately before elective operative procedures to remove calculi because they have a tendency to change their position. A-mode ultrasound has been used to locate the interureteric portion of calculus during operation.

5.4 Consequences of Calculi in the Urinary Tract

5.4.1 Acute Renal Obstruction

Calculi which descend into a ureter can cause colic and the features of acute obstruction to one kidney. Patients with a solitary kidney are especially vulner-

5.4.3 Recurrence of Urinary Infection and Continuing Surveillance

Urinary infection is a common adjunct to calculus disease. After calculi have been cleared by operation

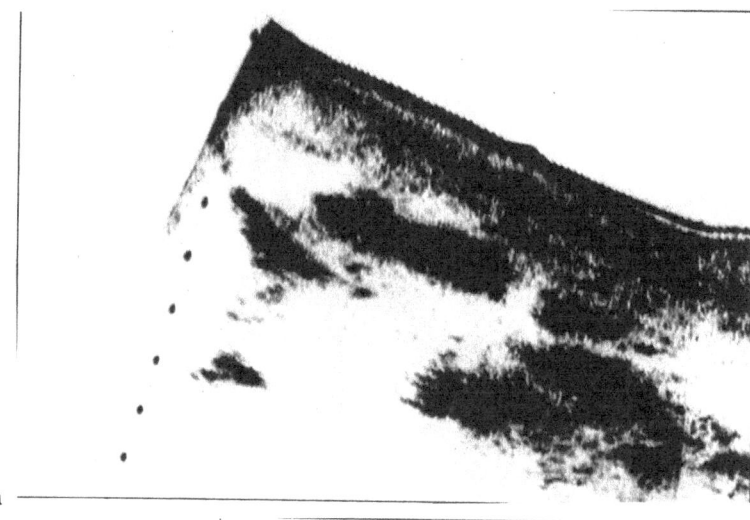

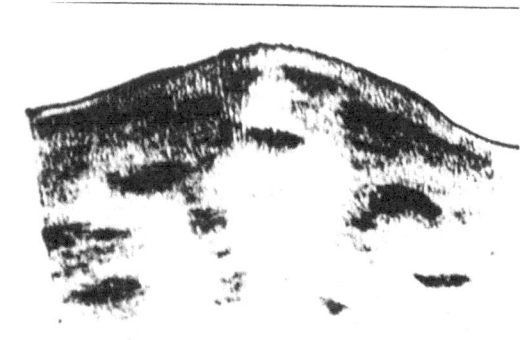

Fig. 5.11 a, b. Age 5. **a** LS prone. The central collecting system echo cluster is replaced by a very strong echogenic region casting an acoustic shadow. This is the typical appearance of a calculus, in this case a large stag-horn. Note the dilated calyces superiorly and inferiorly and the thickness of remaining cortex. **b** TS prone showing that there are bilateral stag-horn calculi. Note the acoustic shadows either side of the spine

a

b

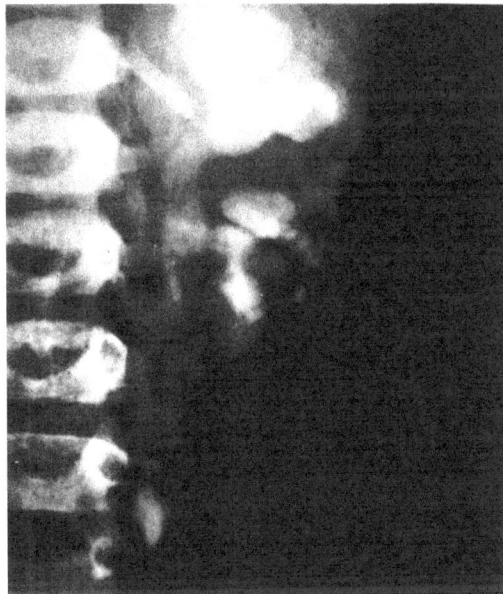

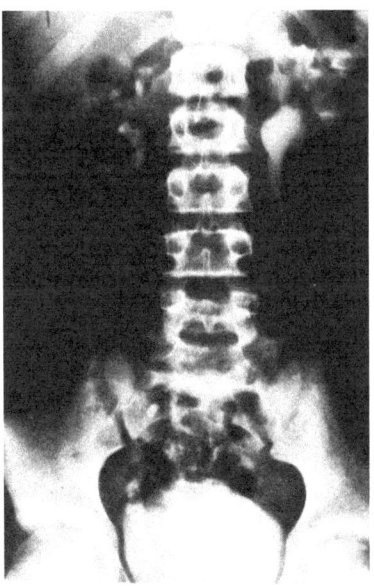

Fig. 5.12. Opaque calculi in the calyces and in the ureter. At IVU the calculus in the ureter obstructs urinary drainage and results in calyx dilatation and obstructive atrophy of the renal parenchyma

Fig. 5.13. Severe obstructive atrophy with non-function at IVU. Calculi in the small non-functioning right kidney and in the lower end of the right ureter are shown. The left kidney has undergone compensatory hypertrophy

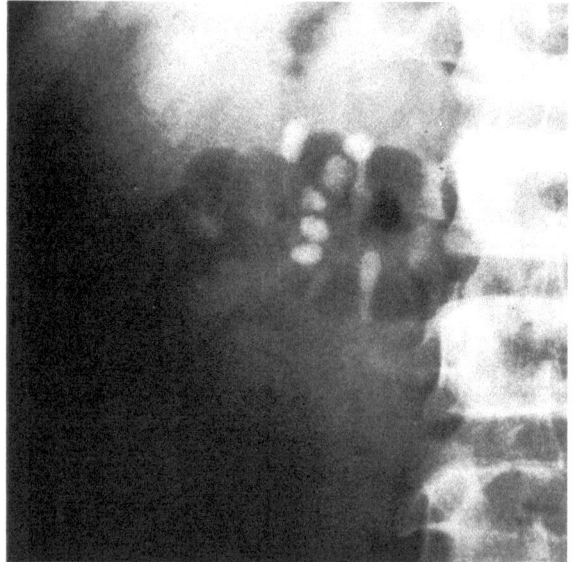

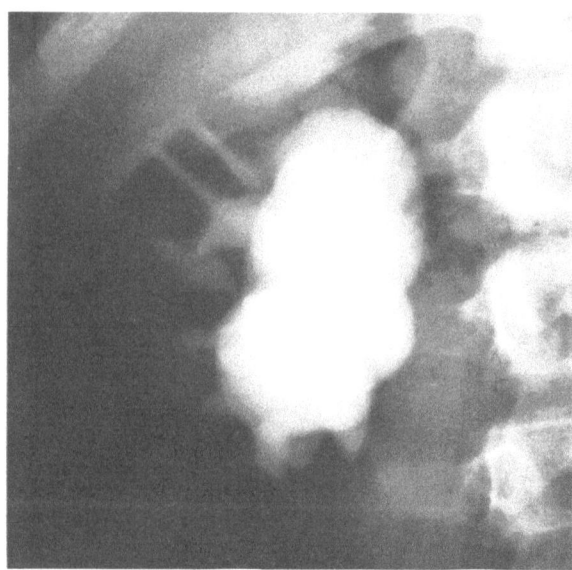

Fig. 5.14 a, b. Calculus formation in an example of congenital anomaly. **a** Small dense calculi shown in the right kidney region. **b** IVU shows the right kidney is malrotated, has a bifid pelvis and there is pelvi-ureteric junction obstruction

a recurrence of infection, especially by *Proteus,* may herald the recurrence of calculus formation in the urinary tract. The potential effects of calculus disease are profound and serious and so continuing follow-up study by plain radiographs is a minimum requirement after calculi have been removed. If the calculus which was present initially was radio-opaque any subsequent calculi tend to be radio-opaque also. Some calculi are exceptionally difficult to remove and small calculus remants may very occasionally be left behind after operation; such

remnants are often stable in their position and may not increase in size over a long time. Even so the status must be periodically checked.

5.4.4 Pyonephrosis

The combination of infection and obstruction to urine flow leads to a non-functioning of the affected kidney – pyonephrosis. Calculi impacted at the pelvi-ureteric junction level or in the ureter are prone to produce that element of obstruction which, when associated with infection, destroys the renal parenchyma and converts the upper tract to a purulent mass. Such masses may be hard and indurated and difficult to distinguish clinically from a renal malignancy. Sonography can differentiate easily between the two conditions; malignancies usually contain an excess of echogenic solid tissue and pyonephrosis deficiency of solid tissue. Clear-cut evidence of a calculus on a radiograph favours pyonephrosis, but calcification in intrarenal malignancies of childhood is usually scanty. Ultrasound may also be used to guide catheters for aspiration and drainage.

5.4.5 Xanthogranulomatous Pyelonephritis

This condition is perhaps appropriately considered in this section. Commonly, but not invariably, it is associated with calculus disease and obstruction. The affected renal parenchyma is transformed into a non-functioning mass consisting of inflammatory xanthogranulomatous tissue which may contain calcium. The calcium in the mass may be demonstrated by sonography or radiography. Ultrasound may also show dilated obstructed calyces. However, the systemic features of fever and polymorphonuclear leucoytosis which are commonly seen in the child with pyonephrosis are very often missing; that is, in xanthogranulomatous pyelonephritis, there may be no systemic reaction to the lesion (*see also* Chapter 9).

5.4.6 Perinephric Abscess

Perinephric abscess may arise as a primary lesion but frequently it is secondary to calculus disease. The combination of calculus obstruction in the kidney and infection may lead to abscess formation. Infection spreading to the perinephric space can be identified by sonography and at IVU when the renal contour and psoas outlines are not visible.

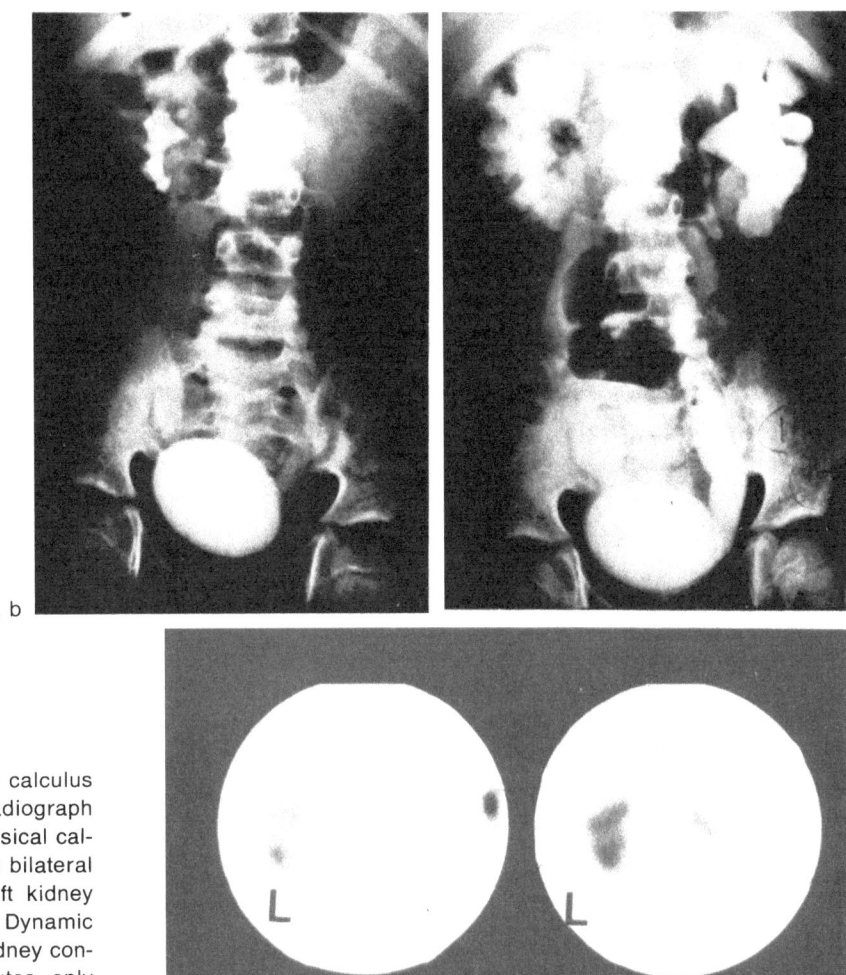

a, b

c

Fig. 5.15 a–c. Staghorn renal calculus and vesical calculus. **a** Plain radiograph shows the right kidney and vesical calculi. **b** Late film at IVU shows bilateral upper tract dilatation, the left kidney being larger than the right. **c** Dynamic DTPA scan shows the right kidney containing the calculus contributes only 15% of the total of renal function

5.5 Miscellaneous Considerations Concerning the Lower Urinary Tract

Calculi which pass through the uretero-vesical junction enter the bladder and because of their small size they may then be voided in the urine. Clearance of such calculi can be observed on serial radiographs, and often recognised clinically. The ureter-vesical junction, after transit of a calculus through it, may be prone to vesico-ureteric reflux, but this is an ill-defined feature and is very often but not always a transient phenomenon. Sometimes oedema at the distal end of a ureter following passage of a calculus, may appear as a filling defect in the contrast medium filled bladder at IVU. The thick, oedematous wall of the ureter serves to distinguish this condition from a ureterocoele in which the wall is characteristically thin.

The vesical calculus presumably develops because not all calculi passing through the uretero-vesical junction are voided. Vesical calculi increase in size by accretion and they may have a lamellar structure visible on radiographs. Ultrasonics study of the bladder is also a decisive and convenient method of investigating possible vesical calculi, particularly those which are radiolucent.

Although most vesical calculi seem likely to start in the upper tract a very small minority develop around a foreign body introduced into the bladder; a variety of foreign objects provide the origin for vesical calculus formation but further details as to their origin need not be considered here. Vesical calculi of any sort tend to produce abdominal pain and haematuria and sometimes strangury on voiding.

Calculi in the course of leaving the bladder may become arrested in the vesico-urethral junction above the narrow male membranous urethra (Fig.

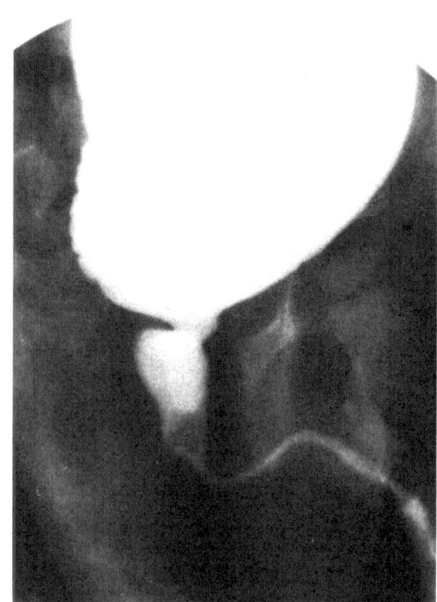

Fig. 5.16. Urethral calculus. MCU in boy with calculus on posterior urethra. The calculus was opaque on the plain radiograph but appears as a radiolucent filling defect in the stream of contrast medium. Diathermy of posterior urethral valves had been carried out early in life and no valve remnant remains, although the posterior urethra is still wide. Urethra calculi may lodge in a urethral diverticulum, above the membranous urethra, distally in the fossa navicularis or in the stump of a closed recto-urethral fistula

5.16). Distally in the male, calculi may impact in the urethra in the vicinity of the fossa navicularis and at the urethral meatus. Calculi impacting in the urethra are a cause of obstruction to vesical emptying and sometimes such obstruction is acute.

Such examples of calculus in the urethra are rare but even rarer are calculi which develop in the vicinity of the male urethra. These are of two types: the first are calculi developing in the urethral end of a fistula which has been operatively closed during surgery for anorectal anomaly; the second is related to calculi which develop in a congenital urethral diverticulum in the male. Both of these conditions give striking radiological features but neither has obstructive sequelae.

5.6 Conclusion

If calcium has been shown to be deposited in the kidney, its collecting system or in the lower urinary tract, it is necessary to search for an underlying cause of this event. This search, as has already been implied, may necessitate a serious and protracted evaluation of metabolic status and turnover even though urinary infection and structural developmental anomalies often provide the basis for urolithiasis. The search for cause is important if progression and recurrence of disease are to be prevented and progressive deterioration in kidney function avoided.

References

1. Wenzl, J. E., Burke, E. C., Stickler, G. B., Utz, D. C.: Nephrolithiasis and nephrocalcinosis in children. Pediatrics **41,** 57 (1968)
2. Epstein, F. H.: Calcium and the kidney. Am. J. Med. **45,** 700 (1968)
3. Eckstein, H. B.: Endemic urinary lithiasis in Turkish children. Arch. Dis. Child. **36,** 137 (1961)
4. Ghazali, S., Barratt, T. M., Williams, D. I.: Urinary calculi in British children. Arch. Dis. Child. **48,** 291 (1973)
5. Hodson, C. J.: Post-obstructive renal atrophy. Br. Med. Bull. **28,** 237 (1972)

6

Innate Abnormalities of Renal Development

6.1 Introduction

In their own ways innate abnormalities of renal development seem to present all the complexities of the coinage of the Common Market countries. But as J. K. Galbraith observed, "there is nothing about money that cannot be understood by the person of reasonable curiosity, diligence and intelligence". And so it is with the innate problems of renal development.

These abnormalities of renal development have exceptionally wide implications for management and prognosis in the individual child. Some lesions have clear-cut genetic determinants which have their expression primarily in the kidney and urinary tract and others comprise part of genetically transmitted syndromes (see Chapter 1). Genetic counselling for parents may follow from the clinical and investigatory findings in their child. When there is a possible genetic basis for the individual child's problem it can be helpful, as in cystic disease of the kidney, to carry out surveys, which include investigation of the family, to try to assess the pattern of inheritance within the family. This having been said, the fact remains that many kidney abnormalities represent idiosyncratic development affecting the individual child only.

It is not the purpose of this book to detail ways in which innate abnormalities might arise, rather it is concerned with identifying the abnormalities. Only after this has been done can the next steps in management of the individual child's problem be realized and the parents advised correctly. The significance of congenital abnormalities lies in the fact that they are responsible for about 20% of all cases of children developing chronic renal failure.

6.2 Abnormalities of Renal Parenchymal Development

6.2.1 Renal Agenesis

Complete agenesis of renal development can be a bilateral or unilateral phenomenon. Bilateral renal agenesis is incompatible with life and soon after delivery anuria leads to investigation. No functioning renal tissue can be shown by either intravenous urography or radioisotope studies (DMSA scan) and no renal structure can be identified by ultrasound examination. It is usually necessary to use more than one mode of examination to establish the diagnosis promptly. The normal neonate, in the first 2 days or so after birth, may not clear contrast medium (and by inference a radioisotope) through a normal kidney and this indicates that precipitate investigation by these means may be unhelpful or even misleading at this early stage. The condition may be associated with urethral atresia or severe stenosis and echography can show there is no kidney structure.

Subsequently, ultrasound study of asymptomatic members of the family of such neonates may bring light developmental abnormalities, such as duplication, amongst family members.

When unilateral aplasia or agenesis occurs the prognosis for the individual child depends on the status of the contralateral kidney [1]. Ordinarily the solitary kidney develops well and is much larger than one of a normal pair of kidneys. Such a kidney may be found as an incidental feature in investigations carried out for a variety of reasons, for example heart disease in the post-angiocardiographic urogram. It may be necessary to confirm there is only one kidney and ultrasonics and micturition cystourethrography may prove there is no sign of a kidney on the one side, not even a small non-functioning one. There may then be recourse to endoscopy; if only one ureteric orifice related to the solitary kidney is seen then that is conclusive but if two orifices are seen then retrograde examination may be the final determinant (Fig. 6.1).

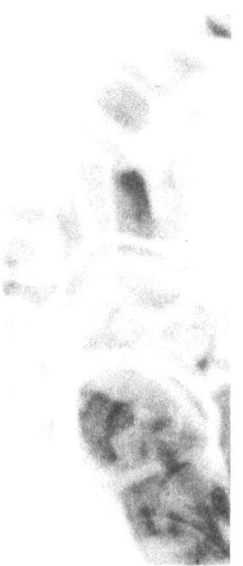

Fig. 6.1. Agenesis. Unilateral renal agenesis is associated with enlargement and compensatory hypertrophy of the contralateral kidney if this normal. IVU, MCU, ultrasound and DMSA scan all may fail to show any kidney tissue on the side of the agenesis. This is usually associated with an absent ureteric orifice, but if one is present retrograde study will show the ureter ends blindly, as in this case

Since a solitary kidney is often large it may be detected as an abdominal mass, especially if it is ectopic [2, 3]. Patients who have only one kidney are vulnerable. Should they suffer trauma and IVU be carried out then there may be unnecessary anxiety until the absence of a kidney is shown by ultrasound. Obviously infection, calculus disease and reflux affecting the one kidney are other reasons for vulnerability.

A variant of renal aplasia is the ureteric bud. This is a canalized ureteric lumen which fails to drain any renal tissue. Such buds may opacify at IVU, since they arise from the ureter and sometimes they are surprisingly long before terminating blindly [4, 5].

6.2.2 Renal Hypoplasia

The infant or young child who has bilateral hypoplasia [6, 7] fails to thrive and grow. For this reason they commonly present in the first year of life. These children have a salt-losing nephropathy and thus hypertension is not seen.

At IVU the hypoplastic kidneys [8] are shown to be small and their lobular contour is accentuated. Within the renal margins lie calyces which vary in size, some being well cupped and others dilated and clubbed. The calyces are irregularly placed within the kidney. Function is poor either qualitatively at IVU or quantiatively on dynamic renal isotope scan (DTPA). These children, commonly presenting in the first year of life, show a slow progressive deterioration in renal function, terminating in end-stage renal failure and renal osteodystrophy between the ages of 8 and 12 years.

Within the differential diagnosis of hypoplasia lie all the causes of small kidneys [9]. In bilateral hypoplasia vesico-ureteric reflux is not present so reflux with reflux nephropathy can confidently be excluded – and this is the principal condition to be differentiated from hypoplasia. Hypoplasia is especially associated with urethral stenosis. Patients with cerebral lesions may have small kidneys [10]. Sometimes hypoplasia is unilateral and if severe may present the same diagnostic problems as aplasia in identifying renal tissue. In these circumstances retrograde study may be the decisive investigation of last resort, but DMSA scan may identify the small, "non-functioning" kidney (Fig. 6.2).

A developmental abnormality which affects one kidney very often affects the other kidney although

Fig. 6.2. Renal hypoplasia. Bilateral renal hypoplasia is associated especially with urethral stenosis. Unilateral renal hypoplasia may be associated with a normal kidney which has undergone compensatory hypertrophy on the contralateral side. Other modes of investigation may fail to show the tiny hypoplastic kidney which is present. This retrograde study shows such a situation, with a tiny non-functioning kidney and a normal-calibre ureter

sometimes in a different way. This principle is exemplified by the fact that multicystic disease of one kidney is quite frequently associated with hypoplasia in the contralateral kidney.

6.2.3 Variants of Renal Rotation and Position

6.2.3.1 Malrotation

There may be unilateral or bilateral malrotation. When there is no associated obstruction or stone formation this variant is of no consequence. Rotation is usually around the long axis of the kidney. At IVU the upper pole of the kidney is usually slightly laterally placed whereas the lower pole appears unduly medial (and so close to the ureter) on antero-posterior projections. Lateral or oblique projections will show whether the pelvis lies anterior or posterior to the renal tissue; such projections can be necessary for the renal pelvis may be difficult to identify on the antero-posterior view. The way in which vessels in the hilum of the kidney are aligned can predispose to pelvi-ureteric junction obstruction. Echography may elucidate these features.

6.2.3.2 Ectopic Kidney

Any kidney in an abnormal position may be described as ectopic, and within this group are a number of variants [2, 3,11]. Very rarely the kidney may be too high, being placed partly in the thorax posteriorly. Sometimes both kidneys are so positioned and then the bilateral "mass lesions" lying posteriorly on the chest radiograph make the diagnosis easier to suspect than when only one kidney lies in the thoracic location (Fig. 6.3). A kidney may lie in the pre-sacral position (Fig. 6.4). In these circumstances it is associated with a short ureter draining to the bladder and the kidney may be dysplastic and subject also to reflux because of incompetence at the uretero-vesical junction. An abnormality of entry of the ureter into the lower urinary tract (for example into the urethra) is often associated with an abnormality of position of the kidney and renal dysplasia.

6.2.3.3 Fused Crossed Ectopia

The two kidney components in fused crossed ectopia lie on one side of the posterior abdominal wall and the lower pole of the one is fused with the upper pole of the other (Fig. 6.5). The ureter from the upper renal component descends on the ipsilateral side to enter the bladder normally, but the ureter from the lower renal component crosses the midline and enters the bladder on the contralateral side. Fused crossed ectopia is one of the commoner urinary tract

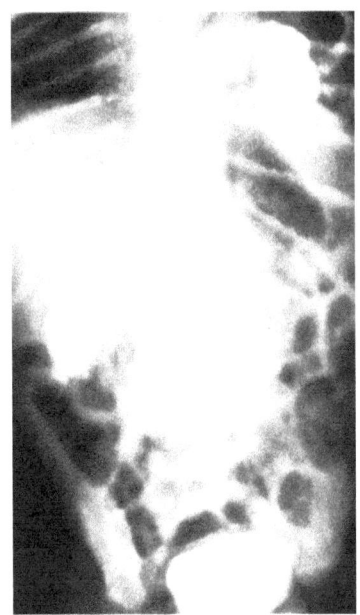

Fig. 6.3. Ectopic kidney. The left kidney presented as a mass lesion in the chest lying behind the heart and posteriorly. At IVU its pelvis is dilated. The right kidney lies in the retroperitoneal space, but it is malrotated with the pelvis dilated and anterior to the parenchyma

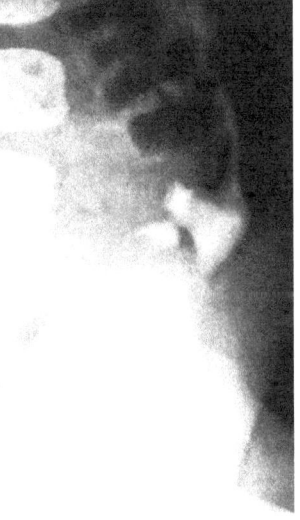

Fig. 6.4. Ectopic kidney. A kidney positioned low on the posterior abdominal wall or in the pelvis can be very difficult to identify at IVU. A lateral projection can be helpful in showing the collecting system which may overlie bone in the AP projection. Isotope scan or sonography may show the location of renal parenchyma in such ectopic kidneys, but MCU can also be informative, for the kidney may be dysplastic and subject to vesico-ureteric reflux

variants associated with ano-rectal anomaly. Concomitant renal dysplasia may occur [12].

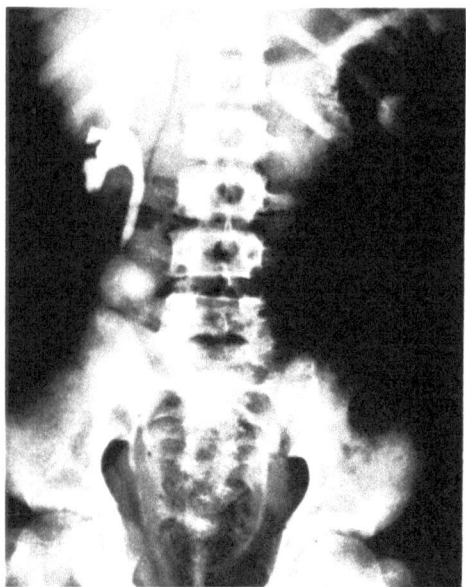

Fig. 6.5. Fused crossed ectopia. There is a right-sided crossed ectopia. The malpositioned lower kidney demonstrates hydronephrosis from a concomitant pelvi-ureteric junction obstruction. The normal course of the ureters within the pelvis is illustrated

6.2.3.4 Horseshoe Kidney

Characterized by fusion at the lower poles of the two kidney components, the horseshoe kidney often lies rather low on the posterior abdominal wall. The hilum of the horseshoe kidney may be a complex structure with a multiplicity of renal vessels dividing rather more proximally than is usual and the major calyces may drain extrarenally to the renal pelves. At IVU each of the renal components appears to lie more vertically than normal with the lower pole calyces being unduly medial in position on the antero-posterior projection. Lateral projections are helpful because they show that both of the lower poles lie unduly forward in relationship to the spine. The lower pole calyces face towards the spine and are medially located in relation to the upper third of the ureter (Fig. 6.6). The precise renal contour of a horseshoe kidney is impossible to define at IVU because renal tissue overlies the spine. An accurate assessment of the renal parenchymal position and function can be obtained by DMSA scan during which an anterior image is essential. At echography the findings are remarkably decisive (Fig. 6.7). The structure of the hilum of the horseshoe kidney almost certainly accounts for the complications such as obstruction to the upper part of the ureter, pelvis or to a major calyx which can lead to hydrocalicosis. These are associated with the symptoms of pain, infection, calculus, and occasionally haematuria-

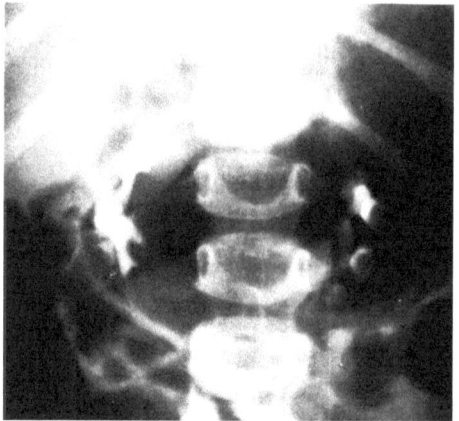

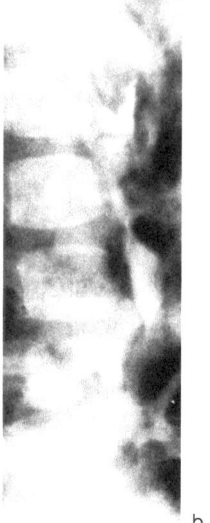

Fig. 6.6 a, b. Horseshoe kidney. When the lower poles of the kidneys are fused, the axis of the kidney alters and renal parenchyma lies in front of the spine. The antero-posterior projection may show kidneys which appear vertically aligned with the lower-most calyces unduly medial (**a**). However, the lateral projection (**b**) shows lower pole calyces and upper ureters are also anteriorly placed and lie in front of the vertebral bodies. The horseshoe kidney may be rather low in position

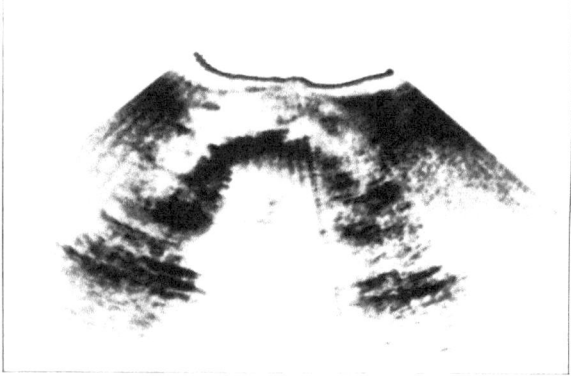

Fig. 6.7. TS supine showing the bridge of tissue of a horseshoe kidney crossing the aorta

which prompt the investigation that leads to the diagnosis. One further complication of horseshoe kidney exists; there is an association between horse shoe kidney and Wilms' tumour. When such a tumour is present there is a gross mass lesion of the kidney, usually affecting one component (*see* Chapter 9).

6.2.4 Dysmorphic Kidney

"Dysmorphic kidney" conveniently describes a range of appearances, usually seen at IVU, with fairly distinctive connotations. The one feature they have in common is that all are associated with a misshapen kidney.

6.2.4.1 Dysplastic Kidney

Frequently, the dysplastic kidney is an abnormally shaped kidney – or kidney component, because dysplasia is very often associated with an ectopic insertion of the ureter into the lower urinary tract [13]. The kidney may have appearances rather like those of hypoplasia and it may be possible to distinguish the two conditions only by histological examination. The dysplastic kidney has tissue (such as fibrous tissue, muscle or cartilage) which are not found in a normal kidney. Small cysts may also be present in a dysplastic kidney and if and when the kidney grows it may become more misshapen (Fig. 6.8 and Fig. 6.12). A dysplastic kidney, since it is very often associated with abnormalities of insertion of the ureter into the lower urinary tract, may be subject to reflux [7, 8]. Kidneys which drain via ureters directly into the urethra, vagina [14] or male

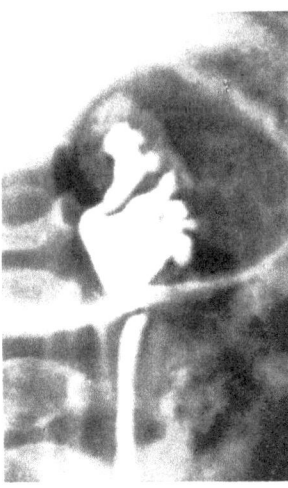

Fig. 6.8. Cystic dysplastic disease with dysmorphism. This marasmic infant failed to concentrate contrast medium at IVU. MCU showed bilateral vesico-ureteric reflux. Calyx opacification shows clubbed calyces crowded together. There is also intrarenal reflux outlining the cysts – the first time this was observed at the Hospital for Sick Children (1967). Renal biopsy proof of the diagnosis followed. No urinary infection was detected

genital tract are frequently dysplastic, small and identifiable by DMSA scan.

6.2.4.2 Segmental Renal Hypoplasia

Changes and abnormalities of development occur in segmental renal hypoplasia which are identifiable by expert nephropathologists [15, 16, 17]. Radiologically the affected kidney has appearances very similar to (or indistinguishable from) the kidney which has chronic pyelonephritic scarring. The indentation of renal contour and the clubbing of the propinquitous minor calyx are seen in the affected segment and this fails to grow. Systemic hypertension is the way in which segmental renal hyperplasia generally manifests its presence (*see* Chapter 11).

Renal dysplasia with its associated propensity to reflux, segmental hypoplasia with its tendency to produce hypertension and chronic pyelonephritic scarred kidneys [18] (where it has been difficult or impossible) to identify an infective episode and reflux may or may not be present) all have, in themselves, provided the backcloth to dramatic controversies. Knowledge of events in the past, the current status and the prospect for the future all contain uncertainties; this is the problem of knowledge itself. Tolstoy's observations in "War and Peace" are especially apt:

It is beyond the power of the human intellect to encompass *all* the causes of any phenomenon. But the impulse to search into causes is inherent in man's very nature. And so the human intellect, without investigating the multiplicity and complexity of circumstances conditioning any event, any one of which taken separately may seem to be the reason for it, snatches at the first most comprehensible approximation to a cause and says: "There is the cause!"

It is surely right to recognise that the causes may sometimes not be definable in the individual child at any one moment in time.

6.2.4.3 Cleft Kidney

A rare maldevelopment, cleft kidney has a deep indentation into the normal convexity of the renal contour. Kidney parenchyma, [19] adjacent to the cleft, drains into calyces which are remote from the cleft itself; they lie deeply within the kidney and the usual distribution of calyces throughout the renal contour is disturbed. At first sight it might be thought there is a space-occupying lesion within the kidney if the cleft has not been shown (Fig. 6.9). Oblique projections of the kidney may clearly show

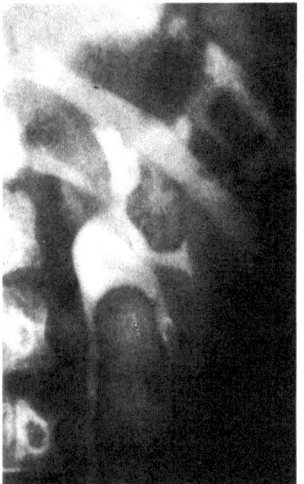

a

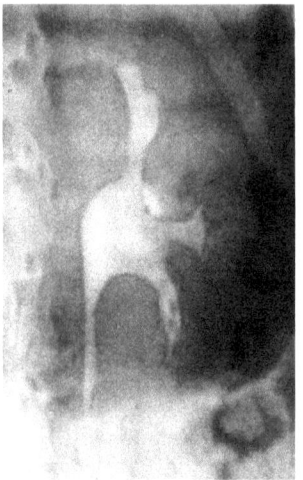

b

Fig. 6.9 a, b. Cleft kidney. The contour of the kidney has a cleft, and an oblique radiograph (**a**) can show the altered contour clearly. The renal window view can also demonstrate (**b**) the deeply placed calyx associated with the cleft

the cleft if it is not seen on antero-posterior projections at IVU. An isotope DMSA scan will demonstrate that there is no space-occupying lesion present and the entire kidney parenchyma functions normally [20, 21]. Likewise sonograms show no space-occupying lesion and indicate that the feature is simply due to altered renal structure (Fig. 6.10) with the indentation of renal margin and the deeply placed columns of Bertin. A familial incidence of the condition has been reported [22].

Unfortunately in former times this entity has been described as "pseudo-tumour" and angiographic studies have been thought by some to be needed to show no tumour is present. The term is unfortunate if for only one reason; it is exceptionally difficult to persuade parents, who are accustomed to debasement of language by a variety of propagandists, that

"pseudo-tumour" is an entirely benign developmental variant which carries no threat to life whatsoever.

6.2.5 Renal Cystic Disease

6.2.5.1 Congenital Renal Dysplasia with Cystic Changes (Potter Type II polycystic kidneys)

This is a group of non-hereditary kidney malformations frequently encountered in infants and children. Its most common manifestation is the *multicystic kidney* and much less common is the *multilocular cystic kidney*. The prognosis depends on the further development of the 'dysplastic' renal tissue as well as on the severity of the co-existing malformations in other organs. This whole group is characterised by "non-function" throughout all or part of a kidney as demonstrated by IVU or isotope scan.

6.2.5.1.1 The Multicystic Kidney

Classically it presents in the neonate as a large abdominal mass and is the most common cause of an abdominal mass in this age group (Fig. 6.11) [23, 24, 25, 26]. Usually there is a large, cystic, "nonfunctioning" kidney, and the proximal end of the ureter is atretic. Conventional radiography by means of an IVU is useful in confirming the diagnosis. Usually there is non-function, but in the neonate there may be sufficient nephrons in the strands of renal tissue between the cystic areas to excrete enough contrast medium for visualization of the walls of the cysts [27]. This visualization was formerly thought to be due to the phenomenon of whole body opacification – seen within the first few minutes of a bolus injection of contrast medium – but the time of optimum visualization was noted to occur much later than this, at about 15 min after the injection. This is thought to confirm the fact that there are functioning nephrons present in the neonate: pools of contrast medium may collect within the cysts ("puddling effect") on delayed films [28]. If the age of presentation is later in childhood then the nephrons have ceased to function and there is no evidence of excretion on the IVU. Not only is the IVU important in indicating the correct diagnosis of a multicystic kidney, but it may demonstrate some abnormality of the opposite kidney or ureter. Contralateral congenital abnormalities associated with a multicystic kidney affect about one-third of patients and the contralateral kidney may be dysplastic or obstructed (Fig. 6.12). Very rarely multicystic disease is bilateral and then the baby presents with renal failure and with Potter-type facies. The bilateral condition is invariably fatal.

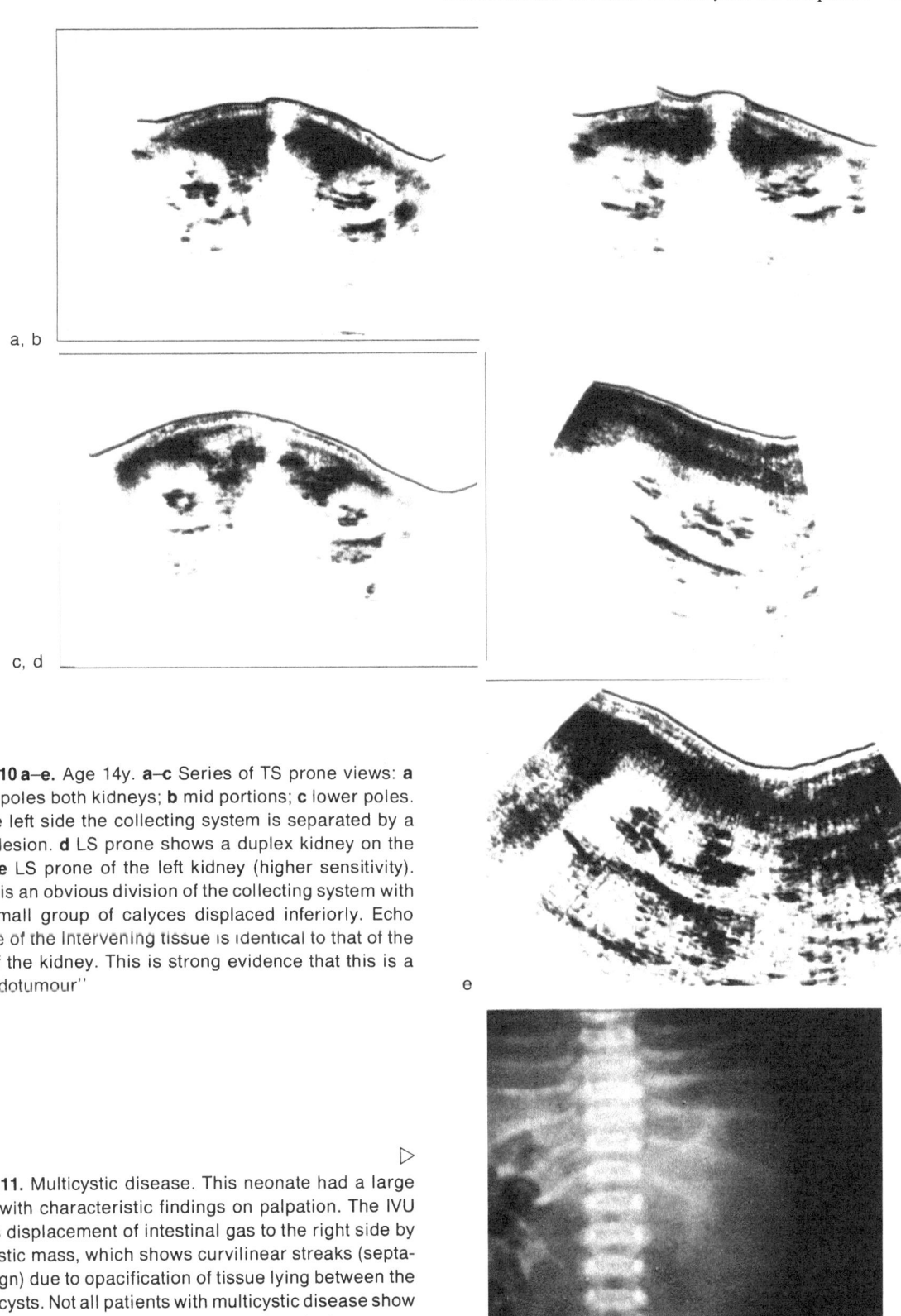

Fig. 6.10 a–e. Age 14y. **a–c** Series of TS prone views: **a** upper poles both kidneys; **b** mid portions; **c** lower poles. On the left side the collecting system is separated by a mass lesion. **d** LS prone shows a duplex kidney on the right. **e** LS prone of the left kidney (higher sensitivity). There is an obvious division of the collecting system with one small group of calyces displaced inferiorly. Echo texture of the intervening tissue is identical to that of the rest of the kidney. This is strong evidence that this is a "pseudotumour"

▷

Fig. 6.11. Multicystic disease. This neonate had a large mass with characteristic findings on palpation. The IVU shows displacement of intestinal gas to the right side by the cystic mass, which shows curvilinear streaks (septation sign) due to opacification of tissue lying between the many cysts. Not all patients with multicystic disease show this; they may simply have a non-functioning mass. Cystadenoma may have identical appearances. Late films may show faint opacification within the cystic spaces (puddling effect) by the contrast medium. The status of the contralateral kidney determines the prognosis

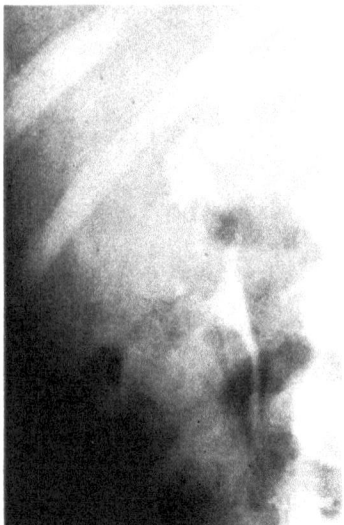

Fig. 6.12. Cystic dysplatic disease. This kidney remained after excision of the contralateral multicystic kidney. The contour of the kidney is irregular and the kidney is dysmorphic. Within the kidney contour calyces of varying size, some of them clubbed, are arranged in sporadic fashion

The differential diagnosis of a unilateral large renal mass presenting in a neonate is: (i) multicystic kidney; (ii) hydronephrosis and (iii) tumors, particularly mesoblastic nephroma. However, at clinical examination of a multicystic kidney usually there is a characteristic finding on palpation.

In any of these three conditions there may be no function on the IVU or radioisotope scan. Strands of tissue may excrete contrast medium in the walls of cysts in a multicystic kidney, but rather similar appearances may be seen in delayed films taken of a severe hydronephrosis. Ultrasound examination will differentiate between solid and cystic areas and should separate a multicystic kidney or hydronephrosis from a tumour. Thus, a triad of investigations may sometimes be thought necessary to confirm the diagnosis of a multicystic kidney; these are; (i) IVU; (ii) rarely a retrograde pyelogram is used to demonstrate an atretic proximal ureter whose distal patent segment above the bladder may be opacified by IVU with reflux from the bladder, or by MCU, and (iii) antegrade studies demonstrating a large cystic area and no communication with the ureter. However, the clinical findings and the size of the mass and the findings at IVU are generally sufficient to warrant operation. Angiography, in the very rare circumstance where it is thought necessary, will demonstrate a hypoplastic renal artery, no pathological vessels and no collateral supply and no evidence of a nephrogram. Provided there is a good measure of confidence about the diagnosis then it is

unnecessary for the patient to undergo urgent surgery. In practice the surgeon finds it difficult to refrain from excising a large abdominal mass speedily.

Not all multicystic kidneys are large and ultrasound examination may then be the sole method of investigation which is then relevant.

6.2.5.1.2 Multilocular Cystic Kidney

The multicystic kidney is an example of renal dysplasia involving the whole kidney. Rarely only part of the kidney may be involved. This is usually at one or other pole. Then there is a non-functioning polar mass with distorition of the pelvicalyceal system shown by the IVU examination. This is a multilocular cyst, or cystadenoma [29, 30]. In contrast to the benign prognosis of the multicystic kidney, the multilocular cystic kidney may have undifferentiated nephroblastoma tissue in the cyst walls and it has the capacity suddenly to enlarge and become malignant at any age. Surgery is therefore indicated and precise pre-operative diagnosis is not essential. In general any focal intrarenal expanding, non-functioning, space-occupying lesion warrants surgery. Other investigations, such as echography, may be necessary to demonstrate the extent of the lesion. Finally, there is always the possible involvement of other organs if malignant change has supervened.

An intermediate condition between the polar multilocular cyst and the non-functioning multicystic kidney seems to exist. In this condition multiple large cysts are seen only within one functioning kidney and usually there are associated renal artery abnormalities with multiple small renal arteries supplying the kidney. Presentation is often later in childhood as a unilateral renal mass, occasionally associated with hypertension. This is often considered to be a form of renal 'dysplasia'.

6.2.5.1.3 Renal Dysplasia with Cystic Manifestations

may be seen in other conditions involving the entire renal tract. The prune belly [3] or triad syndrome may show cystic changes in the renal parenchyma. Posterior urethral valves may be associated with dysplastic cystic changes in the kidneys [32]. These are thought not to be due to the prolonged back pressure changes as a result of the urethral obstructions, but to a primary renal maldevelopment. An example is shown of an infant with a urinoma secondary to fornix rupture due to the raised intrapelvic pressure caused by posterior urethral valves. In theory the rupture should have protected that kidney from gross parenchymal damage and an IVU demonstrated the pelvicalyceal system was of normal proportions with prompt excretion. A sonogram of that same kidney demonstrated multiple small cystic areas within the renal parenchyma. The cysts are usually small and are rarely seen at IVU examination: this shows ultrasonics examination is the method of choice in elucidating the presence of possible cystic areas within such kidneys. Very occasionally the cysts communicate with the pelvicalyceal system and fill with contrast medium either on the IVU or MCU (Fig. 6.13 and see also Figs. 3.39 and 3.40).

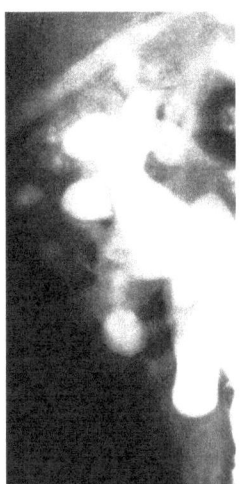

Fig. 6.13. Cystic disease in posterior urethral valves. At MCU a multiplicity of small parenchymal cysts has been opacified by contrast medium entering the collecting system after vesico-ureteric reflux

6.2.5.2 Polycystic Disease

The second large group in cystic disease in children comprises patients with polycystic disease of the kidneys and liver. Radiographically they have one feature in common, that is collections of contrast medium in dilated collecting tubules. Broadly the group consists of (i) patients with *infantile type of polycystic disease,* (ii) *renal tubular ectasia* and (iii) *intermediate forms* [33, 34, 35].

6.2.5.2.1 Infantile Polycystic Disease
and Renal Tubular Ectasia

These variants may be considered as the extreme manifestations of one condition, with an autosomal recessive inheritance. In these two conditions it is the relative degree of involvement of the kidneys and liver and the rapidity of progression that determine the age at which the condition occurs and the mode of presentation. This is more often renal in younger children and hepatic in older children. The findings vary according to the degree of renal and liver involvement.

In *infantile polycystic disease* the renal findings predominate. These patients may present with bilateral renal masses and with renal failure in the neonatal period (Fig. 6.14) or within the first few

months of life. Sometimes detection of the lesion is in early childhood. The long-term prognosis is usually poor. A small percentage die within a few weeks of birht, most of the remainder survive to the age of 5 years or more when they develop hypertension and a progressive deterioration in kidney function. Very occasionally, there has been a gradual normalization of clinical and IVU findings. Typically at IVU the kidneys are enlarged, often grossly so (Fig. 6.15). The renal outline is usually poorly

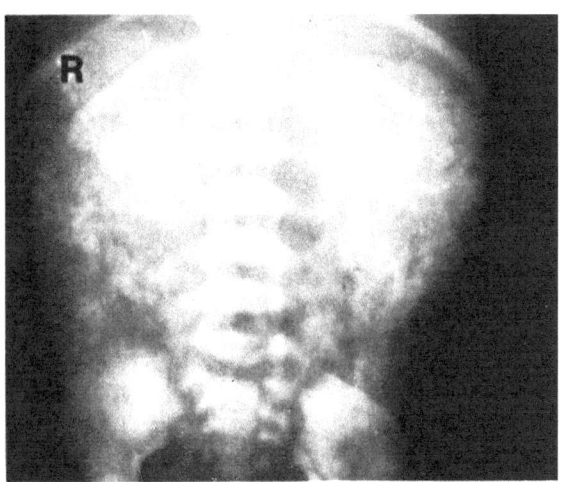

Fig. 6.14. Infantile polycytic disease. This condition has a wide spectrum. In this neonate, large kidneys were palpated and led to IVU. The initial radiographs were not diagnostic, but at 24 h the kidneys show spotty streaky opacities throughout the parenchyma. Abdominal distension was present, although not to a degree to obstruct labour

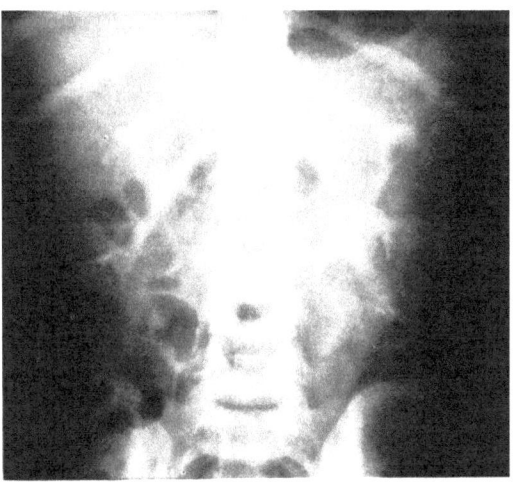

Fig. 6.15. Infantile polycystic disease. This 2-year-old failed to thrive and the kidneys show at IVU gross enlargement and some streaky spotty parenchymal opacification. The calyces are evenly distributed throughout the parenchyma, indicating the diffuse nature of the condition in the kidneys

Fig. 6.16. Infantile polycystic disease – renal tubular ectasia with liver disease. This child had oesophageal varices which led to haematemesis. The liver was enlarged and cystic. The IVU shows only some pyramids in the kidney have a blush, diagnostic of tubular ectasia in this clinical context   ▷

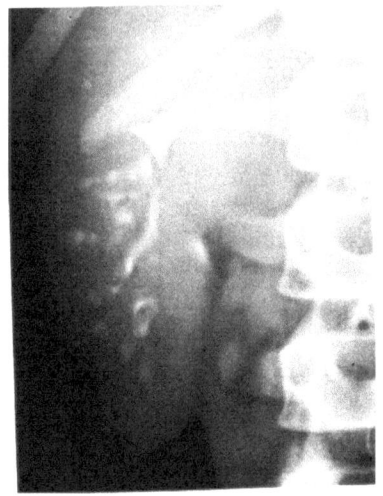

defined, but there may be evidence of multiple small cystic areas within the nephrogram. However, characteristically there is the appearance of radiating streaks or spotty collections of contrast medium in the renal parenchyma. The pelvicalyceal systems are usually poorly opacified, but if seen they may be distorted. Delayed films are often necessary and may show the lesions best.

In older children with *renal tubular ectasia* the fibrotic changes in the liver seem to be progressive and become more severe with time. Presentation is usually a result of one of the complications of portal hypertension, commonly from bleeding oesophageal varices. Liver function tests are usually normal, and other clinical manifestations of liver disease, such as jaundice, ascites and coma, are absent until late in the course of the diasease.

The renal abnormalities may be almost incidental findings and there may be only a barely discernible pyramidal blush at IVU (Fig. 6.16). Fibrotic changes may be present in other organs, such as the salivary glands and pancreas as well as the liver. Differential diagnoses of IVU findings of renal tubular ectasia are a normal pyramidal blush and a dense nephrogram associated with shock, dehydration and medullary necrosis.

Between these two extremes of infantile polycystic disease presenting in the neonate with renal failure and large kidneys, and renal tubular ectasia presenting with liver dysfunction, there is an intermediate group where overt renal and/or hepatic findings may be present clinically and radiologically and where the age of presentation is intermediate between these two groups. This has been termed juvenile polycystic disease. A diagnosis based simply on radiological criteria is not always fully reliable and there must be an integration of the clinical, genetic and imaging information, especially that derived from echography (Fig. 6.17). The liver always shows a histological picture identical to congenital hepatic fibrosis and this pathological data must be included before a final diagnosis may be considered irrefutable.

6.2.5.2.2 Adult Polycystic Disease

This lesion usually presents in the fourth decade with either palpable renal masses, renal failure, hypertension or haematuria. Haematuria is a common presenting childhood symptom. Hypertension when seen in childhood occurs towards the end of the first

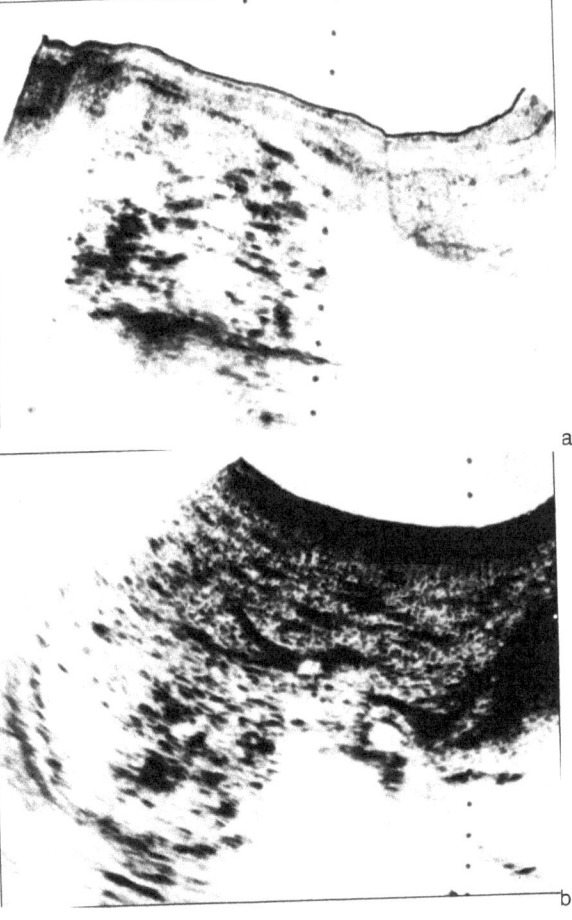

Fig. 6.17. a LS prone. The kidney is so enlarged that the poles are hidden by the acoustic shadows of the ribs and the iliac crest. The collecting cluster cannot be defined and there are several clumps of very high level echoes. **b** (Same case) TS supine showing poor definition between the right enlarged kidney and the liver. Appearance characteristic of infantile polycystic disease

decade. Cysts may be present in other viscera, and there is an increased incidence of intracranial aneurysms. Changes on the IVU have been demonstrated in asymptomatic children investigated because of relatives affected by this lesion with its dominant mode of inheritance.

In children rather large kidneys show a distorted pelivcalyceal system due to compression by cystic areas. The renal outline is smooth in childhood at IVU (Figs. 6.18 and 6.19). Sometimes the kidneys may not be unduly large but on other occasions in later childhood the overall pattern is similar to that seen in adults. The cysts may appear as negative defects on the nephrogram and are transonic at echography (Fig. 6.20). In contrast to the infantile type of polycystic disease the renal outlines and pelvicalyceal systems are usually well seen.

In the not too distant past people were confident they could distinguish between infantile and adult polycystic types of disease on clinical and radiological grounds. This confidence was misplaced [36, 37, 38, 39, 40]. Occasionally, the IVU changes of children with a family history of adult-type polycystic disease are indistinguishable from the classic IVU appearance in infantile-type polycystic disease. To add to the difficulty some young children who showed typical changes of infantile-type polycystic

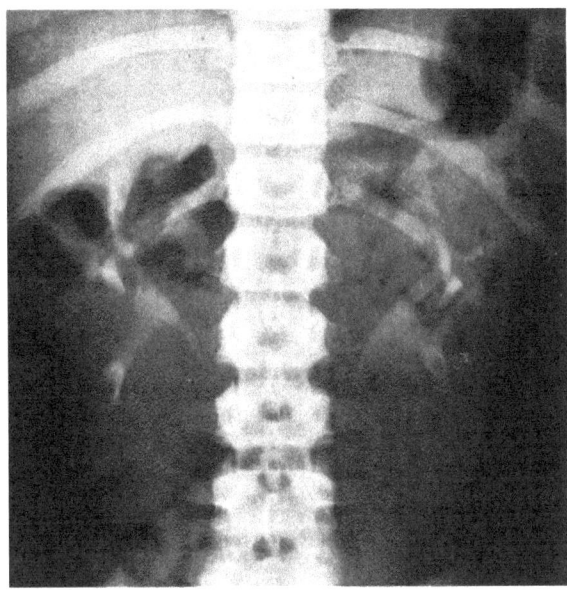

Fig. 6.19. Adult polycystic disease. This child has gross renal enlargement with spidery stretched calyces – the classic pattern seen in adults. Renal osteodystrophy is present in the ribs and spine. Contrast these features with those in Fig. 6.18

disease at IVU in early childhood lose their theoretically specific features and gradually change to an adult-type radiological pattern at IVU as they grow older (Fig. 6.21). Diagnosis is established by means of a percutaneous liver biopsy. The kidneys may be so large, causing displacement of the liver, that accidentally a renal biopsy may be obtained also! In these cases an anterior approach to the liver may be necessary. The importance of arriving at a correct diagnosis relates to prognosis and genetic counselling; infantile polycystic disease must be differentiated from an early presentation of the adult type of polycystic disease. The former has a recessive mode of inheritance, with a one in four chance of subsequent offspring being affected and the latter a dominant inheritance with a one in two risk.

Differential diagnoses of the IVU findings of adult-type polycystic disease presenting in childhood include:

1. Other cystic disease – tuberous sclerosis multiple simple serous cysts (very rare in children)
2. Infiltrations – lymphoma may rarely demonstrate multiple mass-like lesions which may be mistaken for cysts.
3. Infection – multiple pyogenic abscesses which diffusely enlarge the kidney, which may retain good function.
4. Tumour – necrotic areas rarely give rise to confusion in malignant tumours.
5. Obstruction – hydronephrosis.

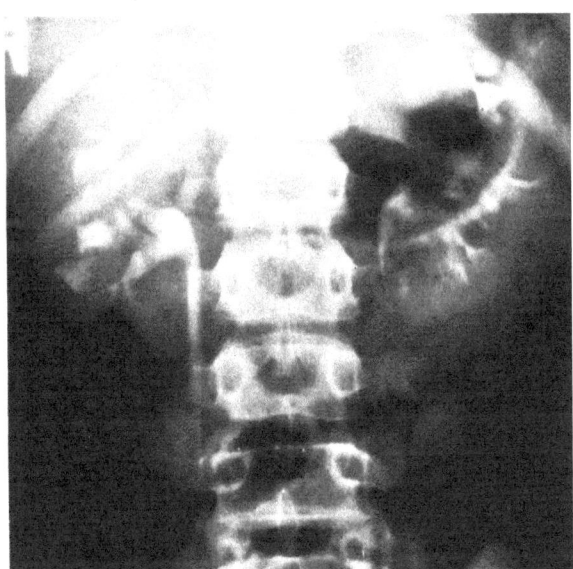

Fig. 6.18. Adult polycystic disease. This midly hypertensive boy had haematuria. The IVU shows slight renal enlargement and smooth contours. Some minor calyces are dilated, others show compression and the calyces are not appropriately distributed within the renal contours. Some young children with infantile polycystic disease may, as they grow older, show transition to adult-type polycystic disease appearances on IVU and the previous parenchymal opacification disappears

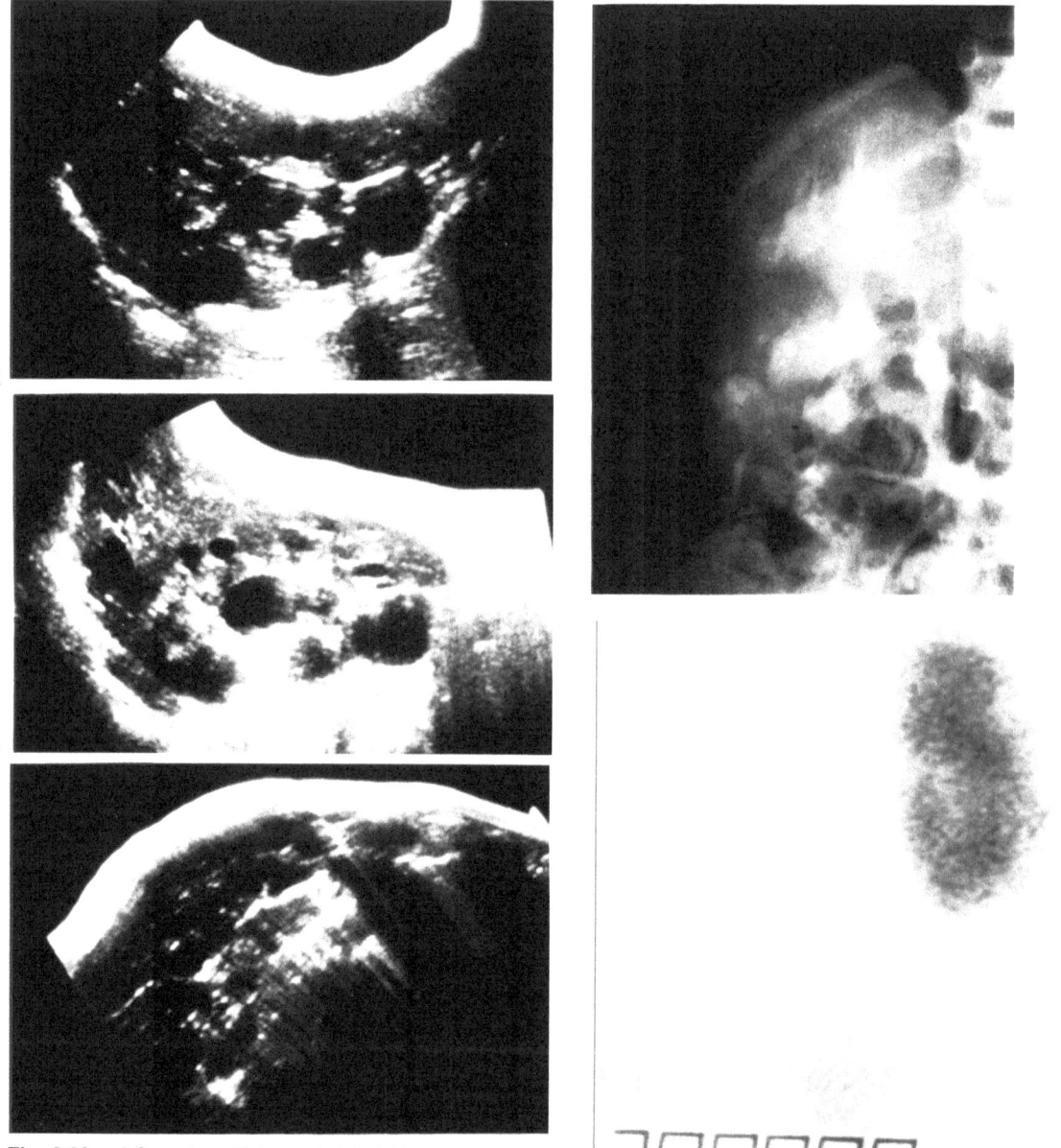

Fig. 6.20. a LS supine. Enlarged right kidney with many cysts of different sizes. **b** (Same case) LS supine. Higher sensitivity to demonstrate the presence of cysts in the liver as well. **c** (Same case) TS supine. Cysts in right kidney and liver can be seen. No obvious cysts in the pancreas. Diagnosis: adult-type polycystic disease in a child

Fig. 6.21 a, b. Transitional form of polycystic disease. The IVU of this child shows a solitary large right kidney (**a**). There is a streaky opacification of the renal parenchyma and the calyces are distended and clubbed. These features are transitional between those of the infantile type and those of adult-type polycystic disease. The DMSA scan (**b**) illustrates the patchy uptake of isotope related to the presence of large cystic areas within the renal parenchyma

High-dose nephrotomography and ultrasound may differentiate between diffuse solid infiltration, as in leukaemia, tumour or infection, and true cystic areas. This differential diagnosis is of practical importance because sometimes adult polycystic disease may predominantly affect only one kidney; it is extremely unfortunate if such a kidney is removed in the mistaken belief that renal enlargement is due to some other lesion.

6.2.5.3 Medullary Sponge Kidney

Medullary sponge kidney is not a renal lesion which has a genetic basis. Sporadic cases occur and the preceding symptoms may be urinary infection, ureteric colic (with complicating calculus disease) or haematuria. Apart from those problems the lesion does not constitute the threat to life which is implicit in, for example, infantile or adult polycystic disease. Medullary sponge kidney is rarely detected during the childhood years [41, 42].

The IVU shows the affected kidney is slightly large and in childhood one kidney only may be predominantly affected. Contrast medium cleared through the nephrons opacifies the small cystic spaces which are closely related to the margin of the pyramids which adjoin the cup of each minor calyx (Figs. 6.22, 6.23). Calculi may develop within the cystic spaces – these concretions may be difficult to identify on plain films but the diagnosis is clarified by IVU. As with other diffuse calcific lesions their high echogenicity should produce a characteristic central echo cluster. When such calculi enter the collecting system and pass down the ureter they may be responsible for an episode of colic and haematuria.

6.2.5.4 Medullary Cystic Disease: Juvenile Nephronophthisis

A rare condition, medullary cystic disease or juvenile nephronophthis may be associated with retinal hypoplasia, mental retardation, cerebellar ataxia and hepatic fibrosis. Because of this mixture of associations it has been suggested, quite rightly,

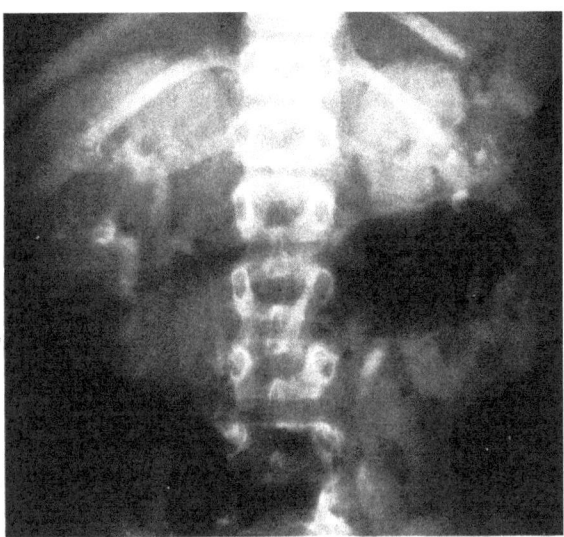

Fig. 6.23. Medullary sponge kidney. The IVU illustrates bilaterally large kidneys. The calyces are large and deeply cupped and there is streaky opacification of renal parenchyma in the region of the pyramids. There was evidence of calculus formation on the plain film of the abdomen

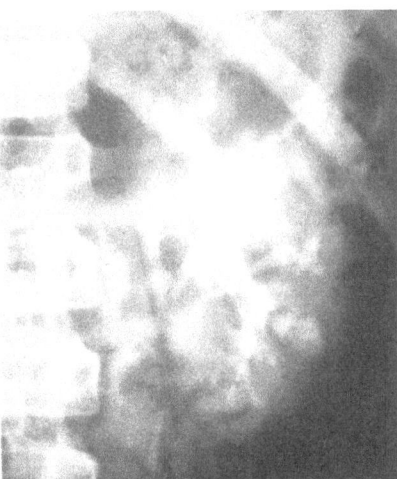

Fig. 6.22. Medullary sponge kidney. At IVU the rather large kidney shows concentrations of contrast medium in the tips of the papillae which are densely opacified. The location of the contrast medium is not quite like that seen in a normal pyramidal blush because it is too dense, variable in the extent of papillary opacification, and is often only along the margin of the papilla. The reason for this IVU was urinary infection, but calculi may collect in the cystic spaces and then pass into the ureter, causing colic; haematuria is another presentation

that juvenile nephronophthis is not a discrete entity [43].

Patients are of very short stature and have anaemia late in the first or second decades. They may, at this stage, have renal failure with polyuria and polydipsia and they die in renal failure [44]. The inheritance is usually autosomal recessive, but autosomal or X-linked dominant inheritances have been reported. Histologically multiple cysts, often no more than 2–3 mm in diameter, are variably present at the corticomedullary junction. Characteristically, the outer rim of cortex is spared of cysts but thinned.

At IVU, as children usually already have renal failure, there is very little or no evidence of opacification of the collecting systems and the nephrograms tends to be faint but of long duration [44]. When failure is severe vicarious clearance of contrast medium through the liver and gut may occur. In relation to the child's small stature the kidneys are not unduly small, they have a smooth, clearly defined outline (Fig. 6.24) and outstandingly poor function for their size. High-dose urograms with nephrotomography may show small cysts [45]. Renal needle biopsy is unwise because of fibrosis in the kidney.

The combination of the clinical, biochemical and radiological findings is usually sufficient to establish the diagnosis. On purely radiological grounds, the IVU of end-stage chronic nephritis is not dissimilar from that of juvenile nephronophthisis.

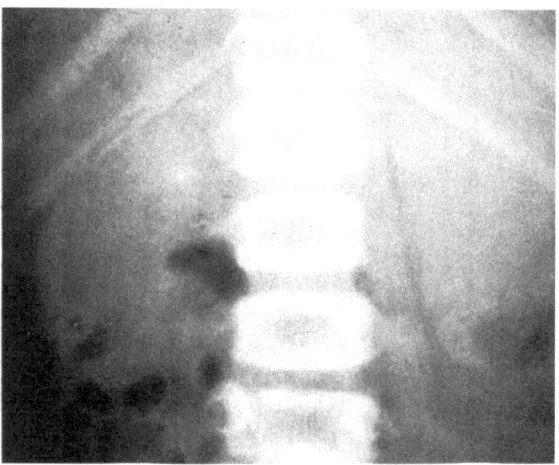

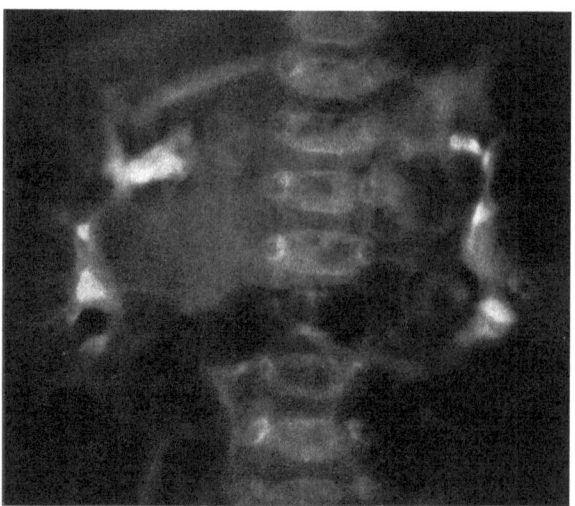

Fig. 6.24. Juvenile nephronophthisis – medullary cystic disease. These small stature children fail to concentrate urine. The 20-min IVU film shows kidneys which are not particularly small in relationship to the child's stature, but for their size they fail to concentrate contrast medium in a remarkable way. Sometimes faintly opacified calyces may be seen and small non-opacified cysts at the cortico-medullary junction may be suspected on nephrotomograms. In the absence of such cysts, the main differentiation on the radiological evidence is from end-stage chronic nephritis

Fig. 6.25. Tuberous sclerosis. This infant, referred for herniotomy, had large kidneys which on IVU showed no abnormal parenchymal opacification. The calyces are evenly distributed within the kidney contour, indicating a diffuse lesion. On biopsy gross dilatation of many Bowman's capsules was held to be consonant with tuberous sclerosis

6.2.5.5 Syndromes Associated with Cystic Kidneys

In summary these include:

1. Neuro-cutaneous
   syndromes: Tuberous sclerosis
                       (Figs. 6.25, 6.26, 6.27)
                       Von Hippel Lindau

2. Multiple malforma-
   tion syndromes: Beckwith-Wiedemann
                       Cerebro-hepato-renal
                       (Zellweger)
                       Dandy-Walker
                       Meckel-Gruber

3. Chromosomal
   anomalies: Trisomy 13
                       Trisomy 18

4. Bone dysplasias: Asphyxiating thoracic
                       dystrophy
                       Lethal short rib poly-
                       dactyly syndromes
                       Hajdu-Cheney
                       syndrome

5. Laurence-Moon-
   Biedl Syndrome
   (Fig. 6.28)

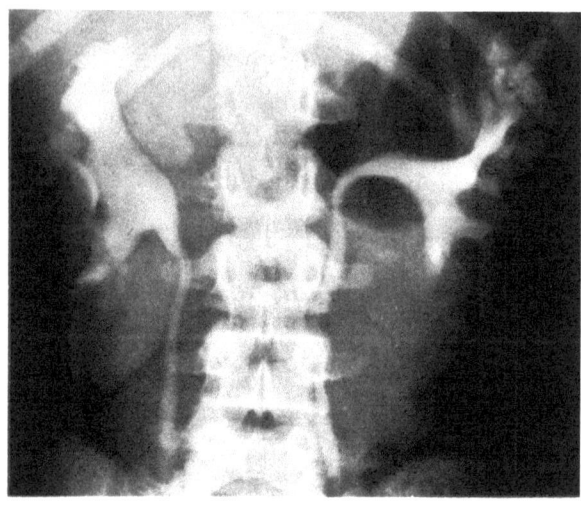

Fig. 6.26. Tuberous sclerosis. This child had clinical stigmata of tuberous sclerosis and the IVU is notably similar to that of the young infant with cystic dilatation of Bowman's capsules

Tuberous sclerosis is an inherited congenital malformation syndrome in which hamartoma may be present in many systems. Radiological abnormalities may be seen in the skull, the skeletal system and in the kidneys. Intracranially, there may be calcification. Skeletal changes consist of ill-defined areas of sclerosis and cystic areas and these changes progress with increasing age. In the kidneys there

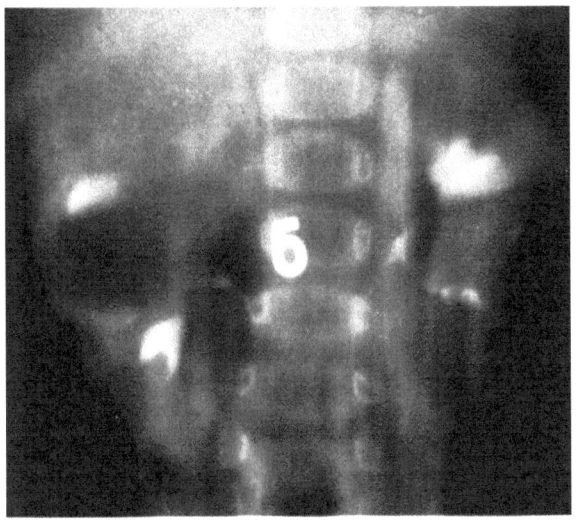

Fig. 6.27. Tuberous sclerosis. At IVU the nephrotomogram shows defects due to cystic spaces in the kidney. In some children with tuberous sclerosis, nephrotomography before the injection of contrast medium may show radiolucent fat within the renal hamartoma. CT scanning can also demonstrate the presence of intrarenal fat

is required to demonstrate the renal artery aneurysms and the vascular hamartomas. These may also be demonstrated in other abdominal organs, such as the adrenals and liver, at angiography.

Cystic dilatation of Bowman's capsules when diffuse results in considerable bilateral renal enlargement and may be a feature of tuberous sclerosis.

Beckwith-Wiedemann syndrome – clinical findings are gigantism, macroglossia, omphalocoele or umbilical hernia, flammeus naevus, neonatal hypoglycaemia and visceromegaly (Fig. 6.29). The importance of recognising the Beckwith-Wiedemann syndrome is threefold: (i) neonatal death; (ii) mental retardation; and (iii) predisposition to malignant diesease.

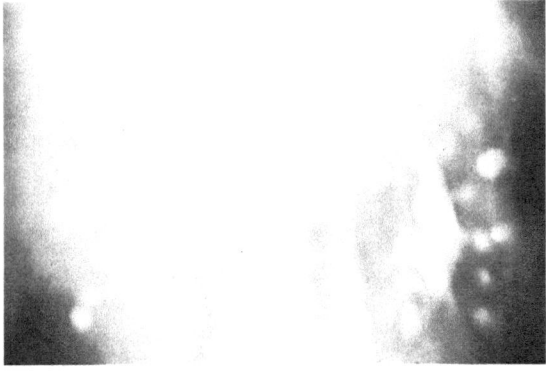

Fig. 6.29. Renal cystic disease in Beckwith-Wiedemann syndrome. The IVU in this young child with bilaterally large kidneys shows pools of contrast medium in cystic spaces scattered widely throughout the renal parenchyma. The child had the other features of the syndrome which include gigantism with macroglossia and visceromegaly, an omphalocoele or unbilicial hernia, neonatal hypoglycaemia and flammeus naevus

Fig. 6.28. Laurence-Moon-Biedl syndrome. At IVU, nephrotomography demonstrates small dysplastic kidneys with irregular outlines and distorted but full pelvicalyceal systems. There is poor concentration of contrast medium. These children often have polyuria and polydipsia

may be multiple hamartomata or cysts and aneurysms may be present arising from the more peripheral renal artery branches.

Plain abdominal views, or plain nephrotomography may demonstrate radiolucent fat within the renal hamartoma. On IVU the kidneys are large, the renal outlines lobulated and the pelvicalyceal systems distorted. Cystic areas may also be seen and taken in isolation, these changes make differentiation from adult-type polycystic disease difficult. Angiography

6.2.5.6 Simple Cysts

In children the simple cyst [46] is excessively rare and when seen it is commonly associated with distal obstruction in the urinary tract. An ultrasound examination is the definitive investigation when IVU has demonstrated the space-occupying lesion (Fig. 6.30).

6.2.5.7 Calyx Cyst

Simple calyx cysts are very uncommonly seen in both infants and children. The sequence at IVU is characteristic in that on an early radiograph taken as contrast medium is just entering the calyx system no opacification of the cyst occurs. Subsequently, as the pelvi-calyceal system opacifies, the calyx cyst is then opacified (Fig. 6.31). Such cysts really present no diagnostic problems if the film sequence is correctly analyzed.

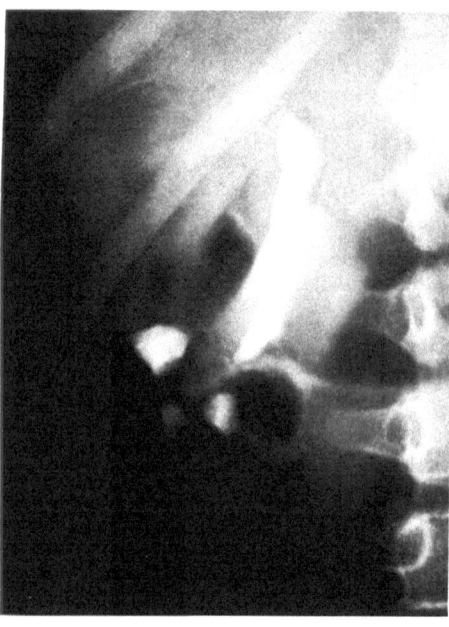

Fig. 6.30. Serous cyst. At IVU this child had bilateral pelvi-ureteric obstruction. A simple serous cyst with a calcified wall is present in the right kidney. Such cysts are uncommon in children and the possibility of echinococcosis must always be considered in the differential diagnosis

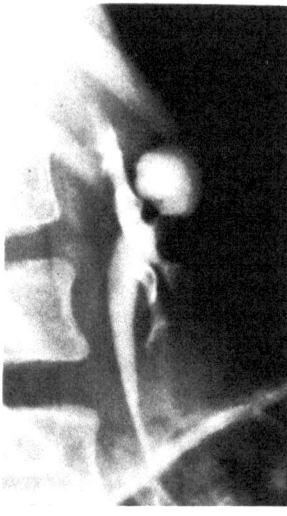

Fig. 6.31. Calyx cyst. The rounded cystic space connects with the calyx system. Five minutes after injecting the contrast medium the cyst was not opacified, but subsequently it was. This oblique view of the kidney shows its smooth contour and the sequence excluded a localised pyelonephritic scar

6.3 Absent Abdominal Muscles (Prune Belly) Syndrome and Variants

This disorder affects males and is diagnosed clinically because of the absence or severe deficiency in muscle development of the lower part of the abdominal wall [31]. The skin over the abdomen is wrinkled and hence the synonym "prune belly" syndrome. The testes are undescended and there is an abnormality of varying degrees of severity in the urinary tract.

The severest form is incompatible with life and this is because there is complete obstruction in the urethra associated with gross bladder enlargement and small grossly abnormal kidneys. Pulmonary hypoplasia and pulmonary infection may contribute to early death. Ultrasonics studies demonstrating oligohydramnious and vesical enlargement could suggest the possibility of this condition prenatally.

Amongst those who survive the neonatal period [31, 47, 48,] there will be found, in varying degrees, dysplastic kidneys draining into markedly dilated non-peristaltic ureters (Fig. 6.32). The vesico-ureteric junction may be incompetent with severe reflux complicating the picture. The bladder is enlarged (Fig. 6.33) and fails to empty completely at micturition, even though there is no obstruction. The urachus may be patent or simply a urachal diverticulum may exist. In the urethra are a variety of abnormalities: the bladder neck urethral junction tends to be conical in shape at micturition; there may be a diverticulum or large "prostatic urtricle" arising

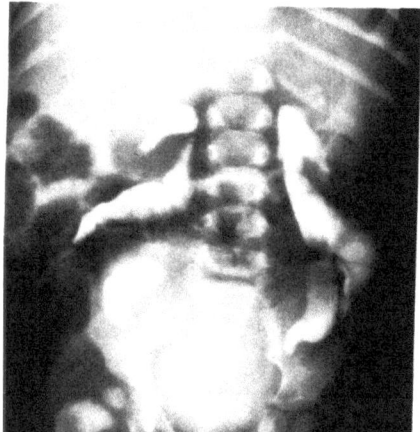

Fig. 6.32. Prune belly syndrome. In this IVU the kidneys show dysmorphic contours and drain into dilated pelvic-alyceal system. The ureters slowly opacify and are dilated, tortuous and aperistaltic. The large bladder is faintly opacified. It may be several hours before the whole urinary tract is opacified

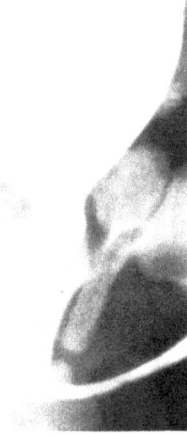

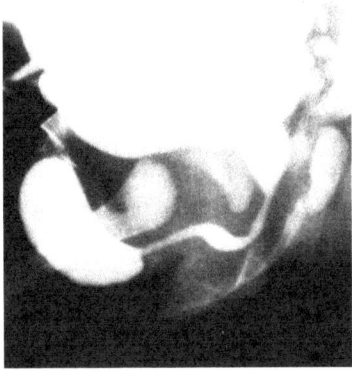

Fig. 6.34. Prune belly syndrome. At MCU the large bladder empties into a urethra which is dilated distally – a feature of megalopenis

Fig. 6.33. Prune belly syndrome. At MCU the large bladder empties through a wide bladder neck, but there is a suggestion of a contraction ring present. The small pocket lying posteriorly in the proximal part of the urethra is at the site of the prostatic utricle – this is a common feature of this condition. There is no reflux in this patient, but this is quite a frequent event

from the proximal part of the posterior urethra; dilatation of the urethra in conjunction with megalopenis may occur distally in the urethra (Fig. 6.34). There is a large undrained residue in the urinary tract. Colonization of the urine by bacteria can occur after urethral catheterization so prophylactic chemotherapy is wise if MCU is carried out. Indeed it is best to try to avoid MCU for so long as is reasonably possible and rely on IVU (often with films taken after an interval of several hours) and isotope studies to monitor progress. Echographic studies of vesical volume will show the extent of the undrained residue. Inevitably renal growth and function are compromised, sometimes to the extent that one kidney may be "non-functioning". The significance of any reflux and obstruction is difficult to estimate in these patients with urinary tract dysplasia. Although some boys continue surprisingly well (despite abdominal distension) into their childhood years, urinary diversion may be necessary.

Variants of the syndrome of absent abdominal muscles do occur. Abdominal musculature may be normal and yet the renal and urinary components of total dysplasia are present [49]. There is the non-obstructive dilatation of the proximal part of the urethra, the unvoided vesical residue after micturition and the uretero-vesical, ureteric and renal features present (Fig. 6.35). These are rare entities. It is important to differentiate such patients from those with *an adynamic syndrome* [50]. Again, this is a rare disorder, but in addition to the dilatation of

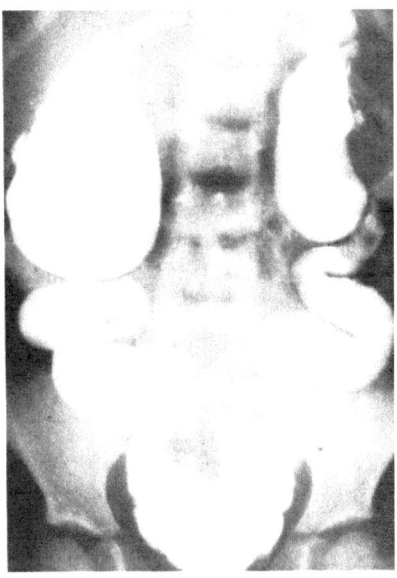

Fig. 6.35. Pseudo-prune-belly syndrome. In this boy the film taken at the end of MCU shows the previously large bladder incompletely empty and bilateral reflux into dilated tortuous aperistaltic ureters. In the collecting systems there are changes compatible with dysplasia. The urethra had the configuration commonly seen in the absent abdominal muscles syndrome, except that the prostatic utricle did not fill. A further "variant" is the "adynamic syndrome" in which the gut is adynamic in addition to the frequently affected urinary tract

urinary tract the alimentary system (particularly the small intestine and large intestine) may show little sign of peristalsis, providing an ileus-like syndrome. In this condition examining biopsy material from the intestine can be helpful in diagnosis, but on radiographs studies of the gut gas pattern is an important pointer.

6.4 Duplication in the Kidney and Ureters

Although in embryological terms the variants and problems which are found in duplication begin in the lower urinary tract it is easier in diagnostic terms to evaluate the problem from the kidney downwards. The reason is simply that the first diagnostic clues generally lie in the upper tract as investigation begins and proceeds.

When there is no parenchymal damage the duplex kidney may be longer than a normal single kidney. The two renal components drain into separate collecting systems. Generally the upper component is the smaller – and it may be very small indeed – and its collecting system has no true renal pelvis. The large component, lying inferiorly, has a pelvis and so it may be subject to pelvi-ureteric junction obstruction. If the pelvi-ureteric junction obstruction is marked then the lower renal component may become severely hydronephrotic and even non-functioning; in these circumstances it presents as a renal mass which can be differentiated from a tumour by echography and its nature confirmed by either retrograde or antegrade pyelography.

There is a relationship between the status of a renal component and the site of insertion of its ureter into the lower urinary tract. Ectopic ureters are frequently associated with dysplasia of the related kidney component. Reflux into such a ureter may lead to pyelonephritic changes in the parenchyma and obstruction produces atrophy or hydronephrosis of varying degrees. In general the more remote is the site of ureteric insertion from the normal location the greater the changes in the parenchyma of the associated renal segment [13].

6.4.1 Simple Duplication

The undamaged parenchyma of each component in a duplex kidney drains into its own collecting system. When the two collecting systems join proximally there may be little more than a bifid renal pelvis draining into a single ureter. The two collecting systems may drain into separate ureters which join to form one ureter at a point proximal to the bladder (Fig. 6.36). The single lower ureter enters the bladder orthotopically and is not particularly susceptible to reflux. Ureteric duplication may be complete and both ureters may enter the bladder orthotopically and in close proximity. In uncomplicated duplication the point where the two ureters join may be difficult to identify on radiographs; the reason is that peristalsis in the two ureters is not

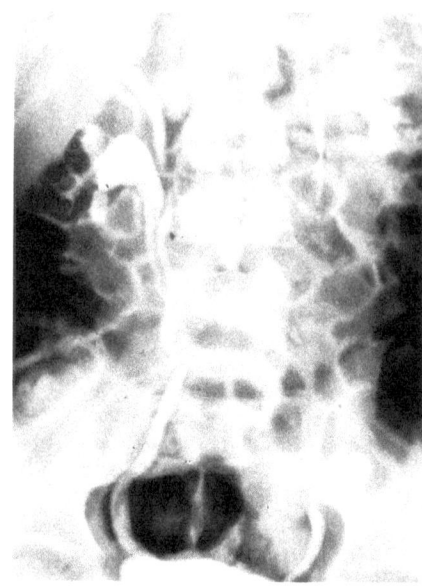

Fig. 6.36. Simple duplication. At IVU a right-sided duplex system has been demonstrated. The classical appearance of fewer calyces in the upper moiety is shown. The ureters unite just above the level of the pelvic brim. Rarely, when the ureters join proximally, there may be interureteric reflux with more dilatation proximally than is seen in this case. Again, and very rarely, calyces may drain extrarenally into three or more ureters

synchronous and one ureter tends to contain no contrast medium when the other is opacified.

6.4.2 Simple Duplication with Complications

Dilatation of the two ureters proximal to the point where they join to form one ureter may develop. In the two ureters peristalsis is discordant and contractions in the one ureter fill the other. Thus, interureteric reflux occurs and with each peristaltic wave only a little contrast-medium-laden urine enters the undilated single ureter which drains into the bladder. When the ureters are duplicated throughout their course to the bladder they may obstruct at the ureterovesical junction and dilatation of both ureters is present.

6.4.3 Complete Duplication with Small or Poorly Functioning Upper Component

When the upper renal component of a duplex system shows very poor function or non-function then the likelihood is that there is a complete ureteric duplication with ectopic entry of the ureter into the lower urinary tract. There are two common variants of insertion – ectopic ureterocoele formation and urethral ectopic ureter.

6.4.3.1 Ectopic Ureterocoele

The ureter draining the upper renal component enters the bladder in the vicinity of the bladder neck and it is obstructed at its point of entry. The ureter is dilated throughout its long intramural course and forms a ureterocoele which is ectopic and lies in the base of the bladder (Fig. 6.37) [51, 52, 53, 54, 55]. Proximal to the ureterocoele the individual ureter is dilated and drains an upper renal component which is generally small and "non-functioning" at IVU. The lower renal component may have a normal parenchyma, but its ureter which enters the bladder at the normal site often tends to have a rather tortuous course (Fig. 6.38).

Usually ectopic ureterocoele is an anomaly found on one side only. However, both sides may be affected where two ureterocoeles then lie in the base of the bladder.

The ectopic ureterocoele can vary in size as intravesical pressure rises (as at MCU) and the ureterocoele

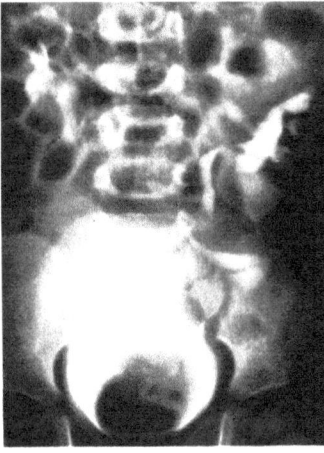

Fig. 6.38. Ectopic ureterocoele. The right kidney is normal. On the left side the upper non-functioning hydronephrotic element displaces downward and laterally, and also rotates, the collecting system of the lower element. The lower element's ureter runs a tortuous course since it is clearly related to the dilated non-opacified ureter which continues down to the ureterocoele

may then empty its content backward into the upper tract and so the ureterocoele transiently becomes invisible or difficult ot see (Figs. 6.39 and 6.40). It is a mistake to think that the ureterocoele is always easily seen in antero-posterior radiographs showing

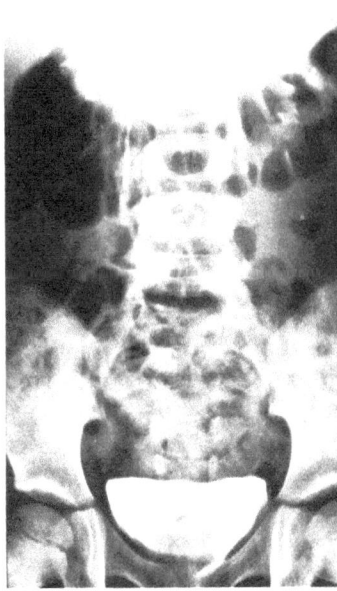

Fig. 6.37. Ectopic ureterocoele. The left kidney is normal and drains by a single ureter to the bladder. The double right kidney has a well opacified collecting system in its lower element with a classic "dropping flower" appearance produced by the fact that the upper element's collecting system is not opacified. However, the upper element shows a faint nephrogram and clears urine into a dilated ureter which terminates in the ectopic ureterocoele. This shows as a non-opacified filling defect in the base of the bladder

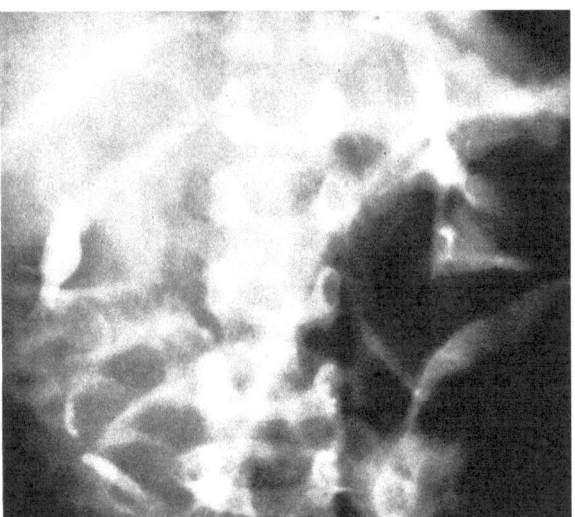

Fig. 6.39. Ectopic ureterocoele. The left kidney is normal, but the IVU shows on the right side the upper element has a rim nephrogram. The collecting system of the lower element is displaced and rotated. Its ureter runs a tortuous downward course – an important factor in radiological terms in differentiating this feature from an adrenal problem. The vesical component of the ureterocoele is not always immediately apparent

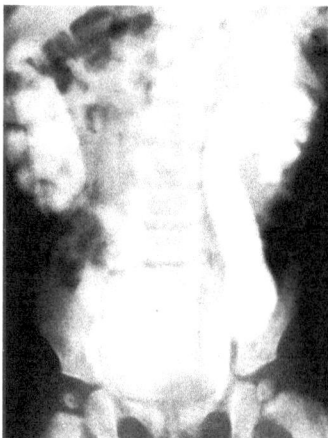

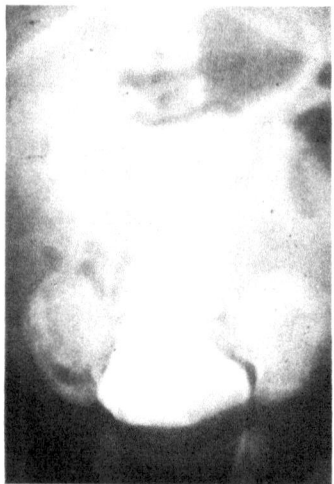

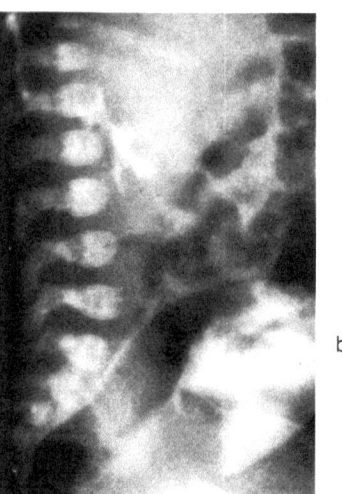

Fig. 6.40. Ectopic ureterocoele with obstruction. This IVU shows bilateral upper tract dilatation caused by a large tense ureterocoele in the bladder base. The ureterocoele is related to the non-functioning upper element on the right side. Note the element of duplication seen in the left kidney and the fact that the ureterocoele is not exactly easy to see

the bladder. Very commonly an ectopic ureterocoele obstructs the ipsilateral orthotopic ureter because of extension within the bladder base. The entire kidney may then become non-functioning and a lateral radiograph can then show the filling defect in the bladder base (Fig. 6.41). However, echography can easily demonstrate a ureterocoele within the bladder, thus avoiding the need for a lateral radiograph of the pelvis and the inevitable gonadal radiation dose in a girl (Fig. 6.42). Such an echographic study will also differentiate an ectopic ureterocoele from gas in the rectum and incidentally demonstrate that the ureterocoele volume varies from moment to moment. On occasion the ectopic ureterocoele extends across the bladder base to obstruct ureter(s) draining the contralateral kidney (Fig. 6.43). It is important to exclude ectopic ureterocoele in all patients who have an initially non-functioning kidney at IVU.

Ectopic ureterocoele may descend into the urethra on voiding (Fig. 6.44) and in girls it may become visible in the perineum if prolapse is a continuing phenomenon. In the male ureterocoele prolapse into the urethra widens the bladder neck and produces a negative image in the posterior aspect of the proximal part of the urethra (Fig. 6.45). It is important to distinguish such a finding from that seen in posterior urethral valves, especially since both lesions can produce considerable upper-tract dilatation and obstruction. Ureterocoeles only very rarely produce that degree of vesical hypertrophy seen in the boy with urethral valves.

Fig. 6.41 a, b. Ectopic ureterocoele with obstruction. The IVU in this neonate shows complete non-function of the left kidney (**a**). Although the bladder appearances are not particularly distinctive in the AP projection, the lateral view (**b**) shows clearly the ureterocoele lying in the base of the bladder and differentiates it from the gas in the rectum

From the foregoing description and given the variation in findings at IVU it is not surprising that the diagnosis of ectopic ureterocoele may prove taxing to the uninitiated. Meticulous anaylsis of the urogram series is needed. In general it is a good policy to think of a possible diagnosis of ectopic ureterocoele in any urographic series which is particularly baffling at first sight. The non-functioning (or occasionally very poorly functioning) upper renal component draining into the ureter leading to the ectopic ureterocoele should not present a problem in itself if the entire urinary tract is studied. Mistaken interpretation of the upper renal component as an adrenal problem almost never occurs in practice.

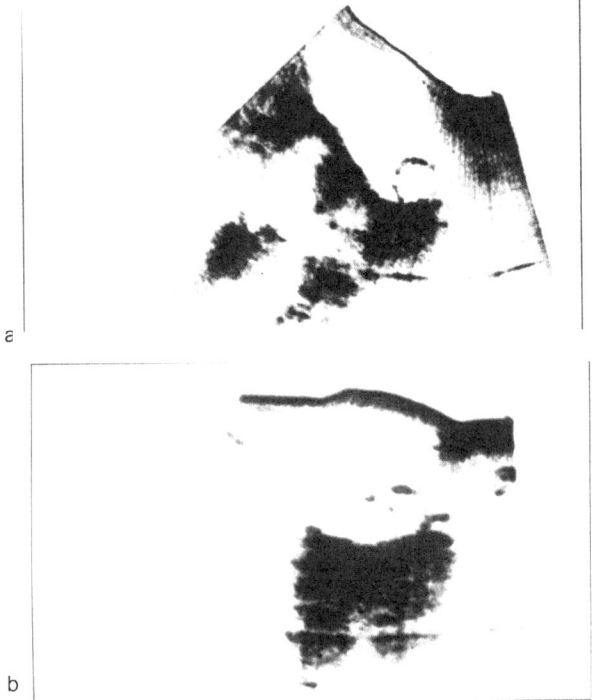

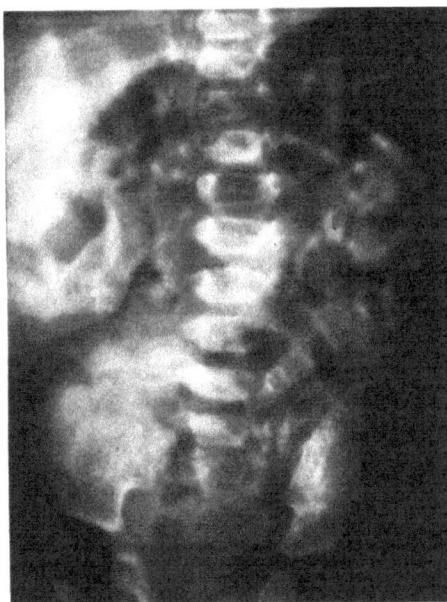

Fig. 6.42 a, b. Age 2. **a** LS supine view of the bladder. Spherical filling defect seen in the base of the bladder. **b** TS supine. This shows that there are a pair of globular structures. Diagnosis: bilateral ureterocoeles

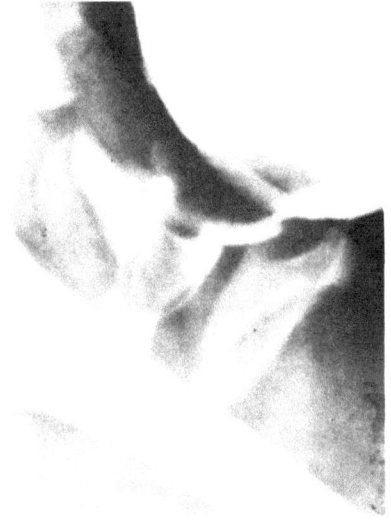

Fig. 6.44. Ectopic ureterocoele. MCU shows a prolapsing ectopic ureterocoele in the urethra in this girl. Not all ectopic ureterocoeles prolapse on voiding. Many ectopic ureterocoeles are not tense and so may not be visible at MCU (or indeed on IVU) because, among other reasons, their content empties backward up the ureter. Tense ureterocoeles obstructing bladder outflow may produce vesical hypertrophy

The combination of ectopic ureterocoele with obstruction to ipsilateral and contralateral ureters and obstruction to vesical emptying can present superficial diagnostic problems when the ureterocoele is difficult to identify on radiographs. Rarely ectopic ureterocoeles rupture spontaneously; when this has happened free reflux through the ureterocoele and into its ureter makes the diagnosis easy.

Surgical uncapping of the ureterocoele and partial nephrectomy and ureterectomy are standard surgical procedures. In follow-up studies it is important to look for complications. If a large flap of mucosa is left behind after uncapping it may obstruct bladder emptying. The bladder base and the proximal part of the urethra may be weakened by a large ureterocoele and incontinence results. Vesico-ureteric reflux into the remaining intact ureters may predispose to urinary infection and inevitably there is reflux into the stump of the ureter (Fig. 6.46) which formerly drained into the ureterocoele. Many of these aspects are illustrated and may be inferred from Fig. 6.46.

6.4.3.2 Urethral Ectopic Ureter

The upper renal component which drains through a ureter direct to the urethra is usually very small and if it functions at all it is opacified very faintly [56]. It is often impossible to be certain that no such upper component is present because it is so small and the

Fig. 6.43. Ectopic ureterocoele with obstruction. This IVU film at 7 h shows severe bilateral obstruction. The large ectopic ureterocoele presents a large negative image occupying most of the bladder, which is faintly opacified by a rim of contrast medium cleared by the only part of the unobstructed upper tract – the left upper renal element. Note contrast medium to right of spine in the obstructed kidney

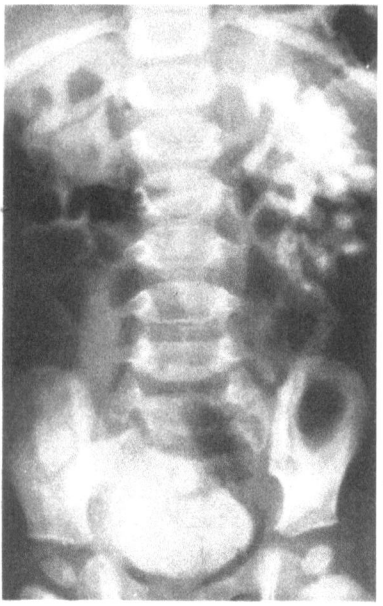
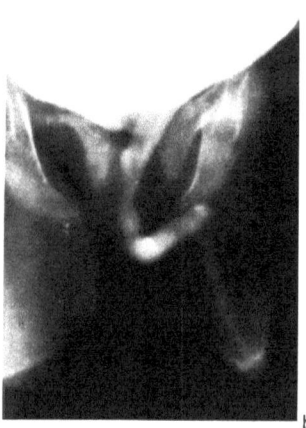

◁ **Fig. 6.45 a, b.** Prolapsing ectopic ureterocoele in a boy. **a** This IVU at 60 min shows a left duplex system with a multiplicity of distended calyces (polycalycosis). On the right side only faint opacification of the dilated right collecting system and its tortuous ureter is shown. The ectopic ureterocoele is very difficult to define within the bladder. **b** At MCU the prolapsing ectopic ureterocoele occupies the proximal part of the posterior urethra and is seen as a negative image in the voided contrast medium. The bladder neck is wide and the proximal urethra has a conical appearance, which must be differentiated from that seen in posterior urethral valves

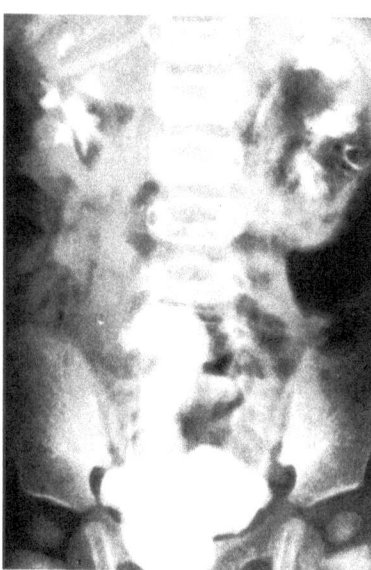

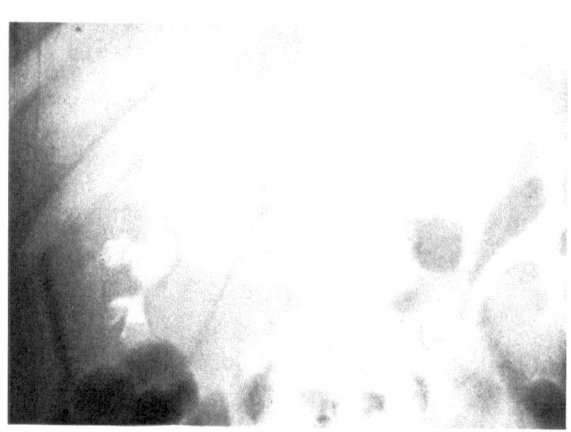

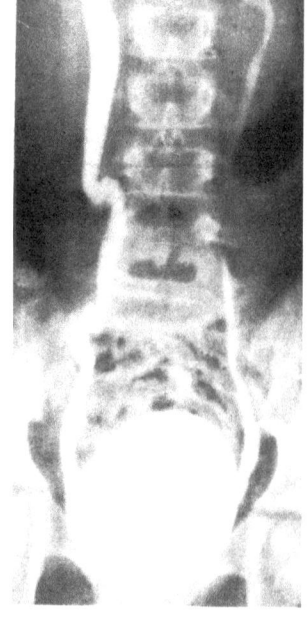

Fig. 6.46. Post-operative IVU in ectopic ureterocoele. This IVU shows several residual features following uncapping of the ureterocoele and partial right nephroureterectomy. The left duplex kidney functions well. The right kidney remnant is rotated. Contrast medium entering the bladder fills the uncapped ectopic ureterocoele lying at the bladder base. There is a reflux into the long ureteric stump associated with the ureterocoele. The changes in the bladder base may be associated either with more generalised reflux shown by MCU with or incontinence

Fig. 6.47 a, b. Duplication with urethral ectopia. **a** IVU shows, in this girl with urinary infectious and perineal dampness, bilateral duplex kidneys with poor excretion in the small upper renal elements. **b** At MCU bilateral reflux into ureters entering the urethra extends up to the small upper renal components   ▷

configuration of the lower renal component can easily be mistaken for normal. The clinical history of continual dampness, often with recurrent urinary infection is an important diagnostic clue (Fig. 6.47). The ureteral orifice is almost invariably incompetent. If the ureter opacifies by reflux during the filling phase of an MCU then the ureteric insertion is proximally located in the urethra. When the ureter fills only during voiding the orifice is more distally located in the urethra. The orthotopically located orifices related to ureters draining the lower poles are usually not incompetent or subject to reflux.

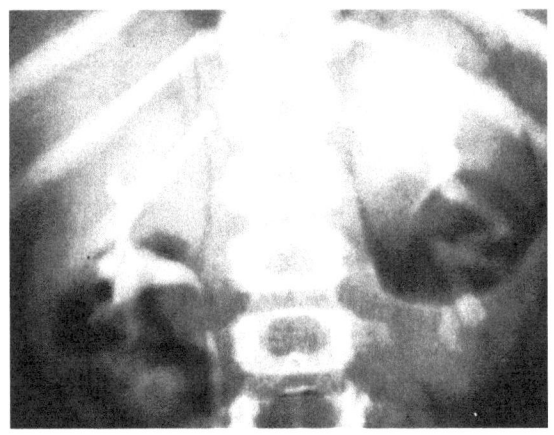

6.4.4 Duplex Kidney with Atrophic Features in the Lower Renal Component

(Williams, 1962 Variant) [57]

In this variant the upper renal component has a normal parenchyma but the lower component shows parenchymal thinning and calyx clubbing at IVU (Fig. 6.48). The ureter draining the lower component is invariably subject to reflux. Ureters draining other renal components may sometimes be subject to reflux although they almost always have a normal parenchymal structure.

Historically (in modern medicine a time interval of 18 years is an historic interval) this was held to be an important entity with general implications. Renal atrophy with features like those of chronic pyelonephritis, its invariable association with vesicoureteric reflux and the fact that patients with this disorder were investigated for urinary infections of a recurrent type provided a combination of circumstances which did much to establish current concepts of reflux, reflux nephropathy and pyelonephritic scarring.

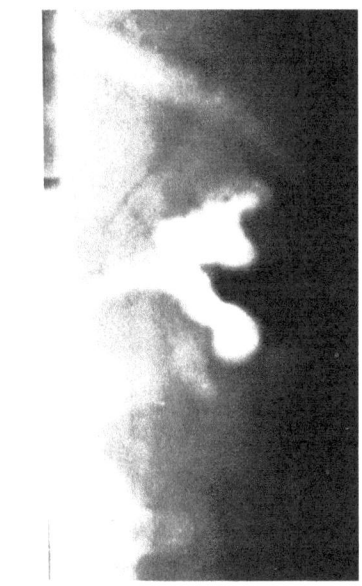

Fig. 6.48 a, b. Duplication with reflux into lower moiety. The IVU (a) demonstrated poor concentration of contrast medium in the lower element of a left-sided duplex kidney. MCU (b) illustrates reflux into the lower element of the left kidney. The calyces are clubbed and intra-renal reflux is present adjacent to the uppermost calyces

References

1. Emanuel, B.: Congenital solitary kidney; a review of 74 cases J. Urol. **111**, 394 (1974)
2. Kelasis, P. P.: Observations on renal ectopia and fusion in children. J. Urol. **110**, 588 (1973)
3. Vereb, J., Tischler, O., Paukovcekova, O.: Differential X-ray diagnosis of renal dysdopias and ectopias in children. Pediatr. Radiol. **7**, 205 (1978)
4. Fillippi, G. de, Forno, S. dal, Bianchi, M.: Blind ureteric buds. Pediatr. Radiol. **5**, 160 (1977)
5. Albers, D. D., Geyer, J. R., Barnes, S. E.: Blind-ending branch of bifid ureter: report of 3 cases. J. Urol. **99**, 160 (1968)
6. Ekström, T.: Renal hypoplasia; a clinical study of 179 cases. Acta Chir. Scand. [Suppl.] 203 (1955)
7. Risdon, R. A.: Renal dysplasia. I. A clinicopathological study of 76 cases II. A necropsy study of 41 cases. J. Clin Pathol. **24**, 57 (1971)
8. Risdon, R. A., Young, L. W., Chrispin, A. R.: Renal hypoplasia and dysplasia: a radiological and pathological correlation. Pediatr. Radiol. **3**, 213 (1975)
9. Habib, R.: Renal dysplasia, hypoplasia and cysts. Pediatr. Nephrol. **1**, 209 (1974)

10. Roosen-Runge, E. C.: Retardation of post-natal development of kidneys with early cerebral lesions. Am. J. Dis. Child. **77**, 185 (1949)

11. Pinckney, L. E., Moskowitz, P. S., Lebowitz, R. L., Fritzsche, P.: Renal malposition associated with omphalocele. Radiology **129**, 677 (1978)

12. Daniel, W. W., Datnow, B.: Crossed fused renal ectopia with renal dysplasia. Am. J. Roentgenol. **128**, 845 (1978)

13. Mackie, G. G., Awang, H., Stephens, F. D.: The ureteric orifice: the embryological key to radiologic status of duplex kidneys. J. Pediatr. Surg. **10**, 473 (1975)

14. Friedland, G. W., Filly, R.: Demonstration of vestibular implantation of ectopic ureters on an excretory urogram. Pediatr. Radiol. **2**, 137 (1974)

15. Ljungquist, A. The Ask-Upmark kidney; a congenital renal anomaly studied by micro angiography and histology. Acta. Pathol. Scand. [A] **56**, 277 (1962)

16. Habib, R., Courtecuisse, V., Ehrenspenger, J., Royer, P.: Hypoplasia segmentaire du rein avec hypertension artérielle chez l'enfant. Ann. Paediatr. (Basel) **41**, 954 (1965)

17. Benz, G., Willich, E., Scharer, K.: Segmental renal hypoplasia in childhood. Pediatr. Radiol. **5**, 86 (1976)

18. Johnston, J. H., Mix, L. W.: The Ask-Upmark kidney; a form of ascending pyelonephritis? Br. J. Urol. **48**, 393 (1976)

19. Flynn, V. J., Gittes, R. F.: Benign cortical rest: "pseudotumor of the kidney". J. Urol. **108**, 54 (1972)

20. Pollack, H. M., Edell, S., Morales, J. O.: Radionucleide imaging in renal pseudotumor. Radiology **111**, 639 (1974)

21. Parker, J. A., Lebowitz, R., Mascatello, V., Treves, S.: Magnification renal scintigraphy in the differential diagnosis of septa of Bertin. Pediatr. Radiol. **4**, 157 (1976)

22. Azimi, F., Bryan, P. J.: Familial occurrence of renal pseudotumour due to enlarged column of Bertin in two brothers and their first cousin. Clin. Radiol. **25**, 467 (1974)

23. Pathak, I. G., Williams, D. I.: Multicystic and cystic dysplastic kidneys. Br. J. Urol. **36**, 318 (1964)

24. Parkkulainen, K. V., Hjelt, L., Sinola, K.: Congenital multicystic dysplasia of the kidney; report of 19 cases with discussion of etiology nomenclature and classification of cystic dysplasias of the kidney. Acta Chir. Scand. [Suppl.] **244**, 1 (1959)

25. Griscom, N. T.; The roentgenology of neonatal abdominal masses. Am. J. Roentgenol. **93**, 447 (1965)

26. Bloom, D. A., Brosman, S.: The multicystic kidney. J. Urol. **120**, 211 (1978)

27. Lachman, R. S., Lindstrom, R. R., Hirose, F. M.: The septation sign in multicystic dysplastic kidney. Pediatr. Radiol. **3**, 117 (1975)

28. Young, L. W., Wood, B. P., Spohr, C. H., Panner, B.: Delayed excretory urographic opacification, a puddling effect, in multicystic renal dysplasia. Ann. Radiol. (Paris) **17**, 391 (1974)

29. Boggs, L. K., Kimmelsteil, P.: Benign multilocular cystic nephroma: a report of two cases of so-called multilocular cyst of the kidney. J. Urol. **76**, 530 (1956)

30. Osanthanondh, V., Potter, E. L.: Pathogenesis of polycystic kidneys. Arch. Pathol. (Chicago) **77**, 459 (1964)

31. Burkholder, G. V., Williams, D. I.: The prune-belly syndrome. J. Urol. **98**, 244 (1967)

32. Williams, D. I., Barrat, T. M., Eckstein, H. B., Kohlinsky, S. M., Newns, G. H., Polani, P. E., Singer, J. D.: Urology in childhood. In: Handbuch der Urologie. Andersson, L., Gittes, R. F., Goodwin, W. E., Lutzeyer, W., Zingg, E. (eds.), Vol. XV Suppl., p. 66 Berlin, Heidelberg, New York: Springer 1974

33. Blyth, H., Ockenden, B. G.: Polycystic disease of kidneys and liver presenting in childhood. J. Med. Genet. **8**, 257 (1971)

34. Gwinn, J. L., Landing, B. H.: Cystic diseases of the kidneys in infants and children. Radiol. Clin. North Am. **6**, 191 (1968)

35. Six, R., Oliphant, M., Grossman, H.: A spectrum of renal tubular ectasia and hepatic fibrosis. Radiology **117**, 117 (1975)

36. Ritter, R., Siafarikas, K.: Hemihypertrophy in a boy with renal polycystic disease: varied patterns of presentation of renal polycystic disease in his family. Pediatr. Radiol. **2**, 98 (1976)

37. Ross, D. G., Travers, H.: Infantile presentation of adult-type polycystic kidney disease in a large kindred. J. Pediatr. **87**, 760 (1975)

38. Fellows, R. A., Leonidas, J. C., Beatty, E. C.: Radiologic features of "adult-type" polycystic kidney disease in the neonate. Pediatr. Radiol. **4**, 87 (1976)

39. Kaye, C., Lewy, P. R.: Congenital appearance of adult-type (autosomal dominant) polycystic kidney disease. J. Pediatr. **85**, 807 (1974)

40. Loh, J. P., Haller, J. O., Kassner, E. G., Aloni, A., Glassberg, K.: Dominantly inherited polycystic kidneys in infants; association with hypertrophic pyloric stenosis. Pediatr. Radiol. **6**, 27 (1977)

41. Snelling, C. E., Brown, N. M., Smythe, C. A.: Medullary sponge kidney in a child. Can. Med. Assoc. J. **102**, 518 (1970)

42. Eisenberg, R. L., Pfister, R. C.: Medullary sponge kidney associated with congenital hemihypertrophy (asymmetry). A case report and survey of literature. Am. J. Roentgenol. **116**, 773 (1972)

43. Nephronophthisis – just a pretty name? (Editorial). Lancet *1979* I, 141

44. Jones, D. N., Risdon, R. A., Hayden, K., Barratt, T. M., Chrispin, A. R.: Juvenile nephronophthisis; clinical, radiological and pathological correlationships. Pediatr. Radiol. **1**, 164 (1973)

45. Spicer, R. D., Ogg, C. S., Saxton, H. M., Cameron, J. S.: Renal medullary cystic disease. Br. Med. J. *1969* I, 824

46. Ahmed, S.: Simple renal cysts in childhood. Br. J. Urol. **44**, 71 (1972)

47. Cremin, B. J.: The urinary anomalies associated with agenesis of the abdominal walls. Br. J. Radiol. **44,** 767 (1971)
48. Welch, K. J., Kearney, G. P.: Abdominal musculature deficiency syndrome: prune belly. J. Urol. **111,** 693 (1974)
49. Williams, D. I., Taylor, J. S.: A rare congenital uropathy: vesico-urethral dysfunction with upper tract anomalies. Br. J. Urol. **41,** 307 (1969)
50. Kapila, L., Haberkorn, S., Nixon, H. H.: J. Pediatr. Surg. **10,** 885 (1975)
51. Eklöf, O., Mükinen, E.; Ectopic ureterocoele; a radiological appraisal of 66 consecutive cases. Pediatr. Radiol. **2,** 111 (1974)

52. Eklöf, O., Löhr, G., Ringertz, H., Thomasson, B.: Ectopic ureterocoele in the male infant. Acta. Radiol. [Diagn.] (Stockh) **19,** 145 (1978)
53. Williams, D. I., Royle, M.: Ectopic ureterocoele in the male. Br. J. Urol. **41,** 412 (1972)
54. Firedland, G. W., Cunningham, J.: The elusive ectopic ureteroceles. Am. J. Roentgenol. **116,** 792 (1972)
55. Williams, D. I., Fay, R., Lillie, J. G.: The functional radiology of ectopic ureterocoele. Br. J. Urol. **44,** 417 (1972)
56. Williams, D. I., Lightwood, R. G.: Bilateral single ectopic ureters. Br. J. Urol. **44,** 267 (1972)
57. Williams, D. I.: Vesico-ureteric reflux. Postgrad. Med. J. **38,** 520 (1962)

7

Vesical and Urethral Problems

7.1 Introduction

In introducing the subjet of vesical and urethral abnormalities it is essential first to mention a few points which can cause perplexity.

The rectal content affects studies of the bladder. Gas in the rectum can mimic either an ectopic ureterocoele or a non-opaque calculus on contrast medium studies (Fig. 7.1); a post-micturition film taken when the bladder is empty will show nothing within the bladder. If the bladder is full of contrast medium and a post-voiding film cannot be obtained, ectopic ureterocoele can be excluded because gas in the rectum does not produce the convex impression in the base of the bladder characteristic of ectopic

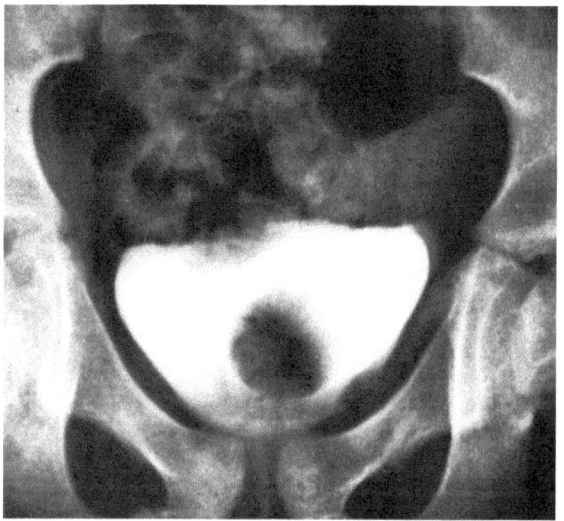

Fig. 7.1. Gas in rectum at IVU producing an image lying within the bladder contour. This feature must be differentiated from a non-opaque calculus and a ureterocoele

ureterocoele. The other alternatives are to get the patient to empty his bowel (which may not be easy) or do a brief ultrasound study.

Large amounts of faecal material in the rectum can occupy the pelvic cavity and displace the bladder. In infants and young children the sigmoid loop very often lies in the right iliac fossa and a loaded gut frequently displaces the bladder (which in young patients is an abdominal viscus) to the left side (Fig. 7.2). Changes in contour in the bladder can produce curious appearances such as bladder ears (Fig. 7.3) which are of no significance in either medical or surgical terms.

Voiding cystograms can cause anxieties in interpretation. In a young girl the distal part of the urethral lumen may, when she micturates rapidly, not open so widely as the greater degree of widening seen proximally, and below the bladder neck. This is the so-called spinning top appearance and it indicates neither a distal urethral stenosis nor a bladder neck problem. Intrinsic urethral stenosis in girls is very rare indeed. Boys quite often have a zone or zones of increased transradiancy in the vicinity of the posterior urethra and this is a normal event (*see* Chapter 2). His urethra proximally is not dilated and the urethra distally is not narrowed; this phenomenon is not pathological and is common in boys beyond the age of early infancy. None of the features in the vicinity are those of obstruction and there is no hypertrophy or sacculation of the bladder.

Sometimes the bladder contracts in an asynchronous way. When this happens the upper part of the bladder is of wider calibre than the ring-like constriction with the ring appearing to divide, incompletely, the vesical lumen into an upper and lower part. There is little difficulty in recognising this phenomenon for what it is, if fluoroscopy is used, at MCU except for one circumstance (Fig. 7.4). When

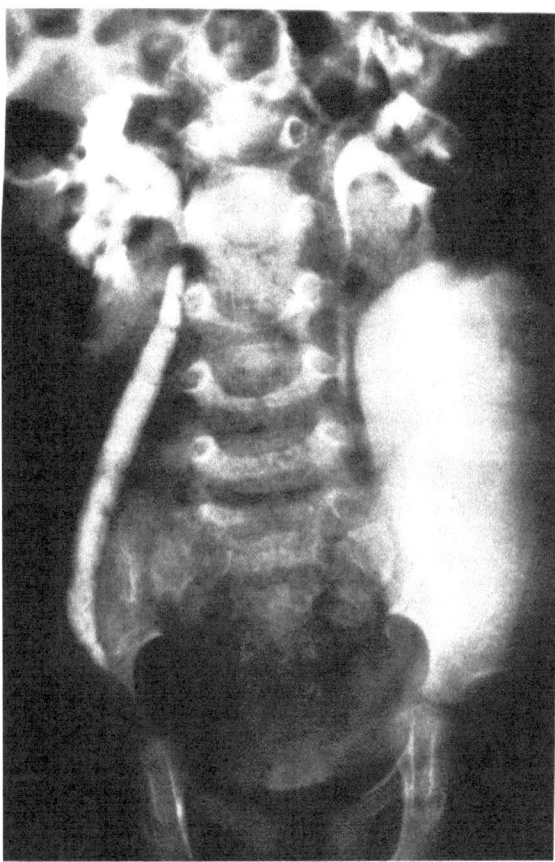

Fig. 7.2. Bladder displacement. The bladder is displaced to the left and the lower part of its lumen compressed by gross faecal retention in the rectum caused by a rectal stricture. There is also some compression of the right ureter as it descends across the pelvic brim. Bladder displacement of this sort is quite common in infants and young children (although seldom quite to this degree). Such displacement need not imply a malignant or benign mass lesion in the pelvis

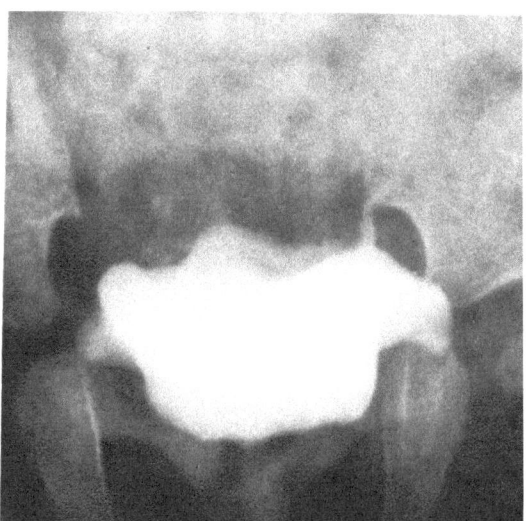

Fig. 7.3. Bladder ears on IVU. The curious configuration of the bladder which is sometimes seen in infancy. It is of no significance, but is related to inguinal herniation

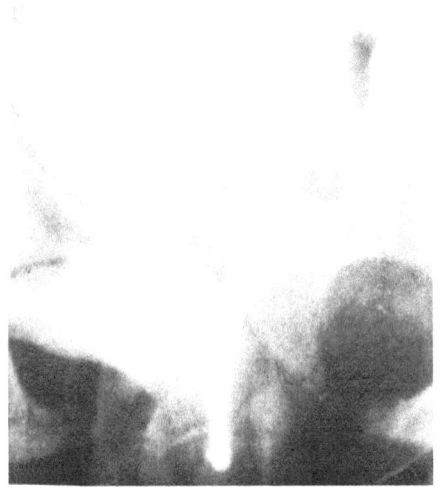

Fig. 7.4. Vesical contraction ring. The bladder contracts asynchronously with a constriction developing between the fundus and the base of the bladder. Reflux into the orthotopic left ureter identifies the position of the ureteric orifice. The urethral lumen below the bladder is narrow and normal

reflux into one or other orthotopically inserted ureter occurs then a mistaken impression may arise, namely, that the ureter is inserted ectopically into the urethra. However, careful fluoroscopy at the time of filling and voiding of contrast medium will make it clear what is happening and when the videotape record or films are studied it is very clear that the bladder neck lies in the appropriate lower location and the contraction ring is too high to be a bladder neck. Lateral or steep oblique projections may avoid such misinterpretation, but the radiation doses at MCU must be kept to a minimum and such projections do not help in achieving this objective. Periodically patients are studied because of persistent enuresis and there is only one point of specific relevance to make for the moment. A very small number of boys will, on voiding cystography, show an exceptionally wide urethral lumen (Fig. 7.5). They can void quickly and there is no sign of any distal urethral obstruction. Why enuresis is related to a wide urethra in these youths is not clear [1]. Diverticulum formation in the bladder may be a feature of obstruction to emptying or associated with vesico-ureteric reflux or ureteric obstruction.

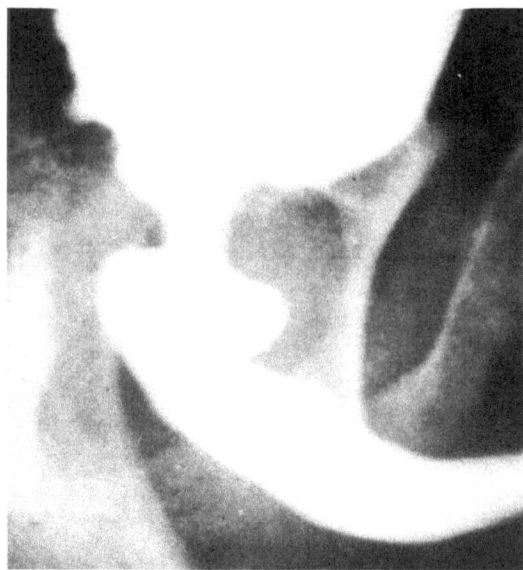

Fig. 7.5. Grossly dilated urethra in an enuretic boy who was otherwise normal. The reason why the dilatation is associated with enuresis is not clear, but sphincteric function is essentially normal

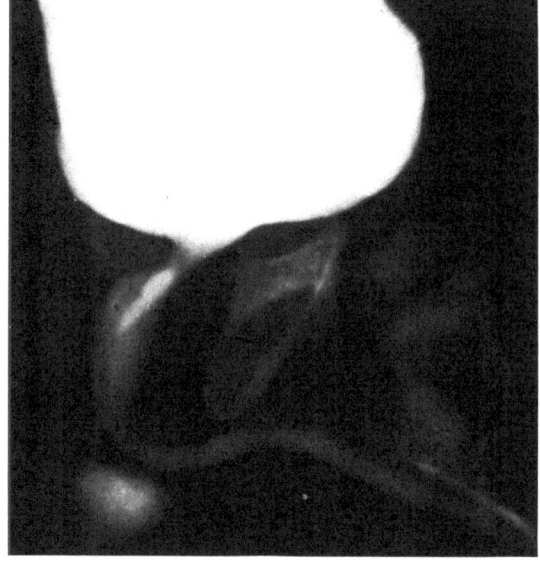

Fig. 7.6. Urethral diverticulum. Small diverticulum arising from the urethra shown on MCU. Calculi can collect in such a diverticulum

Sometimes there appears to be no particular reason for a diverticulum to develop. A posteriorly located large diverticulum may obstruct the urethra at micturition and there may then also be an associated reflux and upper tract dilatation. Large vesical diverticula always mean there is an unvoided vesical residue because the diverticulum empties its content back into the bladder after micturition. Urethral diverticula (except for anterior urethral diverticulum *see* Chapter 3) are exceptionally rare. When they are of the type shown in Fig. 7.6 calculi may develop within them.

Reflux of contrast medium from the urethra into the prostatic ducts is most often found either in neuropathic bladder or in boys with posterior urethral valves [2]. Such reflux is held by some to be a possible nidus from which the urinary tract, once infected, may become re-infected [3]. Abscess formation may occur (Fig. 7.7). Occasionally more extensive reflux into the male genital tract and seminal vesicles may occur, notably in conjunction with ectopic ureterocoele and also in neuropathic bladder.

In certain intersex states contrast medium entering the lower genital tract passes along circuitous routes (Fig. 7.8). However, the implications of intersex states have limited relevance in the context of this discussion for the subject is dominated by clinical, physical, laboratory and psychosocial considerations.

In the subsequent parts of this section a wide range of developmental problems affecting primarily the lower urinary tract is detailed. Unfortunately neoplastic disease of the region occurs and much of it is distinctly malignant. Lower urinary tract infection can lead to specific problems in the bladder especially. Finally, neuropathic bladder and its cryptogenic variants are described. The problems of obstruction and vesico-ureteric reflux have been considered at various points previously in this volume.

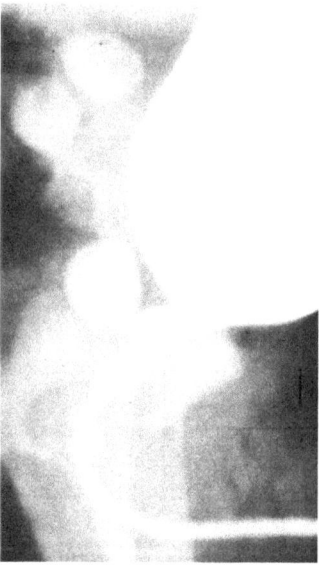

Fig. 7.7. Prostatic abscess. Boy with fever, retention and urinary infection. MCU shows prostatic filling posteriorly. On rectal examination pus passed down the urethra

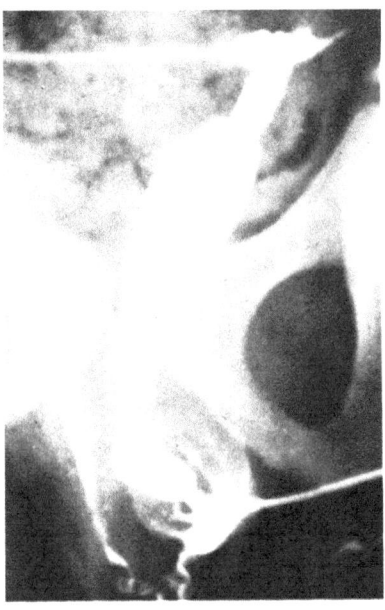

Fig. 7.8. Catheterisation of an intersex case. Catheter has passed along urethra into a "utricle". Contrast medium has then passed through a uterus along a "Fallopian tube" which extends into a vas deferens to the epididymis

7.2 Developmental Variants

7.2.1 Absence of Ureteric Orifice in the Normal Location

Generally this feature is characteristic of renal agenesis. Rarely it is because the ureter from the kidney drains ectopically. Both ureters may drain single dysplastic kidneys and the ureters may enter the urethra. In these circumstances the bladder is poorly developed and cystourethrography shows reflux (Figs. 7.9 and 7.10).

Ureters which drain outside the urinary tract *may* enter the vagina, the vas or seminal vesicle or rectum. These rare congenital anomalies are generally associated with very poorly functioning dysplastic or pyelonephritic kidneys. A DMSA scan can demonstrate such kidneys, perhaps more effectively than other modes of investigation.

7.2.2 Exstrophy and Epispadias

Exstrophy affects both males and females. The defect is typified by separation at the symphysis pubis, abnormalities of rectus muscle development and, of course, a failure of closure of the anterior wall of the bladder. Sometimes this anterior defect is covered by skin, but usually the bladder mucosa is exposed. Genital development in the male is defective.

IVU shows the kidneys and upper parts of the ureters are normal at the outset (Fig. 7.11). As time progresses and treatment initiated, pyelonephritic scarring or features of obstruction in the upper tract may develop. The course of the lower part of the ureters is abnormal – they sweep downwards to enter the bladder (after reconstruction) from the inferior aspect (Fig. 7.12). The uretero-vesical junction is

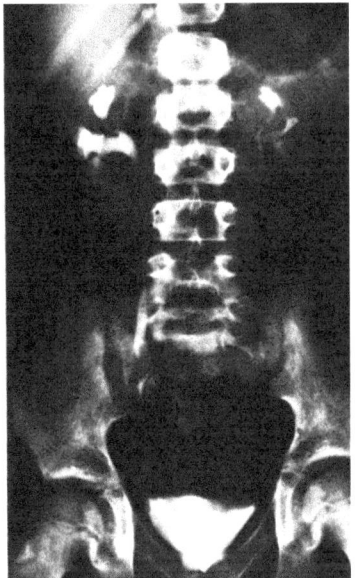
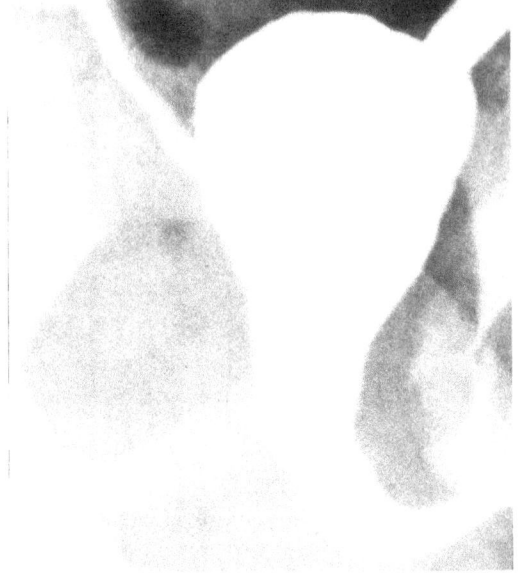

a, b

Fig. 7.9 a, b. Ectopic ureter. The IVU in this boy (**a**) shows the right kidney is well developed, but the left kidney is small. The ureters from the kidney drain into the proximal part of the urethra and so the bladder fills. MCU (**b**) shows the small bladder capacity and the bilateral ureteric reflux

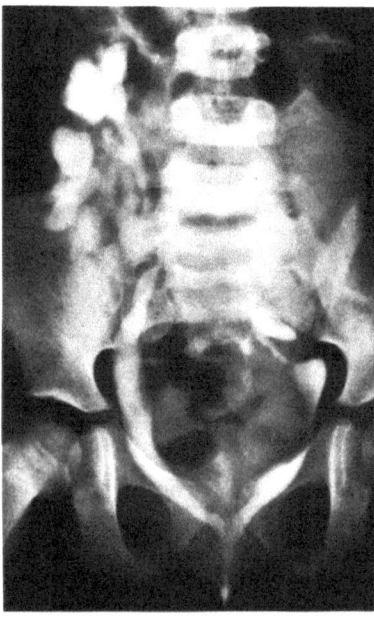
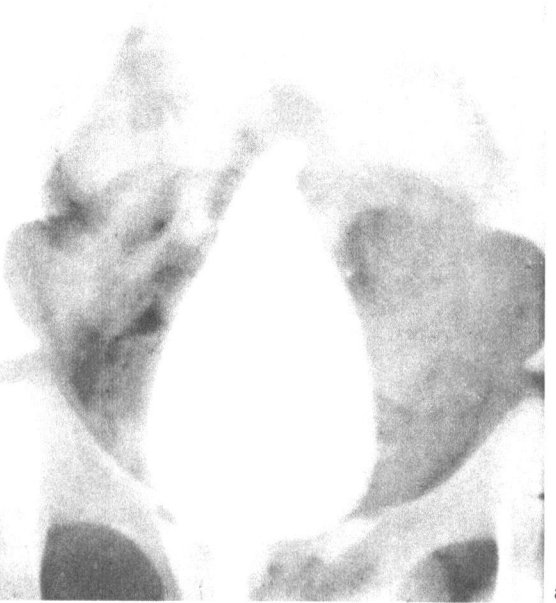

a, b

Fig. 7.10 a, b. Ectopic ureteral drainage. IVU (**a**) in girl with both ureters entering the distal part of the urethra. No vesical filling occurs. The right kidney lies low in position with clubbed calyces and an irregular contour. The left kidney is grossly abnormal and lies in front of the sacrum. Cystogram (**b**) carried out as part of an endoscopy shows how very small the bladder is

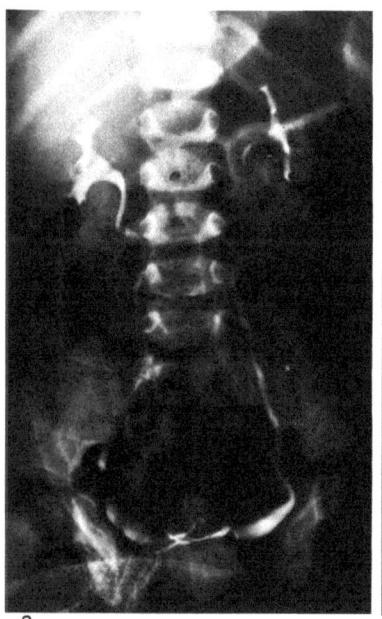
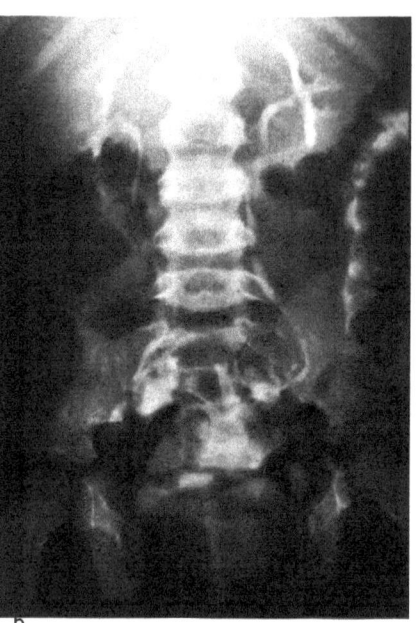
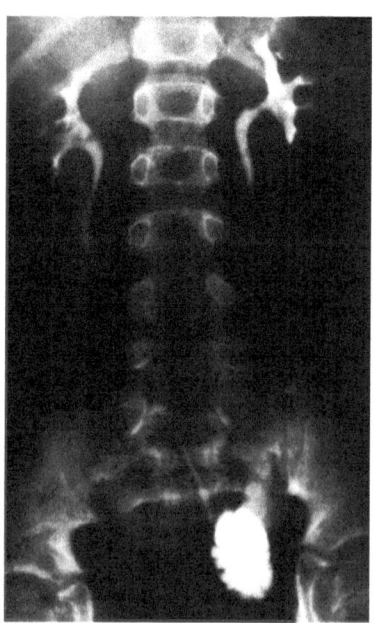

a   b   c

Fig. 7.11 a–c. Ectopia vesicae. **a** Male with ectopia vesicae. Both kidneys are normal at IVU and the ureters pass towards the ectopic bladder with its deficient anterior wall. The defect in the symphysis is clearly shown. **b** Diversion procedure to the sigmoid colon has been carried out. IVU shows the kidneys remain normal. Contrast medium enters the large intestine opacifying the descending colon, the sigmoid and rectum. **c** The boy now aged 9 years had the sigmoid diversion exteriorized to the skin surface. His IVU shows his kidneys are of normal structure and his ureters are undilated. Thus, he has avoided the possible complications of vesico-ureteric reflux and pyelonephritic scarring, obstruction and obstructive renal atrophy, calculus disease and pyonephrosis

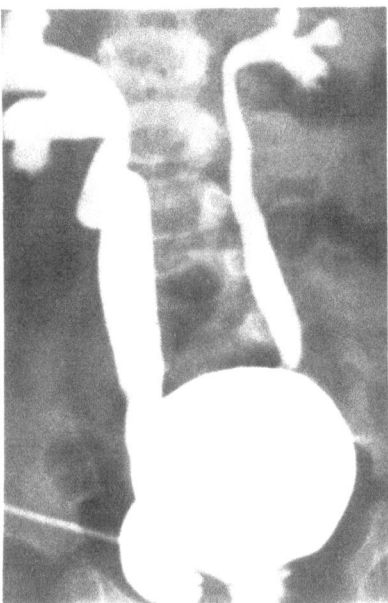

Fig. 7.12. Ectopia vesicae. MCU in girl who had the anterior vesical defect closed. The bladder contour is smooth but the capacity is small. There is no sphincteric control, so contrast medium and urine leak down the urethra. Bilateral reflux occurs because of the abnormality of insertion of the ureters into the base of the bladder. The information on this radiograph indicates serious potentialities for the future. Incontinence may be the most socially deleterious but reflux nephropathy and renal scarring and obstructive uropathy presage renal failure in later life unless these problems can be countered

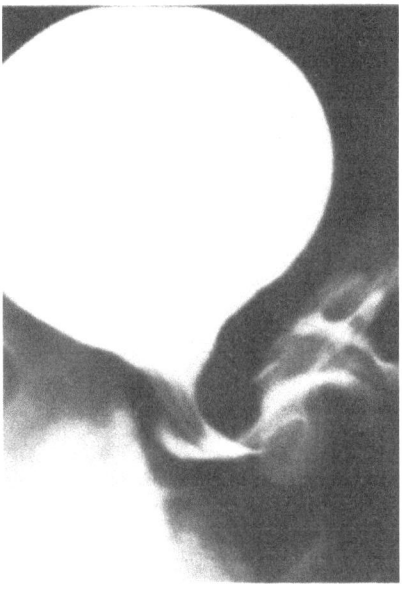

Fig. 7.13. Epispadias. Boy with incontinence. Sphincteric function is inadequate and the urine leaks from the meatus. Bladder capacity is not unduly small

prone to allow reflux which may be correctable [4]. Even after reconstruction the bladder capacity is small and the absence of adequate sphincteric development results in incontinence. A variety of operations can be carried out to improve continence, but these carry the risk of obstruction of the bladder and there may be also upper tract distension. The fact is exstrophy is an exceedingly difficult problem to treat whith corrective measures and many children have a urinary diversion ultimately [5]. If diversion to the sigmoid is contemplated, it may be wise to ensure that anal sphincteric control is adequate to prevent incontinence of urine; this can be done simply by injecting contrast medium into the rectum and seeing if there is leakage through the anal canal.

Epispadias is a less severe form of the combination of defects which constitute exstrophy. In epispadias bladder capacity is rather small, the uretero-vesical junction frequently permits reflux and inadequate sphincteric development tends to make the patient incontinent (Fig. 7.13). Reconstruction of the male urethral lumen along the shaft of the penis can be

carried out but as with exstrophy patients there is need to maintain continuing surveillance to ensure the upper tract is not damaged irrevocably.

7.2.3 Hypospadias

In this abnormality in boys the lumen of the urethra is defective along its ventral aspect. The principal problem requiring radiological study is the possibility of stricture which may sometimes develop after plastic surgical repair as well as being part of the basic lesion (Fig. 7.14). Upper tract problems, such as unilateral renal agenesis may occur.
"Female hypospadias" is an unrelated disorder in which the urethral meatus enters the anterior wall of the vagina. This developmental variant makes it impossible to catheterise the bladder without anaesthesia because the meatus cannot be seen.

7.2.4 Persistent Cloaca

This developmental failure is observed soon after delivery. In essence the intestine and urinary tract drain through a common orifice. Before undertaking any reconstruction or diversion, studies may show that the infant has a short alimentary tract which is incompatible with an independent existence. Variants of cloacal anomaly present with varying degrees of concatenation of urinary, genital and hindgut components in the cloacal problem (Fig. 7.15) overall.

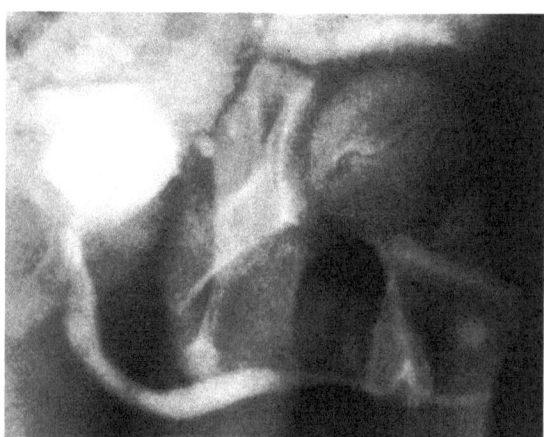

Fig. 7.14. Hypospadias. Boy with hypospadias shows on MCU a stenosis of the urethral meatus which is located on the ventral aspect of the penis. There is slight dilatation of the urethra proximally and some sacculation of the bladder whose emptying is partially obstructed

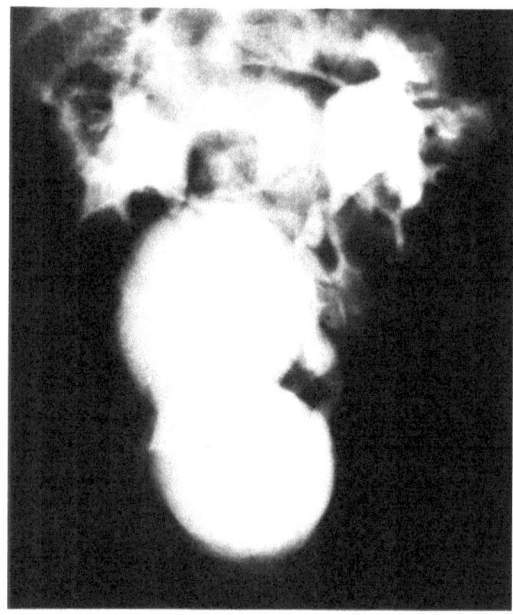

a, b

Fig. 7.15 a, b. Urogenital sinus anomaly. Female infant with imperforate anus. In the urogenital sinus, three orifices catheterised in sequence show double vagina (**a**) and small bladder without vesico-ureteric reflux (**b**)

7.2.5 Persistent Urachus and Urachal Cyst

As everyone minimally conversant with embryological development knows, there is in organogenesis a phase when there is a communication from the apex of the bladder through the umbilicus. Normally this lumen closes before birth. When the lumen is not occluded urine may pass from the bladder via the urethra and also via the patent urachus to the umbilicus. The lesion is sometimes a feature of lower urinary tract obstruction and the absent abdominal muscles syndrome. It may also be found in ventral abdominal wall defects (omphalocoele). Cystography with lateral projections can demonstrate this lesion. It is probable that examples of diverticulum formation at the apex of the bladder (Figs. 7.16 and

Fig. 7.16. Urachal diverticulum. In this post-angiocardiographic urogram, contrast medium cleared through the kidneys has shown the bladder lying inferiorly and above it a large urachal diverticulum. Angiocardiography entails clearance of exceptionally large amounts of contrast medium. Although the kidney calyces are well cupped, the renal pelves are dilated, as is the left ureter; these are features of the diuresis

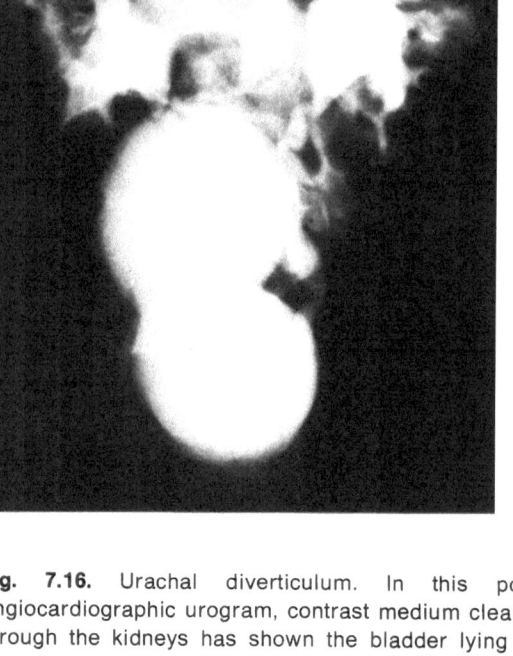

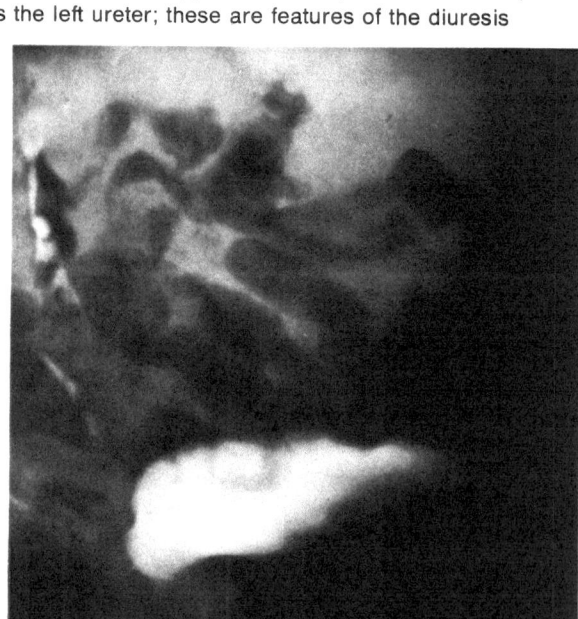

Fig. 7.17. Urachal remnant. Lateral projection at IVU showing the long forward extension of the bladder along the patent urachus

7.17) are really a persisting patency of the lower end of the urachal lumen with occlusion at the umbilical end. Sonography also shows a patent lumen to the umbilicus when the bladder is full.

Urachal cyst denotes an encapsulation of fluid within the urachus which is occluded immediately above the bladder and closed at the umbilicus. Again, sonography can demonstrate the cystic nature of this lesion which forms an anterior, midline abdominal swelling.

7.2.6 Duplication in the Bladder and Urethra

The bladder may be divided by a septum lying in the sagittal plane [6]. The septum may be incomplete, in which case the two parts of the bladder communicate. When septation is complete two separate urinary bladders lie side by side (Fig. 7.18). Such double bladders may each have a urethra providing for egress of urine.

Simple double urethra in a male can be diagnosed by inspection of the genital region. Each urethra has a separate origin in the bladder. One lumen may preferentially conduct urine to the exterior and sphincteric control of each is good. Incomplete double urethra [7] may be associated with stenosis in the male.

One variant of double urethra in the male leaves the narrower channel passing along via naturale, whilst the main conduit is by a channel passing to the anorectal margin [8].

7.2.7 Anorectal Anomaly and the Lower Urinary Tract

The first problem in all variants of this disorder in the male is to define whether a fistulous communication is present between the hindgut and the urinary tract. Air in the bladder is a decisive finding in the initial radiographic study. The fistula may be direct to the bladder (rare), to the prostatic urethra (common), or to the bulbous urethra (less common). MCU is one way of showing such a fistula, but distal loop study (after colostomy and with injection of water soluble contrast medium through the distal stoma) is possibly a more reliable but essentially complementary method (Fig. 7.19).

7.2.8 Vesical Diverticulum

Diverticulum of the bladder may be, in special circumstances, associated with ureteric or urethral obstruction (Chapter 3) or with uretero-vesical reflux (Chapter 4). Leaving these important types of

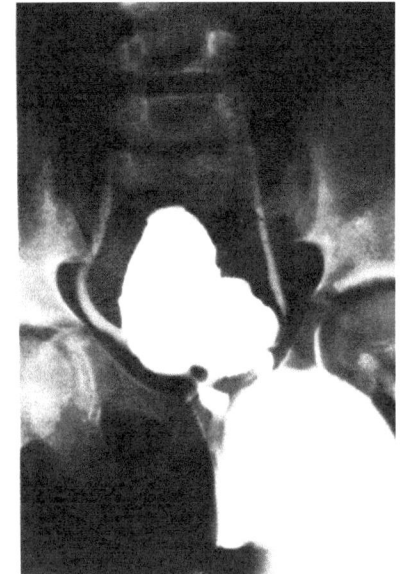

a

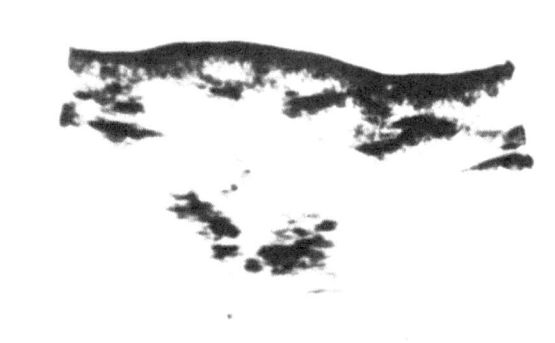

b

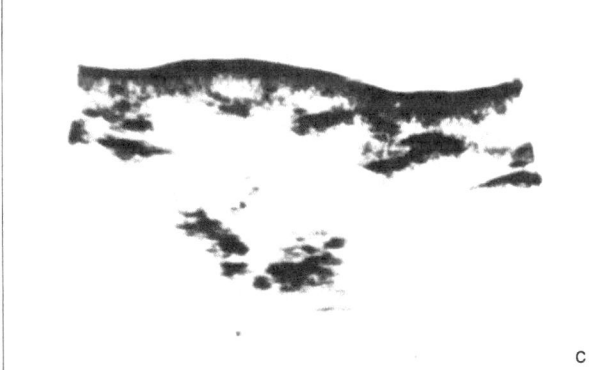

c

Fig. 7.18 a–c. Double bladder and double urethra. **a** At MCU the two bladders communicate, although they empty asynchronously. The left is less full than the right and the two urethras are shown. Bilateral vesico-ureteric reflux is present, with a small saccule visible on the lateral margin of the left bladder. **b** At ultrasound (different case), TS supine view of bladder shows a central filling defect resembling a papillary mass. **c** (Same case as in **b**) LS supine shows that the filling defect is a septum completely dividing the cystic space. The presence of a double bladder was confirmed by contrast radiology

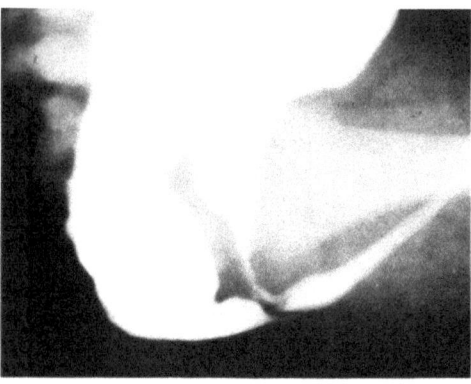

Fig. 7.19. Rectourethral fistula. Water-soluble contrast medium injected into the distal loop (via a colostomy) in an infant with ano-rectal anomaly. The rectum drains via a fistulous communication to the bulb of the urethra. Contrast medium in the urethra has passed distally down the urethra and retrogradely into the bladder. If the urethra is catheterised, the catheter may pass directly into the rectum. Such a fistula may enter the urethra more proximally, or the bladder. Note the associated sacral anomaly

diverticulum to one side, the main problem of vesical diverticulum is that when large it inevitably contains a sizeable urinary residue after micturition has ceased and the bladder has emptied [9]. Diverticula distend as the bladder contracts. Small diverticula may only be visible late in a voiding series. Occasionally a calculus forms in a diverticulum.

As small children cry curious alterations in vesical contour can occur – these may be localised and give the impression of bladder herniation, sometimes called "bladder ears". If the operator can con-

centrate on both looking at the image and listening to the sound it soon becomes clear what the nature of this feature really is.

Diverticula of the bladder are found in a number of rare syndromes [11, 12, 13].

7.3 Neoplastic Disease

7.3.1 Rhabdomyosarcoma

Embryonic sarcoma or rhabdomyosarcoma arises around the base of the bladder [14, 15]. There are two principal forms – the polypoid and solid types (Figs. 7.20, 7.21, 7.22). The prognosis in the polypoid variety which generally presents in the younger age group is much better for it tends to be localised to the bladder base, and the prostate in boys, and the vagina in girls. The solid variety of tumour is usually found in a rather older age group; this tumour has usually infiltrated the pelvic structures widely before diagnosis is made and treatment started. The prospect for complete surgical excision is thereby handicapped. Both lesions can be diagnosed in a presumptive way on IVU although accurate interpretation of biopsy material obtained by endoscopy is essential. It is quite unnecessary to carry out MCU. Echography can help in identifying the extent of the lesion; particularly in the solid variety of the tumour where this and CT scanning can be especially useful. The IVU in either type of lesion is characteristic. There is a tendency for the calyces and ureters to be rather distended proximally because the tumour

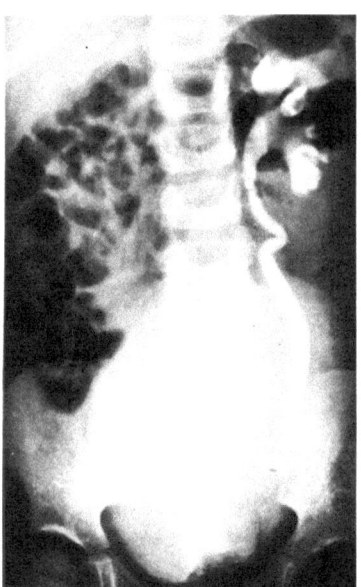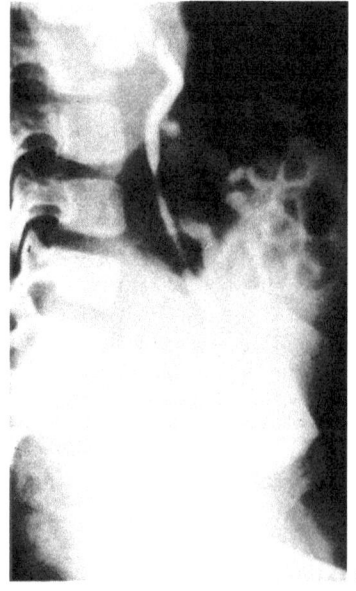

Fig. 7.20 a, b. Rhabdomyosarcoma. **a** Patient had retention and a palpable mass. IVU shows at $1\frac{1}{2}$ h the left kidney calyces are cupped but distended and the left ureter is slightly distended. The right kidney shows a faint nephrogram but no opacification of its collecting system. The bladder is large and faintly opacified with an indentation of its base on the left side. Note the urogram has features suggesting acute and recent obstruction – this is a common feature of rhabdomyosarcoma. **b** Lateral projection at IVU shows the large pelvic mass which elevated the base of the bladder and displaces the left ureter forward

Fig. 7.21 a, b. Rhabdomyosarcoma.
a This solid tumour extensively invades the pelvic tissue elevating the base of the bladder slightly but principally distorting the left side of the bladder and partially occluding the left ureteric orifice. Note the parenchyma of the left kidney is well preserved but the calyces are blunted and the ureter filled throughout its length. This upper tract appearance of recent partial obstruction is common in rhabdomyosarcoma. Occasionally ureteric occlusion is complete. **b** Following treatment which included radiotherapy, the obstruction has been relieved, but the left kidney is atrophic. Slip of the left capital epiphysis has developed

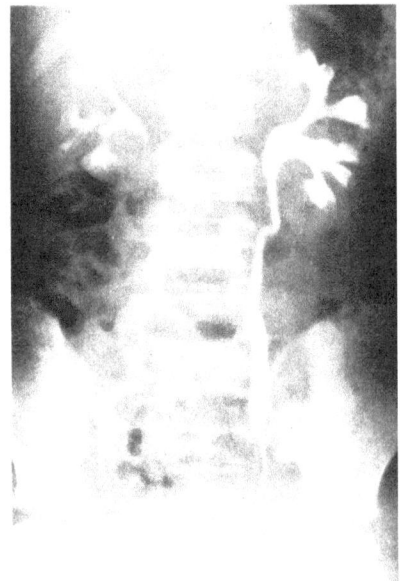 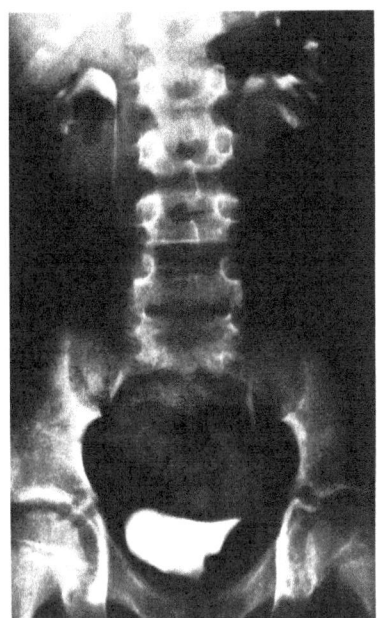

a, b

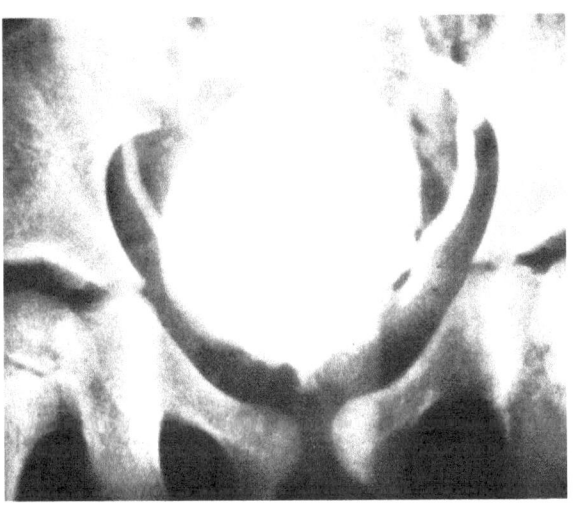

Fig. 7.22. Polypoid rhabdomyosarcoma. On this IVU the base of the bladder is elevated and its contour indented by many polypoid masses. These clearly involve the vicinity of the uretero-vesical junction on both sides

obstructs ureteric and bladder emptying. Complete obstruction of a ureter may occur.

The solid lesion results in marked elevation of the base of the bladder and there may also be displacement of the bladder cavity laterally when the tumour is especially massive. The contour of the bladder is smooth. In boys, in whom the urethra can be seen at voiding after IVU, the posterior urethra is elongated and narrowed.

In the polypoid variety of rhabdomyosarcoma the lesions indent the contour of the bladder lumen. The base is especially affected so that the lumen of the bladder is elevated. The lesion may partially obstruct the lower ends of the ureters and if it prolapses into and through the urethra the lesion may be visible externally in girls.

Symptoms which initiate investigation are straining, frequency, haematuria and pain. Urinary infection is quite a common complication. Findings at IVU explain why these symptoms occur.

The lesion extends directly into surrounding tissues, invades the lymphatics and distant metastases to bone and lung may also occur.

Although these lesions originating in the urogenital region carry the same name as lesions arising in the orbit, sinuses, thorax and abdomen it is doubtful just how much they all have in common with each other and with the like-named tumour of adult life.

Staging of these tumours involves both lymphangiography and ultrasound examination of the retroperitoneal lymph nodes. A chest X-ray is also essential. Bone deposits do occur and a radioisotope bone scan is a sensitive investigation of such deposits. CT scanning may yield much of this necessary information and is essential in complex problems arising during follow-up study (Fig. 7.23).

7.3.2 Other Malignant Lesions

Other types of malignant lesions are exceptionally rare. Transitional cell tumours do occur and phaeochromocytoma may be located in the bladder [16].

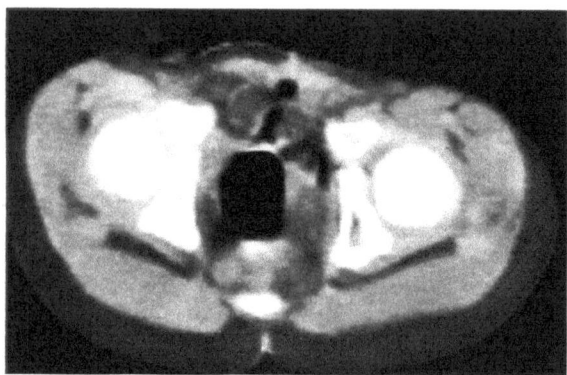

Fig. 7.23. Recurrent rhabdomyosarcoma. This 4-year-old girl had an anterior pelvic exenteration for rhabdomyosarcoma at age 1 year. A local recurrence was detected 3 years later and this was treated by chemotherapy and radiotherapy. CT scan shows a mass in the pelvis and the diagnosis on this examination alone was either necrotic tumour or abscess cavity. This observation underlines the need for correlation between clinical findings and findings from investigation

Commoner are the problems of leukaemia and its treatment. There may be direct leukaemic infiltration of the bladder wall [17]; colonization of the bladder by opportunistic infections, such as moniliasis, may produce cystitis and a small bladder. Cystitis due to cyclophosphamide has been reported [18] and it may be anticipated when the patient has received a dose of 6 g cyclophosphamide per square metre of body surface.

7.3.3 Non-Malignant Mass Lesions

7.3.3.1 Simple Polyps

Haematuria is usually the dominant feature but infection and reflux may also occur. The polyp may lie in the bladder, descend into the bladder neck at micturition or it may originate in the posterior urethra in boys [19, 20]. Such polyps may be very mobile because the stalk to which they are attached can be long (Fig. 7.24)

7.3.3.2 Angioma

The urinary tract may be affected by angiomatous malformations at any point and the bladder and urethra are no exception [21]. They may be part of a wider lesion affecting a child and evident on simple external inspection (Figs. 7.25 and 7.26).

7.3.3.3 Myomas

Myomas are rare. One characteristic of these and other non-malignant lesions is their tendency to present with haematuria (Fig. 7.27). They may be visible on a film with the bladder partially opacified with contrast medium. They may be best seen on a film taken after voiding at IVU; in children who have haematuria a post voiding radiograph is essential. Such intravesical lesions should be amenable to investigation and identification by sonography which will show their localised nature. Accurate interpretation of biopsy findings (or the specimen itself) is essential if mistakes are to be avoided,

a, b

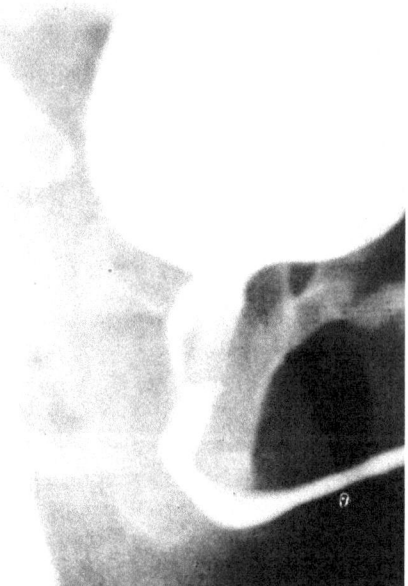
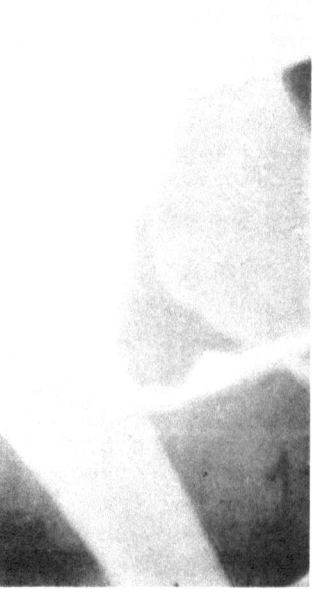

Fig. 7.24 a, b. Simple urethral polyp. Boy with haematuria who shows on this MCU a polyp arising from a stalk in the posterior urethra. The polyp is mobile, changing position as voiding proceeds

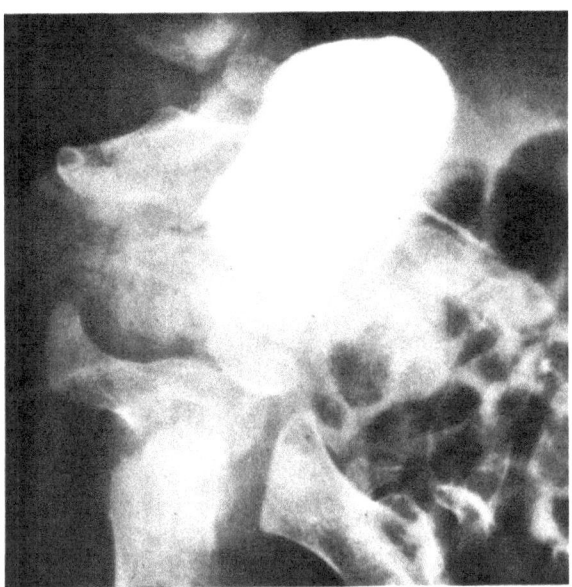

Fig. 7.25. Angioma. IVU in this 1-year-old girl shows the massive angioma of the left buttock and thigh extends into the pelvis to produce irregularity of the base of the bladder postero-laterally on the affected side

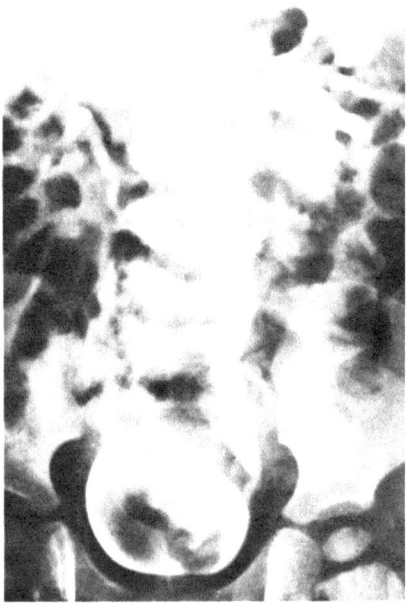

Fig. 7.27. Myoma of bladder. Boy, 1 year of age with haematuria and retention. The bladder contour is smooth and the base of the bladder is not elevated. Within the bladder lumen lies the myoma. The left kidney and ureter show features of partial obstruction and the right ureter is filled throughout its length with contrast medium on this IVU

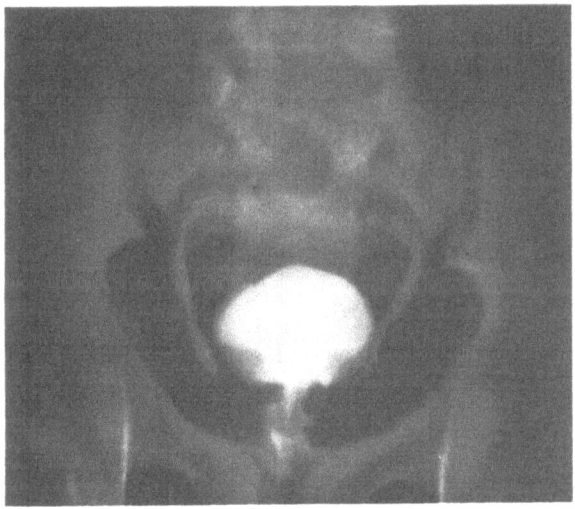

Fig. 7.26. Haemangioma of bladder. Female infant with haematuria. IVU showed a normal upper tract. The fundus of the bladder appears normal but irregularity and narrowing of the lower part of the bladder is produced by the haemangioma

7.4 Cystitis

7.4.1 Simple Cystitis

Sometimes children with *simple cystitis* due to *E. coli* infection are investigated by IVU during the acute phase of infection and when the bladder mucosa is seriously inflamed (Fig. 7.28). The bladder capacity is then small and the contour of the lumen indented by markedly thickened mucosal folds [24]. It is important, in these circumstances, not to rush to a precipitate diagnosis of a malignancy, such as polypoid rhabdomyosarcoma; the clinical context is decisive.

7.4.2 Cystitis Cystica

A condition in which the uro-epithelium develops first invagination and then cystic changes, as [25] the points of invagination become deeply isolated within the bladder mucosa, is known as cystitic cystica. Subsequently the intramural cysts enlarge (Fig. 7.29). This condition is associated with chronic infection. The bladder may be (but not always)

malignancy erroneously diagnosed and the wrong treatment instituted. Of course radiology cannot produce such certainty of diagnosis, but it can suggest in conjunction with echography that a lesion is circumscribed and that it has features which make malignancy an unlikely possibility.

uniformly affected and the underlying cause of protracted infection may be evident.

Opportunistic colonization of the lower urinary tract may occur when immune responses are compromised and antibiotic therapy has been instituted; *Monilia* is one such invader (Fig. 7.30), which may produce indentations of vesical contour due to

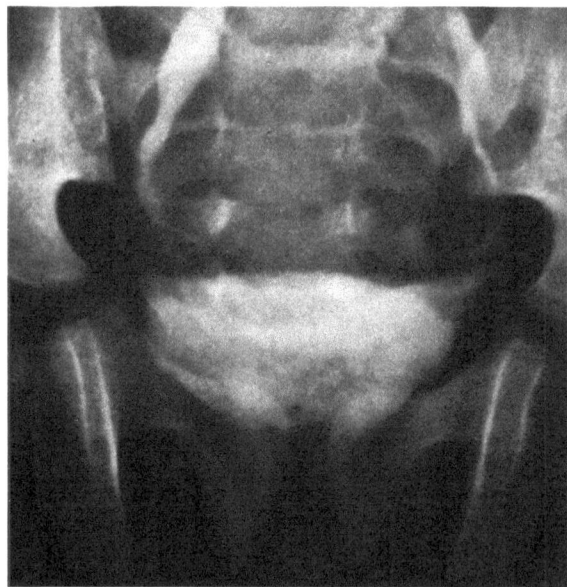

Fig. 7.28. Acute cystitis. Acute urinary tract infection with haematuria. At this IVU the bladder is of small capacity and thick mucosal folds are visible. MCU should not be and was not performed at this stage of management

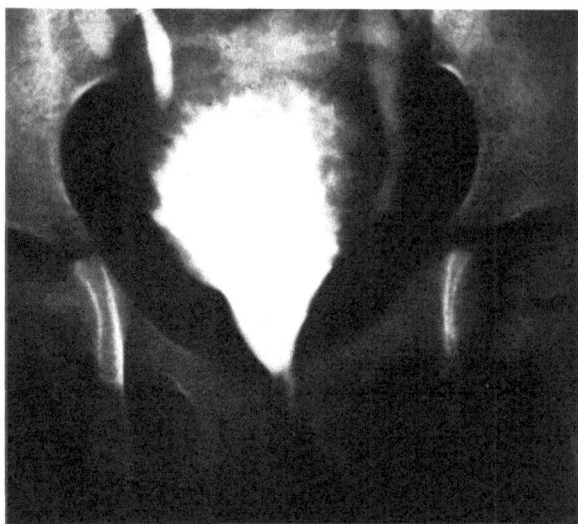

Fig. 7.30. Cystitis due to moniliasis in chronic granulomatous disease. In addition to general manifestations of the disease this boy had frequency and haematuria. The IVU shows a small bladder whose margin is grossly irregular in the vicinity of the fundus. Chronic granulomatous changes in the posterior abdominal wall had obstructed the left ureter and produced deviation of the course of the right ureter. In chronic granulomatous disease the underlying problem is that although polymorphs ingest bacteria they fail to kill them and so a continuing infective inflammatory response occurs. Protracted treatment with antibiotics provides the chance for opportunistic infecting organisms to colonize the urinary tract. Parallels can be found in patients with malignancy treated by chemotherapy, notably children with leukaemia, and sick neonates

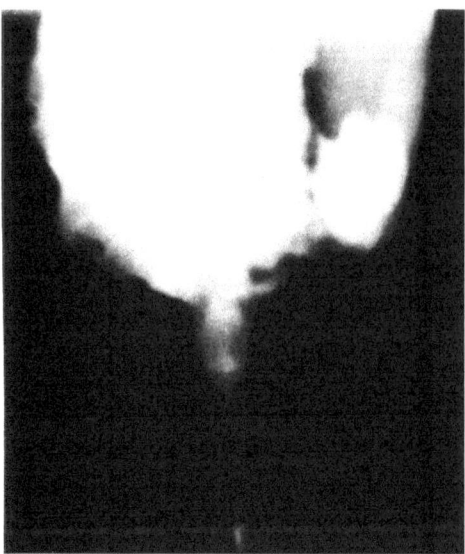

Fig. 7.29. Cystitis cystica. Girl with recurrent and persistent urinary infection. MCU shows the bladder margin indented by a multiplicity of cysts, which do not obstruct the urethra. There is, on the left, reflux into a ureter

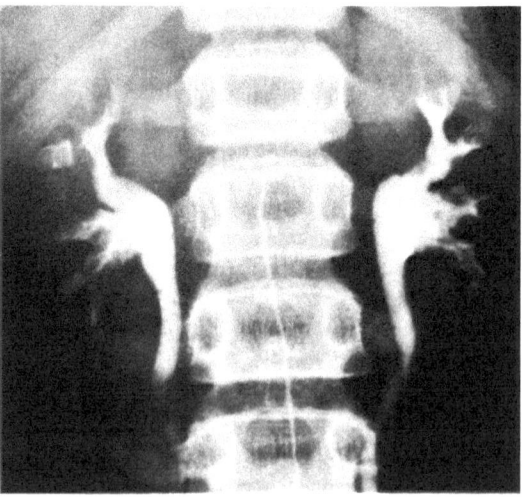

Fig. 7.31. Pyelitis and ureteritis cystica. Within the collecting system, renal pelvis and the ureter there is a multiplicity of small filling defects typical of the condition. Such appearances can be found in moniliasis, Henoch-Schönlein purpura and also ulcerative colitis, which this patient has. This cystic change is not necessarily a feature of urinary infection

clumps of the yeast. As with other benign lesions this condition must be differentiated from malignant polypoid rhabdomyosarcoma.

The entity of ureteritis and pyelitis cystica [26] (Fig. 7.31) is often linked to that of cystitis cystica, with protracted infection being the common factor. This is not always the case for appearances simulating ureteritis cystica and pyelitis cystica may be found in Henoch-Schönlein purpura [27] and in ulcerative colitis. Moniliasis in the upper tract may present rather similar appearances.

7.4.3 Tuberculous Cystitis

Fortunately tuberculous cystitis now is a rare condition. The chronic inflammatory change reduces the bladder capacity considerably so that increased frequency of micturition results. Abnormal and unusual calcification may be seen on the plain film. Fistulae can be demonstrated at MCU, when present, in tuberculous disease. The only other causes of acquired fistulae are Crohn's disease, malignancy and trauma.

7.4.4 Bilharzia

Lesions of the bladder wall in bilharzia reduce its capacity. Late in the disease process intramural calcification may develop. The disease may extend into the wall of the lower ends of the ureters and so produce obstruction to drainage from the upper tract. Calculus disease may be a further complication [28].

7.5 Neuropathic Bladder

7.5.1 Causes

Although spina bifida is a common cause of neuropathic bladder its incidence overall is declining. In preliminary radiographs at the start of an IVU it is important to inspect the spine carefully for clues of spinal dysraphism and sacral dysgenesis may be observed for the first time. Serious trauma to the spine may result in a neuropathic bladder as part of a wider neural deficit. Neuropathic bladder is a rare consequence of certain childhood viral diseases such as measles. Operations in the pelvic region (for Hirschsprung's disease and anorectal anomalies) can be complicated by widespread infection which leads to neuropathic bladder. In patients in whom

there are clinical features which suggest neuropathic bladder it is important always to look for a cause and sometimes this is not immediately self-evident.

One of the most devastating errors can arise if there is confusion in diagnosis between neuropathic bladder and vesical obstruction. Neither vesical shape nor the bladder neck region can in themselves differentiate the neuropathic from the obstructed bladder (Chapter 3) (Fig. 3.31). For example, to describe the bladder as having the shape of a pine cone is not useful because it does not further the diagnosis in the child.

7.5.2 Characteristics

(Figs. 7.32, 7.33, 7.34, 7.35). The functional problems of neuropathic bladder are inextricably linked to the physiological failures in the urethral sphincter [29]. The detrusor muscle of the bladder fails to contract and empty the vesical content and this results in a continuing vesical residue. Furthermore, there is a concomitant failure of sphincter inhibition adding to the vesical emptying problem: incontinence inevitably follows.

The neuropathic bladder may have a large, intermediate or small capacity. Typically there is thickening of the vesical wall and many saccules may develop. Much less commonly the bladder is grossly enlarged and its contour is remarkably smooth. The vesical capacity and the characteristics of the bladder wall can be examined by sonography and by contrast medium studies. As the bladder is filled with contrast medium the most proximal part of the urethra opacifies (an indication of the urethral sphincteric problem) and such opacification can be seen in IVU series and at cystography.

Ultrasound examination demonstrates the presence of diverticula and trabeculation and estimates of bladder wall thickness can be made although allowance has to be given for the degree of filling. Stretching of the bladder wall obviously thins this out and the difference in thickness when there has been partial evacuation can be striking.

Ultrasound is also very useful for estimating the residual volume without resorting to contrast medium studies, and has been used to assess the therapeutic effectiveness of drugs on bladder emptying in attempts to reduce the residual volume.

No normal act of micturition under voluntary control occurs. Usually as filling proceeds the bladder content leaks away through the urethra. Such leakage may be accentuated by coughing, straining or by suprapubic pressure. Manual expression of the bladder is one method of managing the problems of

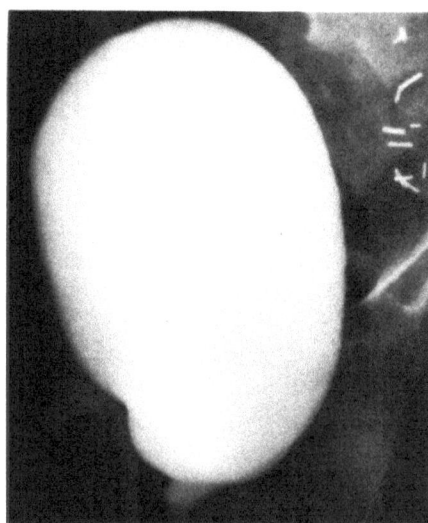

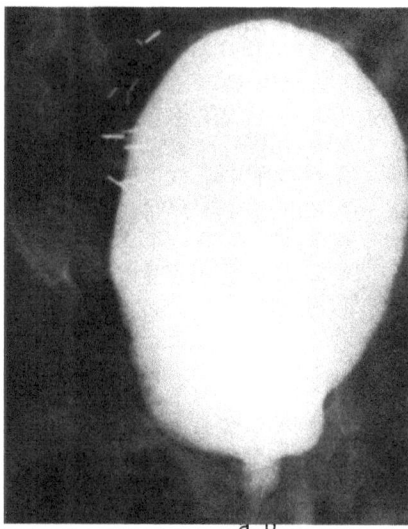

Fig. 7.32 a, b. Neuropathic bladder. Girl with spinal dysraphism (operated) with neuropathic bladder. The bladder has a large capacity and its contour is smooth. As vesical filling proceeds (**a**) the proximal part of the urethra fills, but no vesico-ureteric reflux occurs. Suddenly, after injection of 200 ml into the bladder an automatic contraction starts to empty the bladder (**b**). A large vesical residue remained unvoided, however

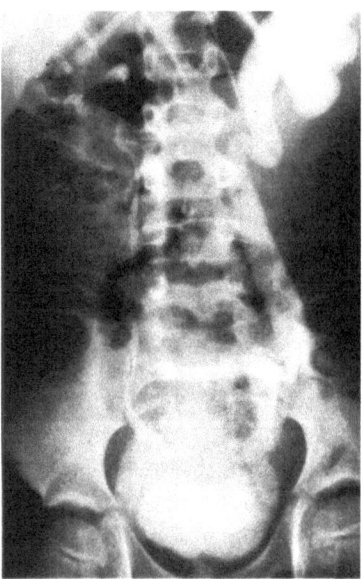

Fig. 7.33. Neuropathic bladder. Boy with sacral dysgenesis. IVU shows that no dilatation affects the right kidney, but the left kidney collecting system and ureter are dilated. Such a dilatation can be consequence of either obstruction at the uretero-vesical junction or vesico-ureteric reflux. The bladder is not large but has a grossly irregular margin because of a multiplicity of saccules

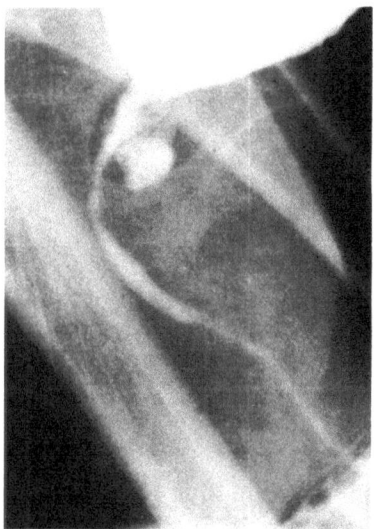

Fig. 7.34. Neuropathic bladder in a boy with sacral agnesis and incontinence. The bladder contour is smooth and the proximal part of the urethra open at all times. On straining, contrast medium is voided down the urethra but prostatic duct and seminal vesicle reflux occurs

patients with neuropathic bladder, but this technique never empties the bladder completely.

Complications of neuropathic bladder of great importance are related to problems which may arise in the upper tract. The predilection for urinary infection in neuropathic bladder is always present. The advent of vesico-ureteric reflux can be associated with the development of pyelonephritic scarring in the kidneys and a large undrained residue in the calyces, renal pelves and bladder. Obstruction at the uretero-vesical junction is associated with progressive dilatation in the upper tract and renal atrophy. Neither vesico-ureteric reflux nor uretero-vesical obstruction are necessarily related to saccules form-

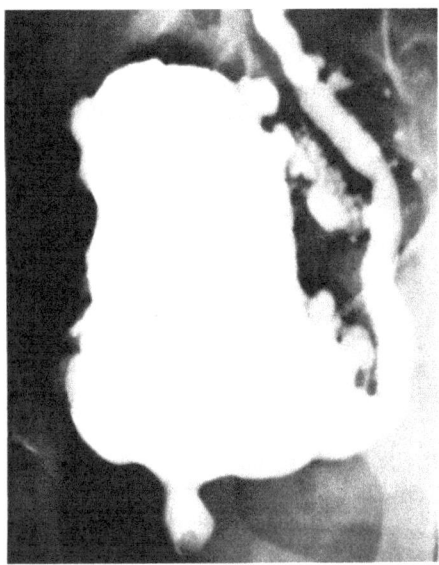

Fig. 7.35. Neuropathic bladder. Boy with spinal dysraphism. Contrast medium residues are seen in the subarachnoid space – a residue of former times. On MCU the proximal part of the urethra fills with contrast medium, the bladder is heavily sacculated and reflux into the left ureter occurs

ing in the bladder in the vicinity of the uretero-vesical junction. Sometimes individual saccules may be very large, amounting to diverticula. The

complications are the prime reasons for urinary diversion at an early stage for only by such diversion can renal function be preserved. Urine flow from the stoma of a diversion is easier to control in a socially acceptable way than urethral incontinence.

7.5.3 Cryptogenic Neuropathic Bladder (Fig. 7.36)

Almost invariably the cause of neuropathic bladder is identifiable. There is a tiny minority of patients in whom this is not so [30]. These children have all the functional and radiological features of the child with the classic neuropathic bladder. As with other children who have neuropathic bladder the urethra is often singularly insensitive at catheterization; this can be an important clue for it distinguishes the child with cryptogenic neuropathic bladder from the infant or child who has vesical obstruction. Finally, doubtful cases can be resolved by cystometrograms.

References

1. Stanton, S., Williams, D. I.: Wide bladder neck anomaly. Br. J. Urol. **45,** 60 (1973)

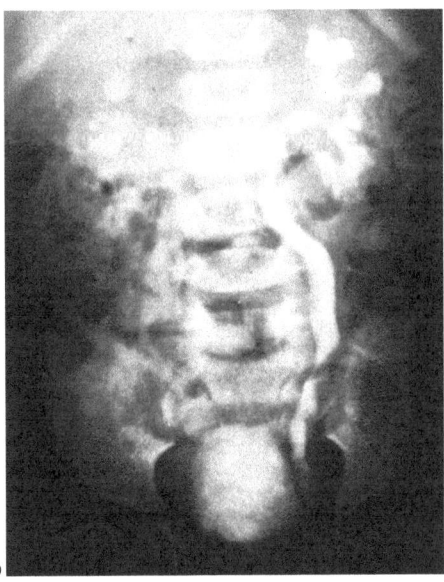
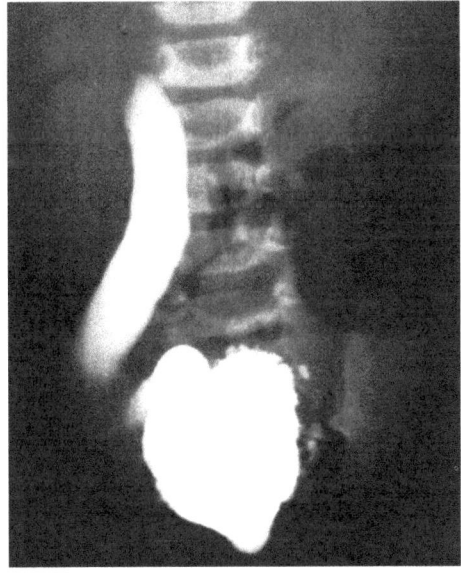

a, b

Fig. 7.36 a, b. Cryptogenic neuropathic bladder. **a** IVU shows the poor concentration in the collecting system of the right kidney and through the length of the dilated right ureter. The left kidney concentrates well, but its ureter and calyces are dilated. **b** At MCU the catheter was passed into the bladder without any sense of discomfort or perception of transit of the catheter into the bladder. Contrast medium injected has confirmed that the bladder is thick-walled, sacculated and not of large volume. There is no reflux into the left ureter, but reflux into the dilated right ureter occurs, where there is also a dilution effect; this indicates a combination of reflux and obstruction on the right side where function is clearly the poorer

2. Theander, G.: The prostate in pediatric radiology. In: Current diagnostic pediatrics. Vol. 1: Current concepts in pediatric radiology. Eklöf, O. (ed.), p. 106. Berlin, Heidelberg, New York: Springer 1977

3. Theander, G.: Relationship between urinary infection and orificial insufficiency of prostatic ducts in infancy and childhood. Pediatr. Radiol. 3, 158 (1975)

4. Williams, D. I., Keaton, J.: Vesical exstrophy – 20 years experience. Br. J. Surg. 60, 203 (1973)

5. Williams, D. I., Savage, J.: Reconstruction of bladder exstrophy. Br. J. Surg. 53, 168 (1966)

6. Wegenke, J. D. Congenital bladder duplication and diverticulum. J. Urol. 117, 800 (1977)

7. Moulsdale, J. E., Marshall, F. F.: Partial duplication of the male urethra. J. Urol. 118, 336 (1977)

8. Williams, D. I., Barratt, T. M., Eckstein, H. B., Kohlinsky, S. M., Newns, G. H., Polani, P. E., Singer, J. D.: Urology in childhood. In: Handbuch der Urologie. Andersson, L., Gittes, R. F., Goodwin, W. E., Lutzeyer, W., Zingg, E. (eds.), Vol. XV Suppl., p. 226. Berlin, Heidelberg, New York: Springer 1974

9. Boechat, M. I., Lebowitz, R. L.: Diverticula of the bladder in children. Pediatr. Radiol. 7, 22–28 (1978)

10. Bauer, S. B., Retik, A. B.: Bladder diverticula in infants and children. Urology 3, 712 (1974)

11. Goltz, R. W., Hult, A. M.: Generalized elastosis (cutis laxa) and Ehlers-Danlos syndrome (cutis hyperelastica). South. Med. J. 58, 848 (1965)

12. Babbitt, D. P., Dobbs, J., Good, T.: Multiple bladder diverticula in Williams elfin facies syndrome Pediatr. Radiol. 8, 29 (1979)

13. Harke, H. T., Capitano, M. A., Grover, W. D., Valdes-Dapena, M.: Bladder diverticula and Menkes' syndrome. Radiology 124, 459 (1976)

14. Ghazali, S.: Embryonic rhabdomyosarcoma of the urogenital tract. Br. J. Surg. 60, 124 (1973)

15. Eklöf. O., Brun, B., Claesson, I., Heikel, P.-E., Stake, G.: Tumours of the lower urinary tract in children. Acta Radiol. [Diagn.] (Stockh.) 19, 171 (1978)

16. Leestma, J. E., Price, E. B.: Paraganglioma of the urinary bladder. Cancer 28, 1063 (1971)

17. Troup, C. W., Thatcher, G., Hodgson, N. B.: Infiltrative lesion of the bladder presenting as gross hematuria in a child with leukemia. J. Urol. 107, 314 (1972)

18. Renart, W. A., Berdon, W. E., Baker, D. H.: Hemorrhagic cystitis and vesico-ureteral reflux secondary to cytotoxic therapy for childhood malignancies. Am. J. Roentgenol. 117, 664 (1973)

19. Downs, R. A.: Congenital polyps of the prostatic urethra. Br. J. Urol. 42, 76 (1970)

20. Williams, D. I. Abbassian, A.: Solitary pedunculated polyp of the posterior urethra in children. J. Urol. 96, 483 (1966)

21. Fuleihan, F. M., Cordonnier, J. J.: Haemangioma of the bladder; report of a case and review of literature. J. Urol. 102, 581 (1969)

22. Ganem, E. J., Ainsworth, L. B.: Benign neoplasms of the urinary bladder in children. J. Urol. 73, 1032 (1955)

23. Williams, D. I., Barratt, T. M., Eckstein, H. B., Kohlinsky, S. M., Newns, G. H., Polani, P. E., Singer, J. D.: Urology in childhood. In: Handbuch der Urologie. Andersson, L., Gittes, R. F., Goodwin, W. E., Lutzeyer, W., Zingg, E. (eds.), Vol. XV Suppl. pp. 314–316. Berlin, Heidelberg, New York: Springer 1974

24. Grunebaum, M., Varsano, I.: Multiple filling defects in children with cystitis. Pediatr. Radiol. 4, 93 (1976)

25. Harris, V. J., Javadpow, N., Fizzotti, G.: Cystitis cystica masquerading as a bladder tumor. Am. J. Roentgenol. 120, 410 (1974)

26. Kohler, R.: Pyeloureteritis cystica. Acta Radiol. [Diagn.] (Stockh.) 4, 123 (1966)

27. Thompson, J. S., Mc Alister, W. H.: Subepithelial hemorrhage in the renal pelvis and ureter simulating pyeloureteritis cystica Pediatr. Radiol. 3, 156 (1975)

28. Ibrahim, A.: Therelationship between urinary bilharziasis and urolithiasis in the Sudan. Br. J. Urol. 50, 294 (1978)

29. Eckstein, H. B.: Neuropathic bladder. In: Handbuch der Urologie. Vol. XV Suppl.: Urology in childhood. Andersson, L., Gittes, R. F., Goodwin, W. E., Lutzeyer, W., Zingg, E. (eds.), pp. 249–265. Berlin, Heidelberg, New York: Springer 1974

30. Allen, T. D.: The non-neurogenic neurogenic bladder. J. Urol. 117, 232 (1977)

31. Williams, D. I., Hirst, D., Doyle, D.: The occult neuropathic bladder. J. Pediatr. Surg. 9, 35 (1974)

8 Acute Kidney Lesions

8.1 Introduction

Like every other organ in the body the kidney has a blood supply which sutains the life of its cells. The structure of the kidney enables it to perform its cardinal role of excretion. When the blood supply to the kidney is reduced because of a reduction in blood flow and perfusion pressure, then function is compromised and the viabilitiy of the cells of the parenchyma endangered. Falling cardiac output and occlusion of the blood vessels of the kidney have, inevitably, serious and deleterious effects.

The parenchymal tissue can sustain, directly, cellular damage which may be manifest as nephritis or the nephrotic syndrome. It is no part of our purpose to present the latest classification of such disorders, but we do describe the role of imaging techniques to further diagnosis, especially by securing the appropriate tissue for biopsy.

Renal disease may be a part of wider symptom complexes, such as in systemic lupus erythematosus, malaria, familial Mediterranean fever, and thalassemia. Infection of the kidney leads to inflammatory changes and haematogenous bacterial pyelonephritis and acute bacterial pyelonephritis are discussed appropriately in this section: not all renal infection is a consequence of bacteria invading the kidney by way of vesico-ureteric reflux.

Finally, brief mention is made of a variety of noxious agents and trauma which may damage the kidney. The clinical background against which the kidney incurs this damage is usually clear.

8.2 Shock States and Kidney Damage

8.2.1 Antecedent Factors

A wide variety of clinical conditions can, in young infants and children, precipitate a shock state. These conditions range widely and include gastroenteritis and viral diseases, neonatal hepatitis, congenital heart disease, perinatal asphyxia or pneumonia, maternal diabetes leading to problems in the neonatal period (including hypoglycaemia) severe burns, accidental injury and excessive acetylsalycylic acid ingestion. Each of these clinical conditions can lead to a reduction in the cardiac output and oxygen consumption.

8.2.2 Vulnerability of the Kidney to the Shock State

A falling cardiac output, a reduced oxygen consumption, a diminished circulatory volume all make the kidney vulnerable to injury. In addition increased coagulability of the blood adds to the potential for kidney damage. These are features of the shock state.

Normally the kidney receives a very large fraction of the cardiac output. When this falls blood flow to the kidney falls; inferences from blood pressure measurements about cardiac output can be misleading because vasoconstriction may sustain blood pressure even when the circulatory blood volume has fallen sharply. In these circumstances it is not difficult to see how perfusion of the kidney by blood may fall and compromise the viability of the parenchymal cells of the kidney [1]. Increased blood coagulability may lead to vascular occlusion within the renal blood vessels, as well as in the liver and brain, among other organs [2]. Adrenal haemorrhage may also occur [3, 4].

The clinical context and the implications which the shock state may carry for the kidney of the infant (or much less commonly the child) can be detailed as follows: (i) tubular necrosis; (ii) medullary necrosis; (iii) renal vein thrombosis; (iv) cortical necrosis; and (v) the haemolytic uraemic syndrome.

These types of acute kidney damage may have a common aetiological pathway but they have differing clinical and radiological characteristics.

8.2.3 Tubular Necrosis

Clinically this is a quite uncommon condition in children and, as in adult patients, there is usually a period of several days anuria or oliguria [5]. In the young infant the oliguric or anuric phase is short, lasting only 2–3 days; this phase may lie within the acute phase of the precipitating illness and so the kidney damage may not be immediately apparent [5]. However, as in all cases of acute tubular necrosis, the kidney becomes unable to conserve water and electrolytes and this is a feature of the so-called diuretic phase of the illness.

In previous years, [6] IVU has shown that kidney after injection of contrast medium rapidly accumulates contrast medium within it (Figs. 8.1 and 8.2). This dense nephrogram develops very rapidly and is uniform throughout the rather large kidney contour. The dense nephrogram may persist for

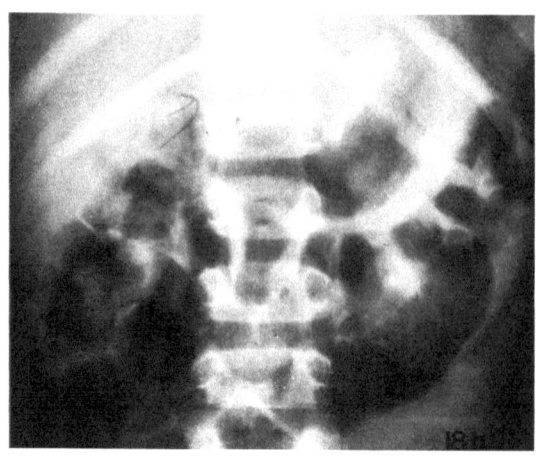

Fig. 8.2. Acute tubular necrosis. This 9-year-old child developed acute tubular necrosis during an infection, probably of viral origin, with symptoms relating to the respiratory and gastrointestinal tract. After a period of low urine output the IVU was carried out and this shows the protracted nature of the dense nephrogram in this radiograph taken at 18 h. Tubular necrosis appears to be a form of kidney damage in which functional recovery can be complete

many hours. It is extremely doubtful if such IVU study is now justifiable in the acute phase of illness. Ultrasonics examination will show that kidney parenchyma is present and that it is not the site of a lesion, such as obstruction, requiring surgical intervention. Renal function can be studied by isotope renography: the kidney may or may not accumulate the DTPA rapidly. However, Bank and co-workers [7] have shown that in tubular necrosis there is leakage from the nephron into the renal interstitial tissues. Such leakage can account for the findings after intravenous injection of agents which are cleared through the glomerulus and then unter the damaged tubule.

As clinical recovery proceeds a check-up IVU, an ultrasound study and a dynamic renogram all become normal.

8.2.4 Medullary Necrosis

Medullary necrosis is rarely a feature of thalassaemia in children [8] but commonly a consequence of the shock state in young infants. The tissue damage is confined to the medulla, especially its central zone where the blood supply is solely that of the long vasa recta.

As with tubular necrosis the first radiological identification of this entity came from IVU study [6, 9, 10]. In the acute phase of damage the medulla is heavily

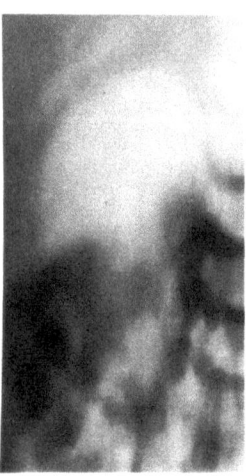

Fig. 8.1. Acute tubular necrosis. This 3-month-old infant developed acute tubular necrosis during an attack of gastroenteritis. Clinically, the renal enlargement needed to be differentiated from obstructive uropathy. IVU shows a very rapid onset (within minutes) of a bilateral very dense and persistent nephoram. The infant cleared dilute contrast medium and urine throughout the procedure. Nephrotomogram at 20 min

opacified by contrast medium very early in the study (Figs. 8.3 and 8.4) although, as with tubular necrosis, contrast medium is cleared through the kidney into the pelvicalyceal system. Again, as with tubular necrosis, it is doubtful if such IVU studies are appropriate with ultrasound examination being able to exclude a surgical cause for excessive water and electrolyte loss and the isotope renogram can assess kidney function.

Intravenous urography some 6 or more weeks after recovery from the acute episode will show the structural damage (of a permanent type) which the medulla has sustained. Total medullary necrosis, although it may not affect all pyramids, leads to

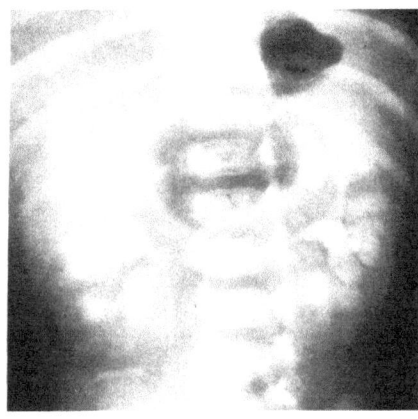

Fig. 8.4. Medullary necrosis − acute phase. This infant had a difficult anaesthetic for congenital pyloric stenosis. After recovery from the acute episode a renal problem became evident. The IVU shows dense medullary opacification indicating medullary necrosis, but there is also increase in density of the cortex adjacent to the corticomedullary junction, suggesting an element of cortical necrosis. Subsequently an IVU was carried out and it appeared normal. However, evaluation of the water and electrolyte losses suggested a continuing functional failure in the medulla

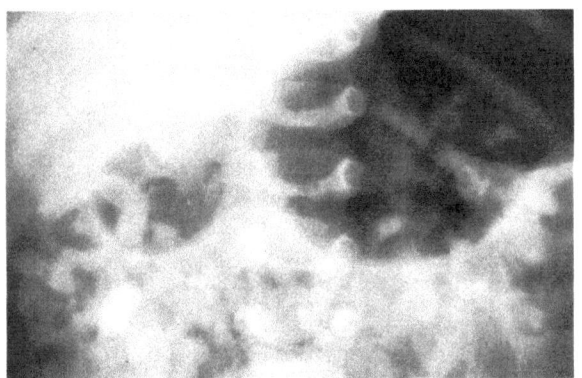

a

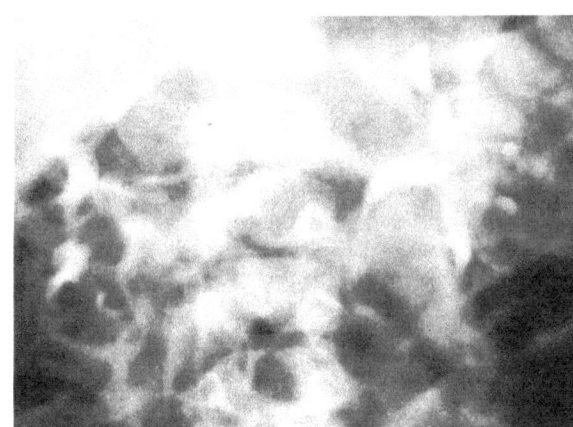

b

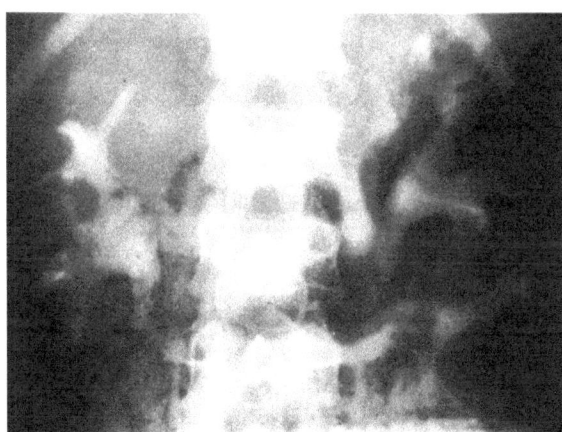

c

caliectasis; the urogram may then look rather like that of chronic pyelonephritic scarring [6, 11]. Partial medullary necrosis is characterised by pools of contrast medium lying within the medulla giving a typical "egg in cup" appearance in relationship to the adjacent and cupped minor calyx. The late

◁

Fig. 8.3 a–c. Medullary necrosis. **a** Acute phase. In this young infant who had severe gastroenterltls the fluid balance was exceptionally difficult to stabilise. The IVU shows an immediate and slight general increase in density of the kidneys, but the medullary zones are especially heavily opacified, indicating medullary necrosis. There was also an element of tubular necrosis in the cortical biopsy. **b** Late phase. After recovery from the acute episode, at this follow-up IVU carried out after an interval of a few months, the onset of the nephrogram was, in general terms, normal. Careful scrutiny shows that some calyces are now clubbed where the medullary damage and loss has been total. Where the medulla has been incompletely damaged there are pools of contrast medium in the tips of the papillae, which have normally cupped calyces adjacent to them. In other parts the medulla now appears completely undamaged and the normal minor calyx cup is retained. **c** Late follow-up. There is still a tendency to excess water and salt loss. This IVU at age 7 years shows the persisting damage to the medulla. The combination of calyx clubbing and adjacent parenchymal thinning might make differentiation from chronic pyelonephritic scarring difficult without knowledge of the preceding story

urogram may be normal, but careful assessment of these patients shows that as they grow older they may have a limited ability to conserve water and electrolytes and this may be as marked as in those who have abnormal urograms.

8.2.5 Renal Venous Thrombosis

A feature of the shock state is the increase in blood coagulability [2]. Renal venous thrombosis is presumably a consequence of this [13]. The extent of the venous occlusion is variable and thrombus may extend centripetally into the renal vein and vena cava. The affected kidney is large and haematuria occurs. If only one kidney is subject to venous thrombosis and the contralateral kidney escapes, urine continues to be cleared [14]. However, extensive bilateral renal venous thrombosis is associated with anuria. Quite surprisingly in some patients the kidney may recover with limited loss of parenchymal tissue. However, when the condition is severe and unilateral the kidney shrinks and atrophies as the undamaged kidney undergoes growth and compensatory hypertrophy.

During the acute phase of renal venous thrombosis the high solute load of an IVU is almost certainly unjustifiable and in the contemporary world studies such as IVU and retrograde examination (Fig. 8.5) which have yielded diagnostic information in times gone by are inappropriate. When recovery of kidney function does occur then an IVU at a later stage will show the extent of kidney parenchymal damage and survival (Fig. 8.6). In unilateral cases the non-

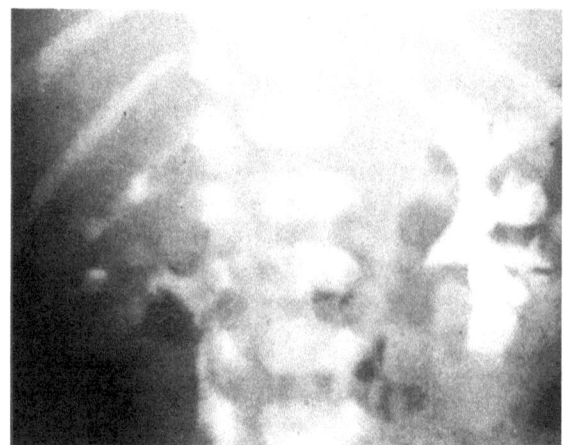

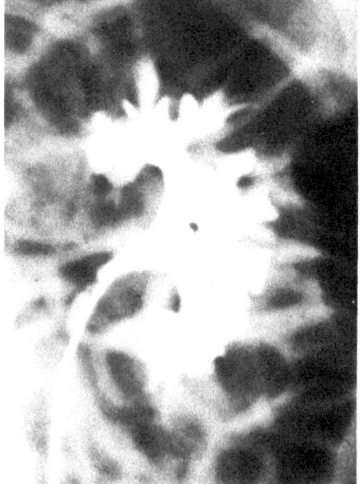

Fig. 8.5 a, b. Renal venous thrombosis – unilateral. **a** This neonate, the son of a diabetic mother, had a left loin mass with haematuria. IVU shows a normal right kidney but no function within the left kidney. **b** Retrograde studies in the acute phase showed the normality of the collecting system of the left kidney. This finding excluded other possible diagnoses, such as mesoblastic nephroma. The haematuria and mass lesion ameliorated quite quickly and no further investigations were performed during the acute stage. Subsequent IVU showed compensatory hypertrophy in the undamaged kidney and a small shrunken left kidney with clubbed calyces

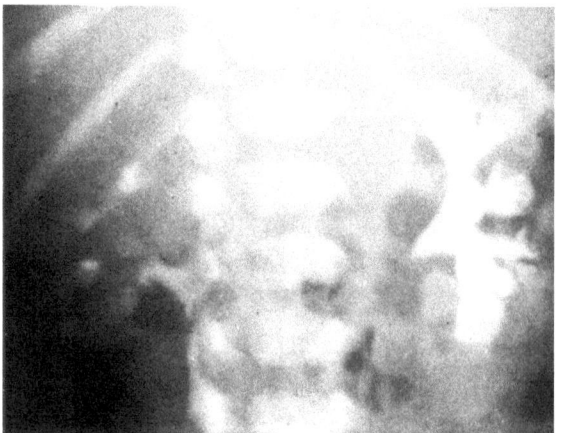

Fig. 8.6. Renal venous thrombosis – unilateral, in an infant. This IVU carried out 1 month after the acute episode of unilateral renal venous thrombosis shows the high speed of shrinkage of the kidney on the affected side and recovery of some function in the damaged kidney

surgical nature of the large kidney associated with haematuria in a young neonate can be identified by ultrasound and the status of the contralateral kidney defined. Dynamic isotope renography will show the function in the unaffected kidney.

Bilateral renal venous thrombosis can be inferred, against the appropriate clinical background, by ultrasound examination. Neither IVU nor renograms will make any further contribution excepting to show there is bilateral "non-function" or poor function (Fig. 8.7). Medical measures, including

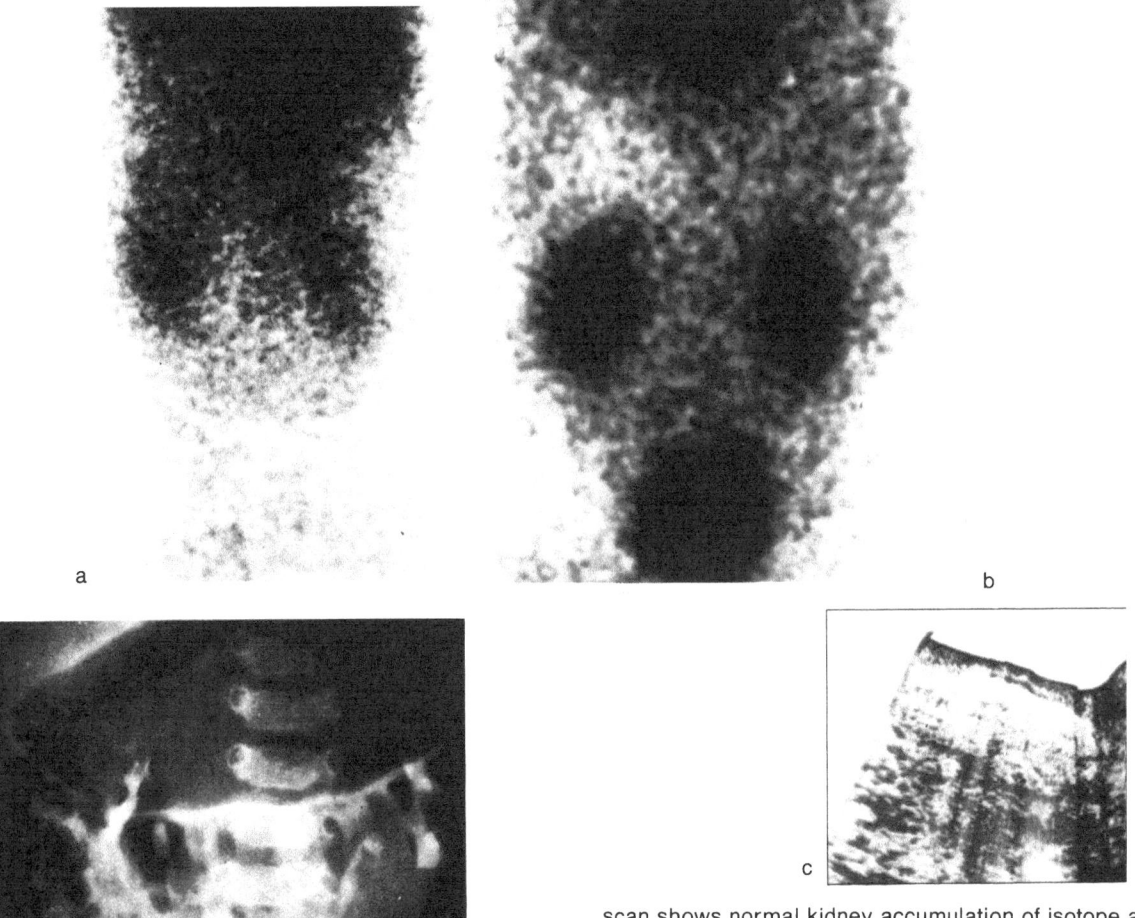

a

b

c

d

Fig. 8.7 a–d. a–c Bilateral renal venous thrombosis. **a** Acute phase. In the acute anuric phase associated with haematuria, this infant, who had been subject to a prolonged labour, had a DTPA scan. Seven minutes after the injection of isotope, exceptionally poor renal accumulation is seen in both kidney areas and none in the bladder. **b** Recovery phase. Five months later the DTPA scan shows normal kidney accumulation of isotope and normal clearance into the bladder 7 min after isotope injection. **c** This IVU, taken concomitantly with the second renogram shows normal function and structure in the kidneys. **d** Renal venous thrombosis in a neonate. LS prone. Initial echographic study of the left kidney shows a compressed central echo cluster and a non-echogenic parenchyma in the acute phase. At repeat study 1 week later the parenchyma was relatively more echogenic. The sequence of ultrasonic or isotope examination in the acute illness (followed by a check-up IVU later) is preferred to that shown in Figs. 8.5 and 8.6. The injection of contrast medium for IVU presents a large solute load to an already sick infant, and the contast medium may conceivably (but not certainly) exacerbate the renal parenchyma damage, be it due to tubular necrosis, medullary necrosis, or renal venous thrombosis

dialysis, can tide the infant with bilateral disease over the acute episode.

8.2.6 Haemolytic Uraemic Syndrome

The central feature of the haemolytic uraemic syndrome is a consumption coagulopathy [15]; this entails the deposition of fibrin and platelets in viscera such as the liver, kidney and brain. Where vascular occlusion occurs tissue damage inevitably ensues [16]. As the blood components needed to maintain haemostasis are lost from the circulation, the infant or young child develops a haemorrhagic diathesis, with intracranial bleeding, gastrointestinal bleeding (perhaps exacerbated by stress ulceration) and haematuria. Progressive kidney damage leads to oliguria and anuria. However, this syndrome has many shades of severity, [17, 18] with some patients being less seriously affected.

If IVU is carried out during the acute phase, the large damaged kidneys develop a faint and late nephrogram with virtually no contrast medium being identifiable in the collecting system or bladder. This is compatible with the widespread patchy renal parenchymal infarction found in the haemolytic uraemic syndrome.

Patients who recover from this form of acute renal failure tend to be hypertensive. A late IVU can then show the apparently normal renal contour with rather poor concentration of contrast medium (Fig. 8.8). However, as with tubular necrosis, medullary necrosis and renal venous thrombosis it is extremely doubtful if an IVU should be carried out until a recovery phase has clearly begun (*see* Chapter 2).

8.2.7 Cortical Necrosis

Of all the tpyes of kidney injury sustained by infants and children as a consequence of the shock state renal cortical necrosis [19, 20, 21] in isolation seems to be by far the least common. At autopsy it is a well recognised finding in conjunction with severe burns. A late sequel to cortical necrosis is calcification in the vicinity of the cortico-medullary junction (*see* Chapter 5).

8.3 Nephritis

8.3.1 Acute Nephritis and its Evolution

In children this lesion starts acutely and there may be frank haematuria; when this happens it is important to exclude a surgical cause, such as tumour. Usually acute nephritis abates within a few weeks at most, with regression of haematuria and excessive proteinuria and loss of oedema and fever, and a return to normal of the erythrocyte sedimentation rate. During the early acute phase there may be mild hypertension with slight cardiomegaly, mild pulmonary congestion and oedema, and small pleural effusions; these may be seen on the chest radiograph (Fig. 8.9), and these features disappear as recovery takes place. The non-surgical nature of the initial clinical problem can be identified by echography (Fig. 8.10).

In a minority of patients progress is not satisfactory; death and renal failure are fortunately rare, but the condition may enter a subacute or chronic phase. As

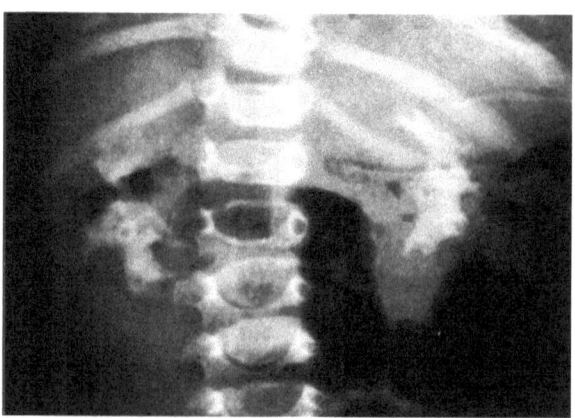

Fig. 8.8. An infant who had haemolytic uraemic syndrome and had hypertension as the prominent clinical finding. In the recovery phase, at IVU the kidneys are rather large but there is no apparent local structural defect with all calyces being comparable

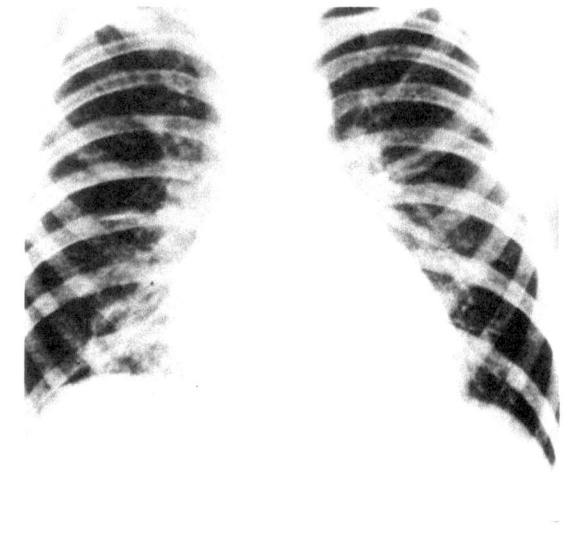

Fig. 8.9. Acute nephritis-chest radiograph. In the acute phase of illness in acute glomerulonephritis the heart is rather large, there are small pleural effusions and signs of mild pulmonary oedema. This chest radiograph distinguished the problem from that of other causes of haematuria of acute onset

the condition becomes more and more protracted the kidneys become smaller and function deteriorates. Chronic nephritis is a cause of symmetrical shrunken kidneys which function poorly at IVU as renal failure develops.

8.3.2 Nephrotic Syndrome

Within the orbit of this entity lie a multiplicity of kidney problems which have in common protracted

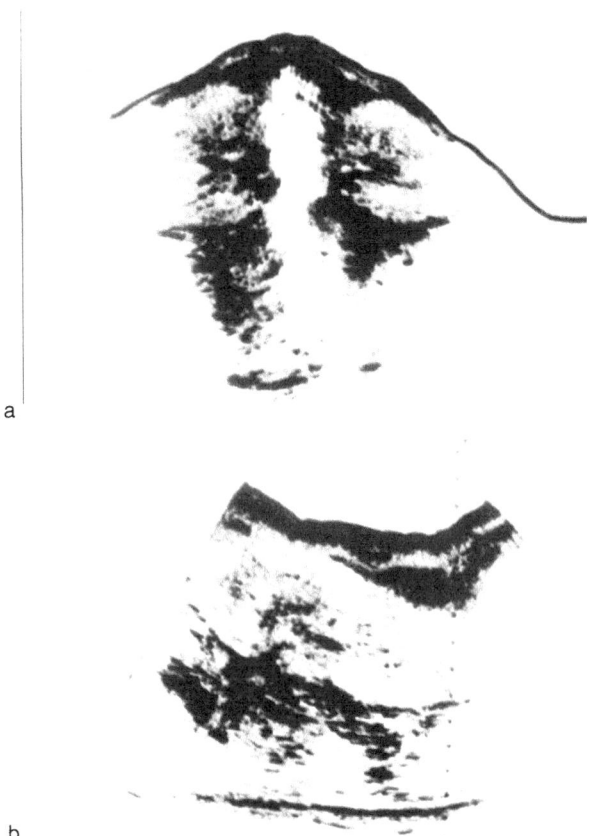

a

b

Fig. 8.10 a TS prone. Bilateral enlarged kidneys. **b** (Same case as in **a)** LS prone showing the enlarged left kidney with some suggestion of lobular architecture and a "squashed" collecting system. This suggests a diagnosis of nephritis or bilateral renal vein thrombosis. Final diagnosis: acute nephritis in a child

oedema and heavy proteinuria. The condition may sometimes be familial. If microscopic haematuria or hypertension are present some underlying form of nephritis may be present. Rarely, the nephrotic syndrome can be induced by toxic chemicals.

In patients with the nephrotic syndrome the kidneys are large and the pelvicalyceal system is normal. Intravenous urograms are carried out as a prelude to needle biopsy of the kidney; this procedure may be carried out either with radiological control using an image intensifier and an intravenous injection of contrast medium or by ultrasonics control. The objective of both techniques is to obtain precision in identifying the site of biopsy, thereby ensuring the biopsy material is adequate for diagnosis and there is no untoward damage to the kidney. Histological examination of the material is directed to defining the nature of the renal lesion and so influencing medical treatment, but also in anticipation of being able to give some indication of prognosis. A prime

concern in biopsy is to ascertain if any "nephritic" component is present in the kidney.

8.3.3 Renal Damage as Part of Generalised Disease

Renal lesions may occur in children who have such non-specific illnesses as juvenile lupoid hepatitis, systemic lupus erythematosis, Henoch-Schönlein purpura and polyarteritis nodosa. Henoch-Schönlein purpura, with a variant of nephritis, may run a protracted course. Polyarteritis nodosa is also characterised by renal arterial lesions which can be occlusive and aneurysmal (see Chapter 11) and lead to patchy renal infarction and to hypertension; a variant of nephritis can also occur as may spontaneous perinephric haematoma.

Generalised infection as in bacterial or subacute bacterial endocarditis can result in renal enlargement due to a focal glomerulonephritis. In children the cardiac lesion is clinically evident and the kidney problem identified because of microscopic haematuria. Rarely the nephritis can be severe but there can be frank haematuria in overwhelming infections such as meningococcal septicaemia. Infectious mononucleosis may be associated with bilateral renal enlargement as part of a wider problem.

8.3.4 Haematogenous Pyelonephritis and Acute Pyelonephritis [22, 23]

In young infants acute pyelonephritis sometimes seems to have its origin in blood-borne bacterial infection (usually *E. coli*) to the kidney. When this happens jaundice may be present as part of the septicaemia; infection in the urine may not be immediately detectable. Alternatively, there seems to be little doubt that acute pyelonephritis, due to *E. coli* urinary infection, can lead to bacteraemia and septicaemia. In all such very sick infants a surgically significant problem, such as obstructive uropathy, needs to be excluded.

When no such lesion is present the kidneys are enlarged at clinical examination. They may be very slow to clear contrast medium injected for the purpose of IVU. The absence of an obstructive lesion can be easily ascertained in such circumstances if an ultrasonics unit is readily accessible in the investigating department. The large kidneys without dilatation of their collecting systems may be surrounded by oedema of the posterior abdominal wall (Figs. 8.11, 8.12, 8.13 and 8.14).

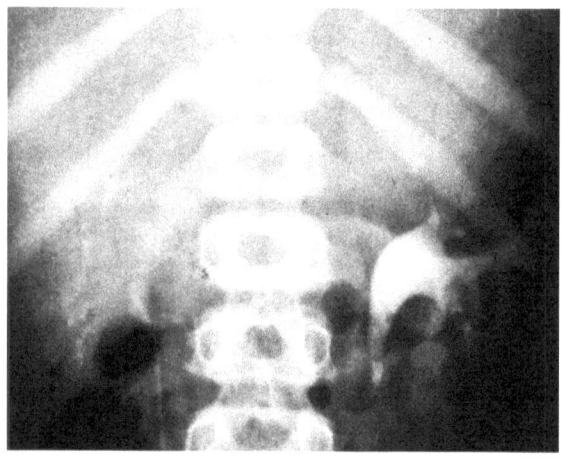
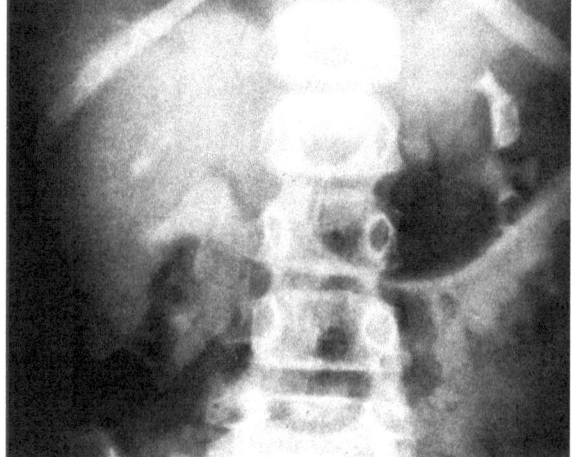
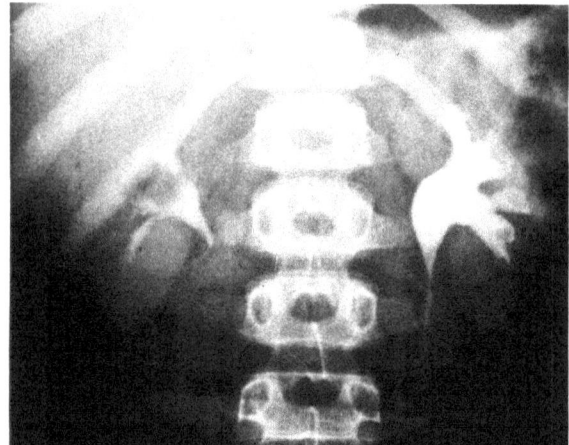
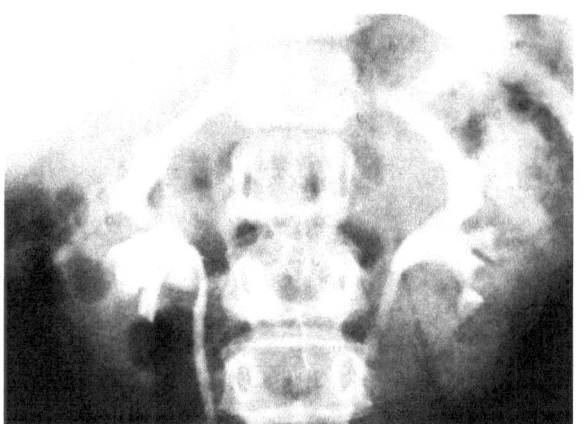

Fig. 8.11 a, b. Acute pyelonephritis. **a** Acute pyeloneph-ritis in a child with local symptome. The right kidney shows enlargement with compressed spidery calyces. The acute pyelonephritis was a concomitant of acute amoebiasis of the alimentary system. **b** IVU 6 months later, with the child now fit, the right kidney is normal. This child was treated with systemically effective chemotherapy. If scarring had been going to develop it should have done so between the two urographic examinations

Fig. 8.12 a, b. Acute pyelonephritis **a** IVU in a 6-year-old girl during an acute episode with *E. coli* in the urine. The right kidney is large and the calyces are compressed. Treatment with a urinary antispetic (not a systemically effective agent) was given. No vesico-ureteric reflux was present 3 weeks later. **b** Follow-up IVU 16 months later shows the right kidney is now small with calyx clubbing especially in the polar regions. Subsequent urograms, despite no further infections, showed almost complete growth failure for 6 years, whilst the left kidney underwent more compensatory hypertrophy

When the infection in the infant is controlled and measures to resuscitate the infant have proved effective the essential normality of the urinary tract can be confirmed by IVU and MCU.

In children acute pyelonephritis is associated with clear-cut evidence of urinary tract infection. Occasionally urograms may be carried out during the acute episode and before treatment has controlled the inflammatory lesion. Kidneys affected in this way show, on IVU, some enlargement with calyx compression – and so apparently poor function. The renal enlargement may be general or sometimes it is confined to only a part of the kidney. Not all such patients may have vesico-ureteric reflux at a subse-quent MCU. This feature does not, of course, preclude the possibility that the kidney became infected by reflux of organisms from the lower urinary tract before infection was controlled – reflux may disappear once infection is controlled. In acute pyelonephritis the lesion is partly within the nephron and partly interstitial; and so antibiotics and chemotherapeutic agents which are effective within tissues (as opposed to, for example, nitrofurantoin, which is solely a urinary antiseptic) can be expected to prevent renal damage such as chronic pyelonephritic scarring and growth failure. Clearly in such children with symptomatic urinary infection follow-up investigations such as were outlined in Chapter 4 are

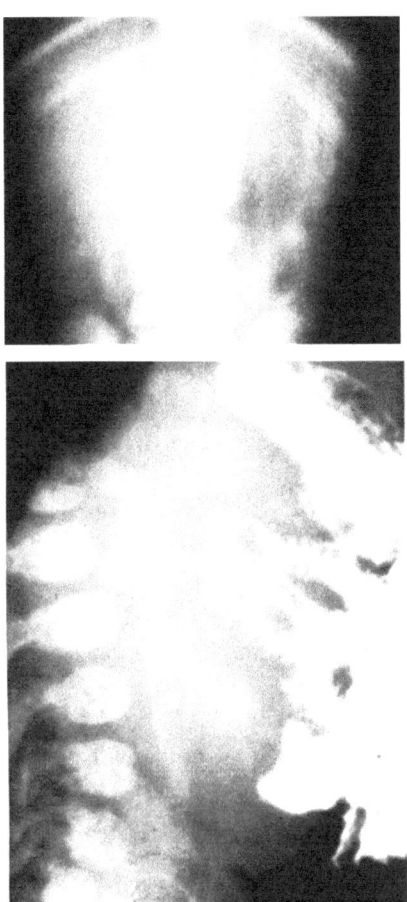
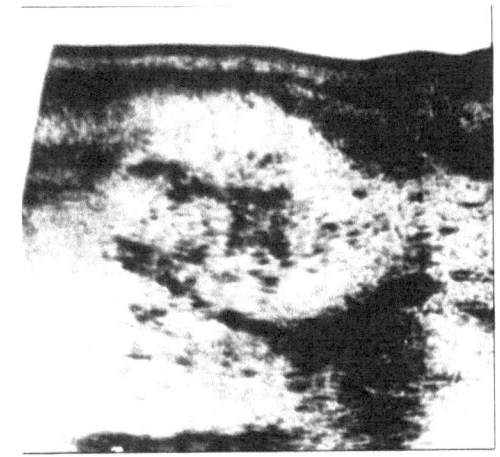
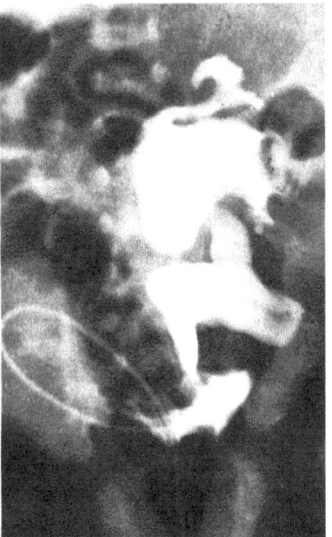
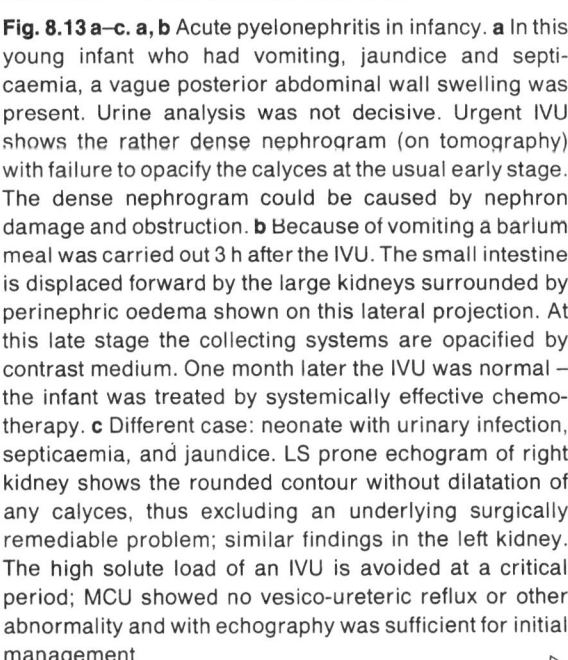
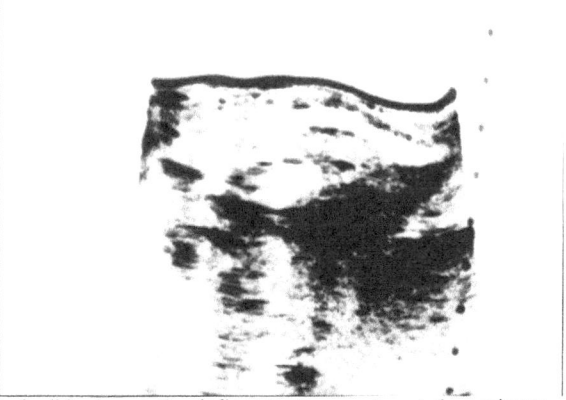

Fig. 8.13 a–c. a, b Acute pyelonephritis in infancy. a In this young infant who had vomiting, jaundice and septicaemia, a vague posterior abdominal wall swelling was present. Urine analysis was not decisive. Urgent IVU shows the rather dense nephrogram (on tomography) with failure to opacify the calyces at the usual early stage. The dense nephrogram could be caused by nephron damage and obstruction. b Because of vomiting a barium meal was carried out 3 h after the IVU. The small intestine is displaced forward by the large kidneys surrounded by perinephric oedema shown on this lateral projection. At this late stage the collecting systems are opacified by contrast medium. One month later the IVU was normal – the infant was treated by systemically effective chemotherapy. c Different case: neonate with urinary infection, septicaemia, and jaundice. LS prone echogram of right kidney shows the rounded contour without dilatation of any calyces, thus excluding an underlying surgically remediable problem; similar findings in the left kidney. The high solute load of an IVU is avoided at a critical period; MCU showed no vesico-ureteric reflux or other abnormality and with echography was sufficient for initial management   ▷

Fig. 8.14 a, b. Acute pyelonephritis with perinephric oedema. This young infant had severe primary reflux (a) and urinary infection with marked ureteric dilatation but normally cupped minor calyces. The initial ultrasonics study (b) shows the inflammatory perinephric oedema confirmed when nephrostomy was carried out to secure good urinary drainage.

A cardinal essential in all young patients who are severely ill with an acute kidney lesion is to separate those who need surgical intervention from those whose treatment is entirely medical: echography, isotope studies, IVU and MCU each has a role in this task essential. The isotope renogram may show protracted depression of function after acute infection even through no structural abnormality is apparent.

8.4 Miscellaneous Types of Kidney Damage

Infants and children subject to trauma (either accidental or non-accidental) may sustain kidney injury. In the overwhelming majority of patients an immediate ultrasonics study and intravenous urogram will determine the following facts: (i) the presence of one or two kidneys; (ii) the extent of the parenchymal damage in a functioning kidney; (iii) the likelihood of avulsion of the kidney from its pedicle in the event of a kidney being non-functioning – and hence the need for angiography and immediate exploration; and (iv) the presence of any additional injury especially to the liver. Late sequelae to parenchymal damage include a localized scar and post-traumatic cyst formation (Fig. 8.15). Systemic hypertension is also a late sequel. Of course kidneys in which there is pre-existing disease, such as hydronephrosis or tumour, are especially vulnerable to minor trauma because of the size of the underlying lesion within the kidney.

Ingestion of a variety of toxic chemicals and potentially toxic drugs (to which the young child may have access or which he may be deliberately given) may cause kidney damage; these chemicals include

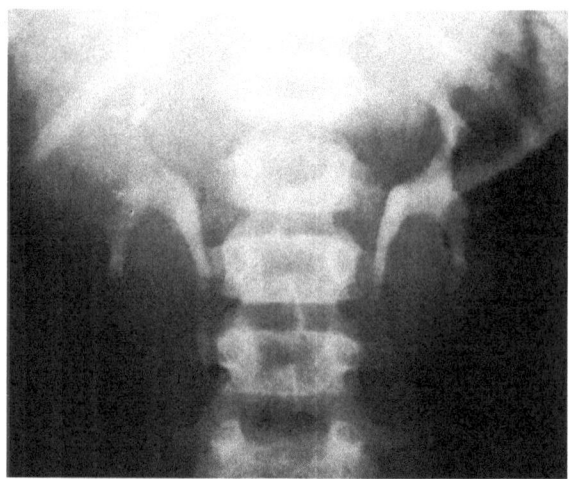

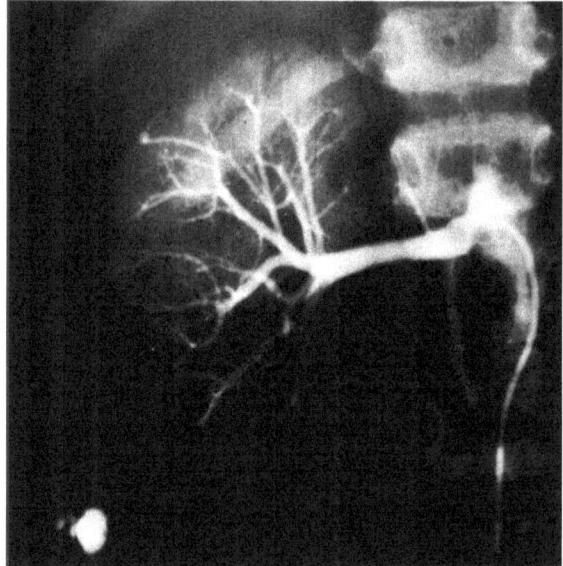

Fig. 8.16 a, b. Polyarteritis nodosa with renal involvement. At IVU (**a**) there are large, but structurally apparently normal kidneys in this child. Selective renal arteriogram, (**b**) shows the multiplicity of tiny aneurysms associated with the small intrarenal arteries. Renal biopsy confirmed the presence of the aneurysms and the nephritis in this boy who had microscopic haematuria, fever, anorexia and weight loss

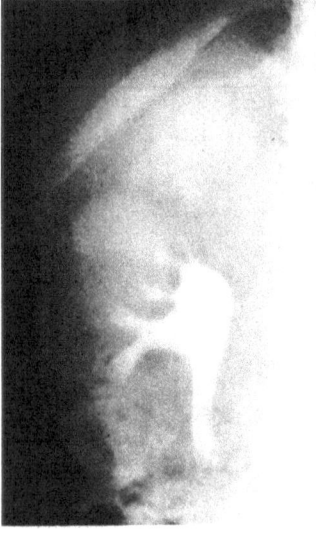

Fig. 8.15. Child investigated for blunt trauma to the loin. Follow-up IVU shows the localised indentation of kidney contour at the injury site with atrophy of the parenchyma associated with the amputated calyx. Hypertension may follow such injury

acetylsalycylic acid, sulphonamides, compounds containing mercury and the miscellany of chemicals around in the environment for agricultural and industrial use.

In the eighteenth century in his novel *Candide,* Voltaire's last advice, in this the best of all possible worlds, was to go and dig in the garden: in the twentieth century before digging in the garden it is also wise to ensure that household drugs are safely locked away, that the various chemicals you are about to use remain under your keen surveillance, and that the children are safely at play or in school.

References

1. Heene, D. L.: Microcirculation, haemostasis and shock, p. 103. Stuttgart: Schattauer 1970
2. Chadd, M. A., Elwood, P. C., Muxworthy, S. M.: Coagulation defectsin hypoxic full term neu born infants. Br. Med. J. *1971 IV* 51b
3. Eklöf, O., Grotte, G., Jonalf, H., Löhr, G., Ringertz, H.: Perinatal haemorrhage necrosis of the adrenal gland: a clinical and radiological evaluation of 24 consecutive cases. Pediatr. Radiol. **4,** 31 (1975)
4. Black, J., Williams, D. I.: Natural history of adrenal haemorrhage in the newborn. Arch. Dis. Child. **48,** 183 (1973)
5. Johnston, J. H.: Renal and adrenal vascular disorders. In: Paediatric urology. Williams, D. I. (ed.), p. 48. London: Butterworth 1968
6. Chrispin, A. R., Hull, D., Lillie, J. G., Risdon, R. A.: Renal tubular necrosis and papillary necrosis after gastroenteritis in infants. Br. Med. J. *1970 I,* 410
7. Bank, N., Mutz, B. F., Aynedijian, H. S.: The role of leakage of tubular fluid in anuria due to mercury poisoning. J. Clin. Invest **46,** 695 (1967)
8. Harris, V. J., Gooneratne, N. S., White, H.: Papillary necrosis in a child with homozygous sickle cell anemia. Radiology **121,** 156 (1976)
9. Mauer, S. M., Nogrady, M. B.: Renal papillary and cortical necrosis in a newborn infant. J. Pediatr. **74,** 750 (1969)
10. Kozlowski, K., Brown, R. W.: Renal medullary necrosis in infants and children. Pediatr. Radiol. **7,** 85 (1978)
11. Mellins, H. Z.: Chronic pyelonephritis and renal medullary necrosis. Semin. Roentgenol. **6,** 303 (1971)
12. Belman, A. B., Susmano, D. F., Burden, J. J., Kaplan, G. W.: Non-operative treatment of unilateral renal vein thrombosis in the newborn. J. Am. Med. Assoc **211,** 1165 (1970)
13. Seigal, A.: Renal vein thrombosis in a newborn. J. Urol. **118,** 464 (1977)
14. Chrispin, A. R.: Aspects of acute kidney injury in young infants. In: Current diagnostic pediatrics. Vol. 1: Current concepts in pediatric radiology. Eklöf, O. (ed.), p. 88. Berlin, Heidelberg, New York: Springer 1977
15. Avalos, J. S., Vitacco, M., Molinas, F., Penalver, J., Gianantonio, C.: Coagulation studies in the hemolytic-uremic syndrome. J. Pediatr. **76,** 538 (1970)
16. Habib, R., Mathieu, H., Royer, P.: Le syndrome hémolytique et urémique de l'enfant. Aspects cliniques et anatomiques dans 27 observations. Nephron 4, 139 (1967)
17. Sorrenti, L. Y., Lewy, P. R.: The hemolytic-uremic syndrome. Am. J. Dis. Child. **132,** 59 (1979)
18. Dolislager, D., Tune, B.: The hemolytic-uremic syndrome. Am. J. Dis. Child. **132,** 55 (1979)
19. Eskeland, G., Skogrand, A.: Bilateral cortical necrosis of the kidneys in infancy. Acta Paediatr. Scand. **48,** 278 (1959)
20. Leonides, J. C., Berdon, W. E., Gribetz, D.: Bilateral renal cortical necrosis in the newborn infant: roentgenographic diagnosis. J. Pediatr. **79,** 623 (1971)
21. Funston, M. R., Cremin, B. J., Tidbury, I. J. K.: Renal cortical necrosis in an infant. Br. J. Radiol. **49,** 94 (1976)
22. Lebowitz, R. L., Fellows, K. E., Colodney, A. H.: Renal parenchymal infection in children. Radiol. Clin. North Am. **15,** 37 (1977)
23. Sgura, J. W., Panayotis, P.: Localised renal parenchymal infection in children. J. Urol. **109,** 1029 (1970)

9 Renal, Abdominal and Pelvic Masses

9.1 Introduction

When investigating mass lesions palpable in the abdomen of an adult it is common to think of studies of the gastrointestinal tract as a first step. However, if in children a similar approach is adopted then very often no definitive diagnosis is likely to be reached. Although mass lesions do arise in the abdomen in children they are relatively uncommon; they can range from teratomas of the stomach to pancreatic pseudocysts through to Crohn's disease of the terminal ileum and so on. Much the commonest causes for a mass palpable in the abdomen of an infant or child are related to posterior abdominal wall structures generally and the kidneys and urinary tract in particular.

Traditionally in infancy and childhood, an IVU has been the first investigatory step when a mass is encountered in the abdomen or arising from the pelvis. This study gives information about the kidneys, the ureters and bladder and shows displacement of these structures.

Ultrasound examination reveals information which is very different with wider, albeit sometimes hazy, diagnostic horizons. Unlike an IVU or barium study which are constricted to a particular system ultrasound can visualize in the same investigation, the urogenital tract retroperitoneum, liver, spleen pancreas, biliary apparatus, major vessels, abnormal fluid collections and many other intra-abdominal details. With ultrasound one can determine whether a mass is present at all. Normal kidneys and palpable liver lobes are found with monotonous frequency. Having identified the anatomical origin of the mass it is not only possible to show whether this is likely to be a normal or abnormal structure but echography can suggest a narrowed differential (cyst, tumour, abscess, etc.) often either not available or not bettered by other diagnostic procedures. As if this is not enough it can sometimes go further and indicate involvement of other systems.

Today every child presenting with a mass lesion should be "insonated" before being irradiated.

Many children are likely to go into IVU because so many abnormalities originate in the kidney and urinary tract and the two examinations are complementary. Ultrasound will have its failures. But no other modality of investigation of disorders within the abdomen is non-invasive, immediately applicable and as decisive in as many areas of the body as is ultrasound. If it does not produce an answer one has at least not harmed the child in any way, or lost time. Angiography was in vogue some years ago, but its diagnostic yield and the extent to which it can influence management has proved circumscribed. CT scanning in children and infants is time consuming, but on occasion it can yield information which provides an important adjunct in certain circumstances. The way in which these various methods of examination are employed is indicated in the following sections. It is important not to subject infants and children to a series of examinations, some of which are unnecessary and may have an infinitesimally small influence on management.

9.2 Renal Neoplasms

9.2.1 Wilms' Tumour – Nephroblastoma

This rather common malignant tumour of childhood has characteristic histological appearances with cells which are foreign to the kidney (such as muscle) comprising the tumour tissue [1]. The tumour is almost invariably located in the kidney but rarely it is found in an extrarenal location.

The tumour is associated with a variety of malformations – some being intrarenal as with horseshoe kidney [2] and others being extrarenal such as aniridia and congenital hemihypertrophy [3, 4, 5]. There is sometimes a tendency for Wilms' tumour to occur in families, [6] but it is doubtful if it is worth extending investigation of siblings of an affected child by any method other than sonography. The first generation of survivors of Wilms' tumour are coming into their reproductive era and skilled counselling about genetic probabilities can be helpful to such ex-patients.

9.2.1.1 Clinical Presentation

[1] At the time of diagnosis abdominal distension and a palpable mass are very commonly present. Accidental trauma may sometimes be the reason for examining the abdomen. Haematuria can occur with quite small renal tumours and the most careful examination and investigation of any patient with haematuria is essential. Vomiting, anorexia, fever, weight loss and pallor are often present. Although young children may seem to have only a short history of being unwell they often look surprisingly ill and it may be that the lesion has been present for a long time. Systemic hypertension is probably commoner than has been recognised but it does not seem to present a threat to life in itself [7, 8].

9.2.1.2 The Renal Lesion

Findings at investigation depend on the way the tumour has grown [9]. Very frequently it originates deep in the kidney and produces a gross distortion of the renal parenchyma and of the calyx pattern at IVU (Fig. 9.1). The mass is often of very considerable size and it displaces the gut containing gas towards the other side of the abdomen. Calcification visible on radiographs can occur in the tumour, but calcium deposits are usually small and localized (Fig. 9.2). The mass may show no function at IVU or there may be a long delay before any calyces opacify. Sometimes when the lesion originates from a pole of the kidney it may then grow and leave the remainder of the intrinsic kidney structure less affected, although perhaps displaced and rotated (Fig. 9.3). Sonography can define the renal origin of the lesion [10]. The tumour has a complex echo pattern on sonograms, but the role of the ultrasonics is much greater than study of the tumour itself, (Fig. 9.4). At IVU there is usually little doubt about the renal

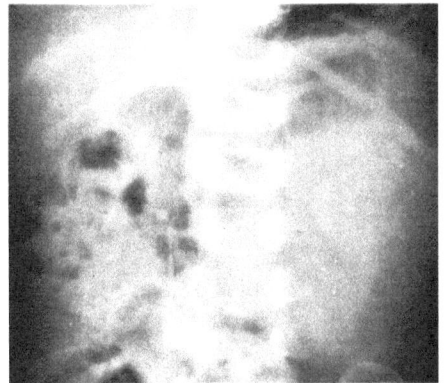

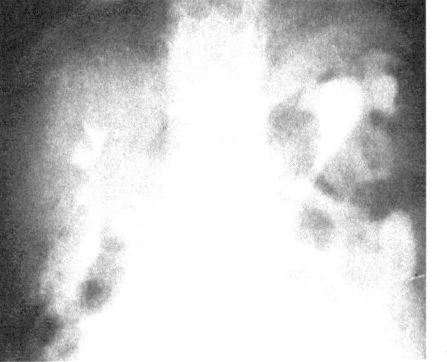

Fig. 9.1 a, b. Wilms' tumour. **a** The mass in the left flank was not functioning initially at IVU and the right kidney image is heavily obscured by superimposed gut shadows. **b** Later on at IVU the tumour mass on the left is seen to function and this renal window view shows the normality of the right kidney

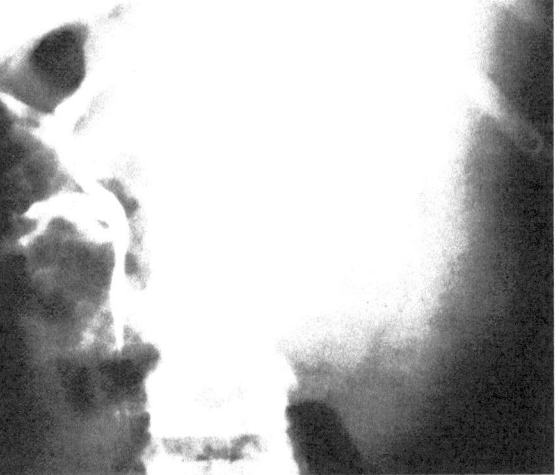

Fig. 9.2. Wilms' tumour. The huge left renal mass is nonfunctioning at IVU and there is a little calcium visible laterally in the tumour in the vicinity of the eleventh rib shadow

origin of the tumour (Fig. 9.5) and lateral radiographs can generally help resolve any uncertainties which may remain. When the tumour is posterior the

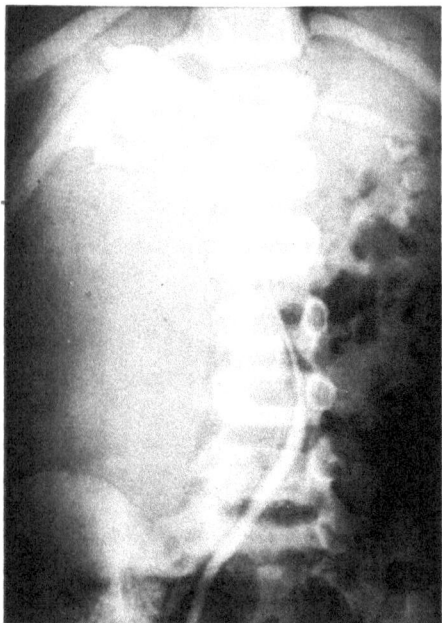

Fig. 9.3. Wilms' tumour. The large right renal mass arises in the lower pole and displaces the functioning renal tissue upward and partially obstructs its drainage into the displaced ureter. The left kidney's position is undisturbed

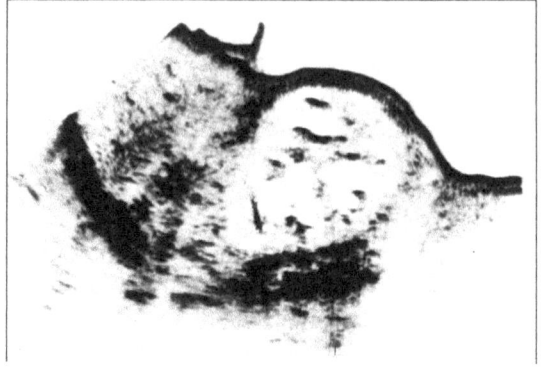

a

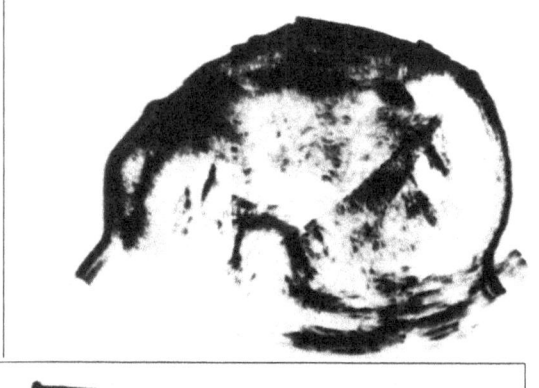

b

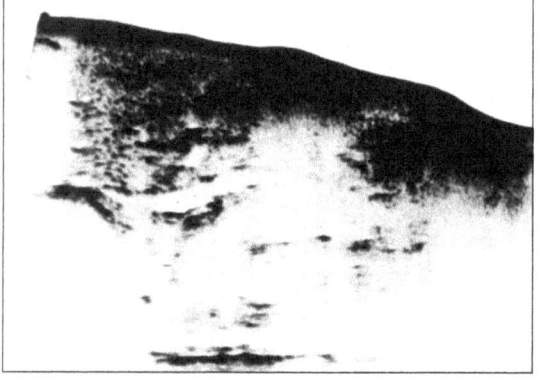

c

Fig. 9.4 a–c. Wilms' tumour. **a** LS supine, left flank. The left kidney is massively enlarged, moderately hydronephrotic and displaced inferiorly by a medially placed tumour, part of which separates the kidney from the spleen. **b** TS supine shows the enlarged kidney laterally with an even larger mass which crosses the midline and even displaces the right kidney, which is otherwise normal. **c** LS showing the inferior vena cava encased and elevated by tumour but not invaded

opacified calyces are displaced forward at IVU, but a tumour originating anteriorly may sometimes produce little sign of calyx distortion (Fig. 9.6). Wilms' tumour may arise in a horseshoe kidney and the precise extent of the tumour must be delineated (Figs. 9.7 and 9.8). The tumour frequently extends into or compresses the renal pelvis and the tumour may occasionally extend down a ureter (Fig. 9. 9). Occasionally, it is not easy to be certain that a kidney with Wilms' tumour is so affected by the lesion on IVU, in which circumstance the echographic findings can be decisive (Fig. 9. 10).

Since the vast majority of patients with Wilms' tumour have a surgical resection of the tumour the contralateral kidney must be studied with care. Wilms' tumour may affect both kidneys [11, 12, 13] and this may be evident at the initial studies.

9.2.1.3 Extension and Dissemination

Posterior abdominal wall structures are often displaced by a large Wilms' tumour. The displaced inferior vena cava (IVC) may be shown radiologically by injection into a foot vein and cavography. Ultrasound examination (Fig. 9.4) and isotope cavograms also give a good demonstration of displacement of the cava. If an injection of 99 m-Tc macroaggregated albumin or microspheres is used for this study the following information will be gained: displacement of the IVC; abnormality of flow in the IVC which could be due to either compression or invasion; an isotope lung scan will be obtained (? tumour emboli); and, colloid may "stick" to the surface of any tumour in the IVC and right atrium and hence the static study may indicate the cause of any abnormal flow pattern seen in the IVC.

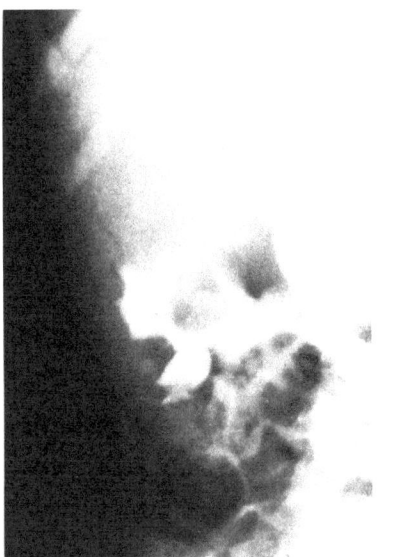

Fig. 9.5. Wilms' tumour. The IVU shows that the right kidney has retained many of its calyces which are displaced downward by the upper pole lesion. At IVU the functioning tissue merges imperceptibly into the tumour, thus excluding an extrarenal lesion

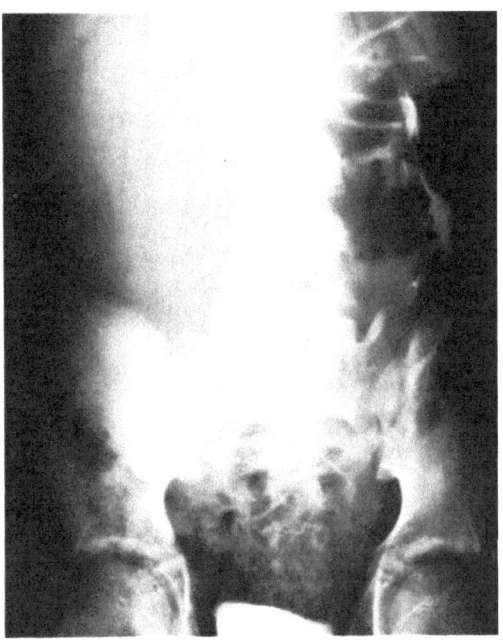

Fig. 9.7. Wilms' tumour in horseshoe kidney. The large right-sided mass, detected 4 days previously, is non-functioning at IVU, but the left component of the kidney functions well. Note the left kidney component is closely apposed to the spine and retains the typical characteristics thereby excluding the diagnosis of neuroblastoma. Angiography confirmed the lesion was confined to the right component

When the tumour is localized to one kidney it usually does not extend across the midline in such a way as to displace the kidney on the other side. This can be important in distinguishing Wilms' tumour from a posterior abdominal wall neuroblastoma at IVU. Ultrasound studies can also be very helpful in distinguishing between these two lesions.

The tumour may extend locally beyond the confines of the capsule and into adjacent viscera; this feature can be detected by ultrasound study as will tumour extending into the renal pelvis and down the ureter [14].

In the ultrasound examination one of the most important objectives for study is the renal vein and the inferior vena cava. The cava is often displaced (Fig. 9.2) but sometimes the tumour grows along the

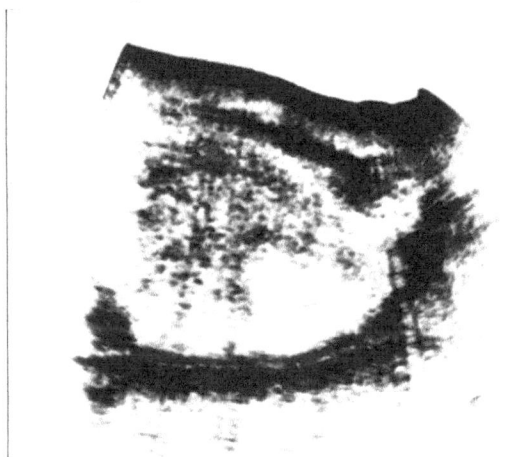

a

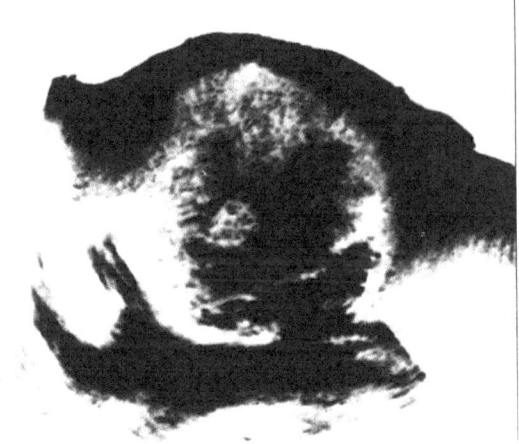

b

◁

Fig. 9.6 a, b. Wilms' tumour. **a** LS prone. A large mass arises from the anterior aspect of the left kidney, squashing the kidney and displacing it inferiorly. **b** LS supine. This shows the squashed kidney and the mass. A high-sensitivity compound scanning motion technique has overwritten and highlighted the entire tumour giving it a spurious resemblance to neuroblastoma

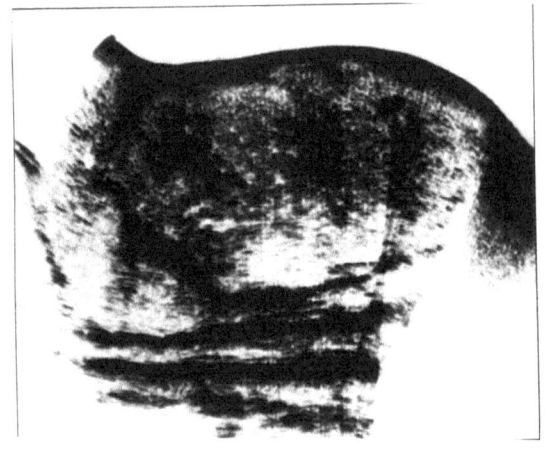

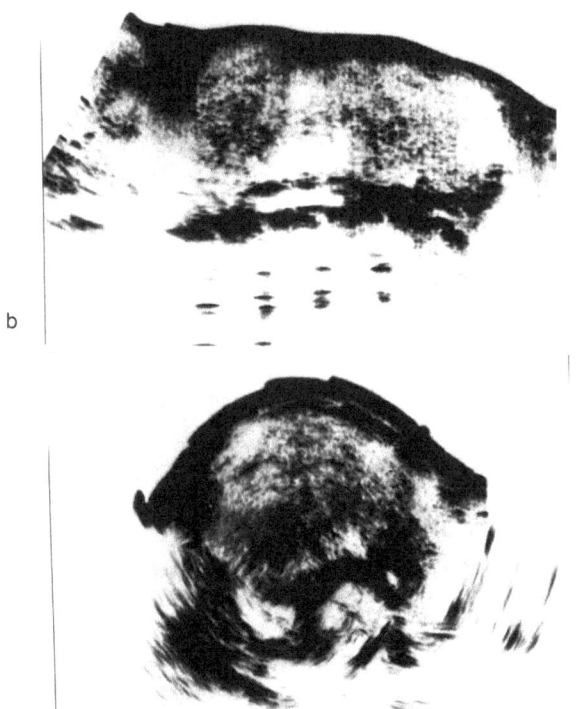

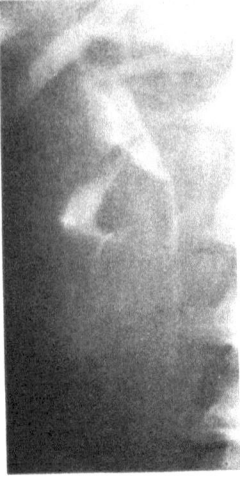

Fig. 9.9. Wilms' tumour. The right renal mass is shown by IVU and there is an irregularity of the lumen of the ureter caused by seeding of Wilms' tumour down the ureter

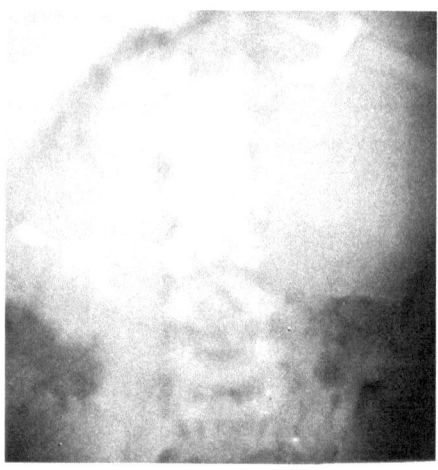

Fig. 9.10. Bilateral Wilms' tumour. The gross alterations in the few opacified calyces are characteristic of the lesion. On the left side the tumour arises in the lower part of the kidney and on the right side the lesion lies especially in the upper part of the kidney

Fig. 9.8 a–c. Wilms' tumour in horseshoe kidney. **a** LS supine. Examined through the right flank, a large homogeneous mass fills the abdomen. **b** LS supine. Above the aorta and spine there is a considerable volume of tumour crossing the midline **c** TS supine. This shows the extent of the tumour and its origin in a horseshoe kidney

renal vein and into the vena cava. When the lumen of the cava is occluded by tumour tissue ultrasound examination, a contrast medium cavogram and an isotope cavogram can all be diagnostic, but sonography is the easiest of these examinations. Any tumour extending into the renal vein and cava may be a rather slow-growing coherent lesion not especially prone to wider dissemination.

Rarely tumour growth extends up the vena cava and into the right atrium [15]. Echography may suggest this has occurred. Confirmation can be obtained by direct contrast medium studies or by the use of 99 m Tc MAA.

9.2.1.3.1 Wilms' Tumour in the Contralateral Kidney [11, 12, 13]. The primary tumour in the one kidney may be accompanied by a second tumour in the contralateral kidney. The second tumour may be discovered at the same time as the first (Fig. 9.11). Alternatively, the second tumour may become apparent on subsequent studies. Intravenous urography, ultrasonics examination (Fig. 9.12) and isotope (DMSA) studies are able to elucidate this development. If a large first tumour has been

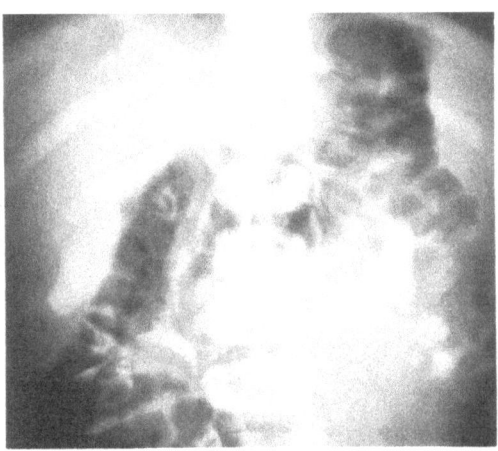

Fig. 9.11. Wilms' tumour. At IVU the bilateral renal masses show a remarkable intrarenal distortion of the collecting systems of the kidneys, reminiscent of cystic disease (but the young age of the patient makes this an unlikely possibility) or tuberous sclerosis

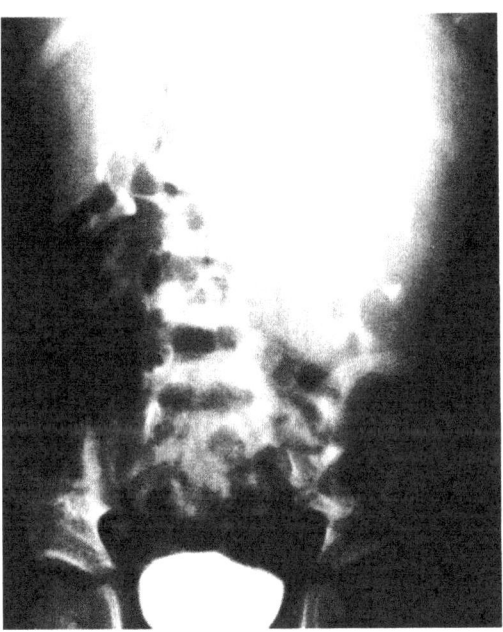

Fig. 9.12. Wilms' tumour. This pyrexial boy had a large left-sided mass with diffuse involvement of the left kidney. The IVU is not especially suggestive of Wilms' tumour, but the ultrasound study confirmed the diagnosis

successfully resected the advent of a second tumour in the contralateral kidney raises special problems. Generally, angiography [16, 17, 18] has little place in the investigation of Wilms' tumour, but when a second tumour is suspected it is essential, and selective renal arteriographic studies are particularly relevant (Fig. 9.13). Such studies can show the

vascular supply to the tumour and that part of the kidney which may not be involved. The vascularity of the tumour itself may be large or it may be small. Often the abnormal blood vessels commonly associated with neoplastic change elsewhere are significantly absent in Wilms' tumour; it follows that it is important not to make a diagnosis of Wilms' tumour solely on the basis of appearances at angiography because if this is done patients who have localized renal dysplasia may be inappropriately treated. Nevertheless knowledge of the blood supply to the affected and non-affected parts of the kidney is derived from angiography. The nephrographic phase will also add information about the extent of the functioning renal tissue which remains. It is on such information that decisions about possible resections of second tumours of the kidney are made.

Very rarely concurrent bilateral Wilms' tumour affects each kidney in a similar way (Fig. 9.14). The extensive bilateral intrarenal masses may then simulate bilateral polycystic disease. However, the patient is too young for such a lesion to be bilateral polycystic disease; and in any one case sonography demonstrates the tumoral nature of the lesion and the absence of a multiplicity of cysts. Very rarely Wilms' tumour is characterised by a multicystic change, but again the distinction from polycystic disease is made likely by the young age of the patient; adult-type polycystic disease is a very rare clinical event in children and in the very young child large bilateral renal masses are not seen with this lesion.

9.2.1.3.2 Liver

Since almost the entire liver is accessible to ultrasound examination any deposit in excess of about 2 cm which lies within the liver should be detectable. The liver is one of the commoner sites for late metastases.

9.2.1.3.3 Chest

In every patient suspected of Wilm's tumour a careful study of the lungs for metastatic deposits is essential. Antero-posterior and lateral chest radiographs are the minimum first requirement. Metastases in the central lung areas are easy to see. The problem is that deposits often lie peripherally in the lung (Fig. 9.15).

On standard radiographs the periphery of the lung must be studied with great care. There are two features which impede this: first, the dome of the diaphragm may be elevated by the abdominal mass and distension and this can make it difficult to see the bases of the lungs posteriorly; secondly, the

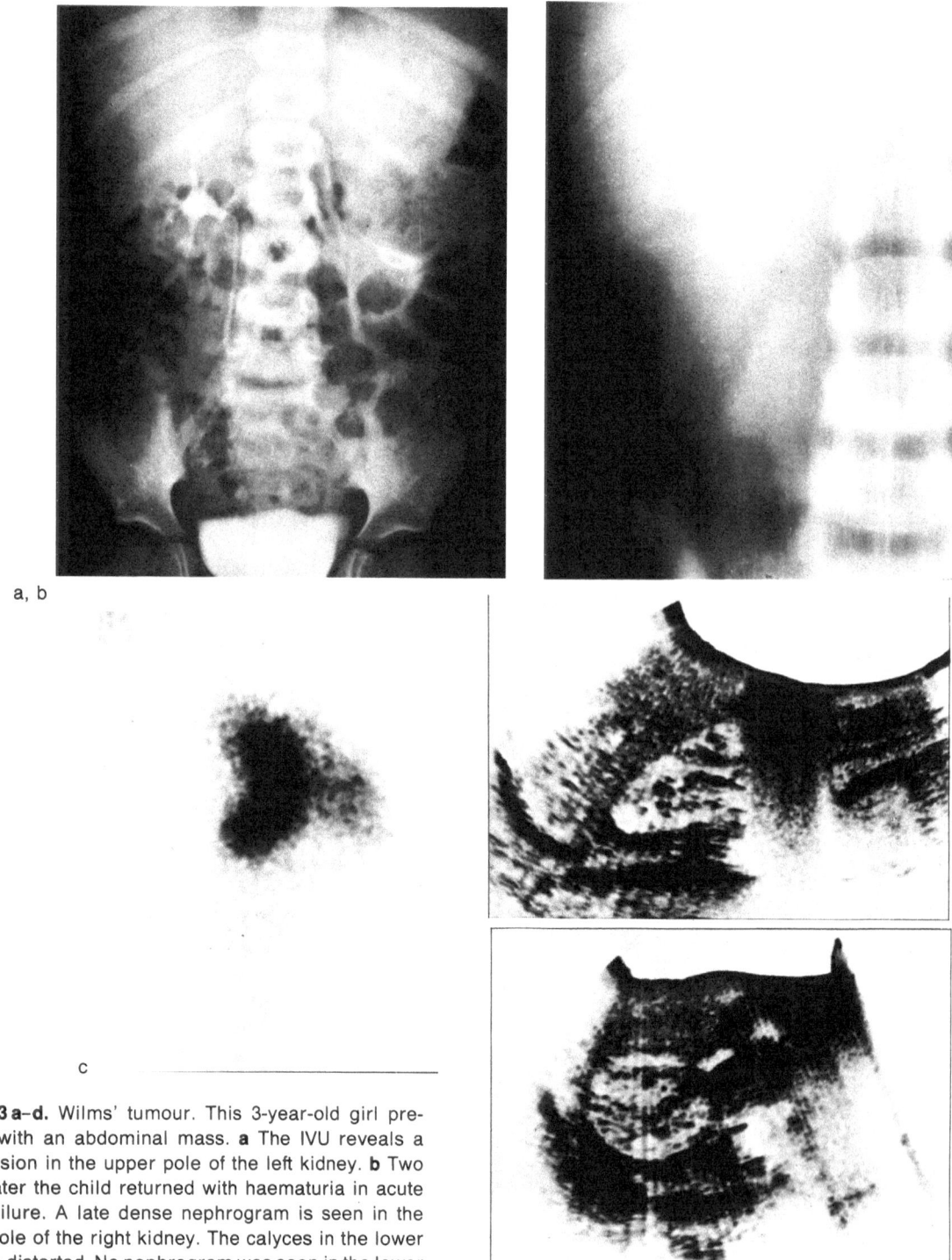

a, b

c

Fig. 9.13 a–d. Wilms' tumour. This 3-year-old girl presented with an abdominal mass. **a** The IVU reveals a mass lesion in the upper pole of the left kidney. **b** Two years later the child returned with haematuria in acute renal failure. A late dense nephrogram is seen in the upper pole of the right kidney. The calyces in the lower pole are distorted. No nephrogram was seen in the lower pole. **c** The DTPA isotope scan shows that only the upper half of the right kidney is functioning, with hold-up in the renal pelvis. **d** Ultrasound: (i) LS supine. The remaining right kidney shows a disrupted collecting system echo cluster. (ii) TS supine. This section confirms the features with a central zone being less echogenic and acoustically different, suggesting there is recurrence of tumour.

scapulae can obscure the upper lateral margins of the lungs on the antero-posterior projection and in the lateral projection the combination of the images of the two scapulae obscures much of the upper chest.

One final handicap to seeing metastases on a radiograph is that the exposure factors needed to display the central lung zones are different from those required to show the bases of the lungs below

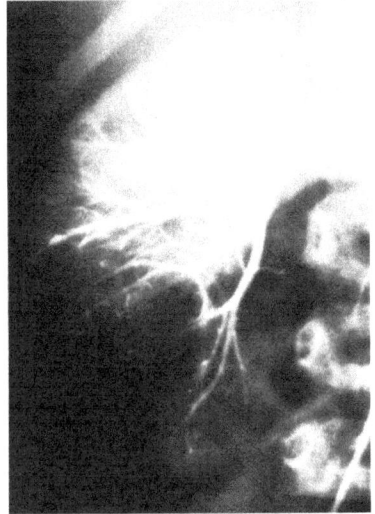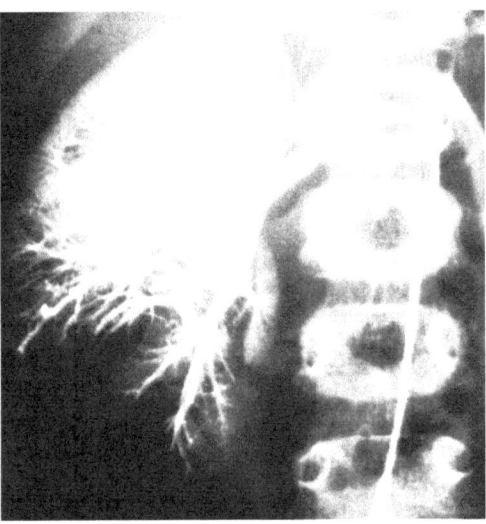

e, f

Fig. 9.13 e, f. e Selective right renal arteriogram shows the avascular tumour in the lower pole. A peripheral filling defect is seen in the mid-portion of the kidney supplied by the upper lobe artery. **f** Repeat selective right renal arteriogram after 6 months of chemotherapy shows the avascular lower pole mass to be much smaller. The second area in the mid-portion is now very poorly seen. Exploration of the kidney after this examination showed a scar in the mid-portion of the kidney. The tumour was enucleated from the lower pole

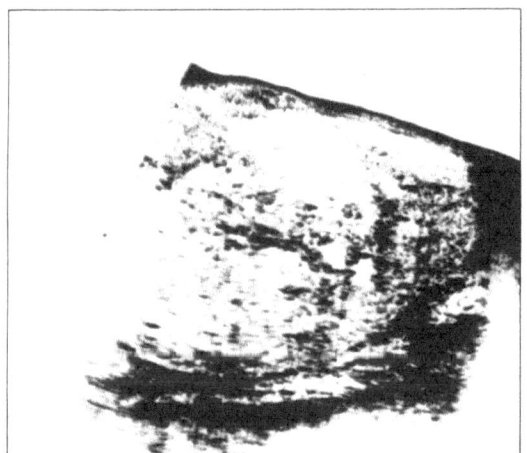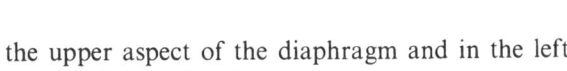

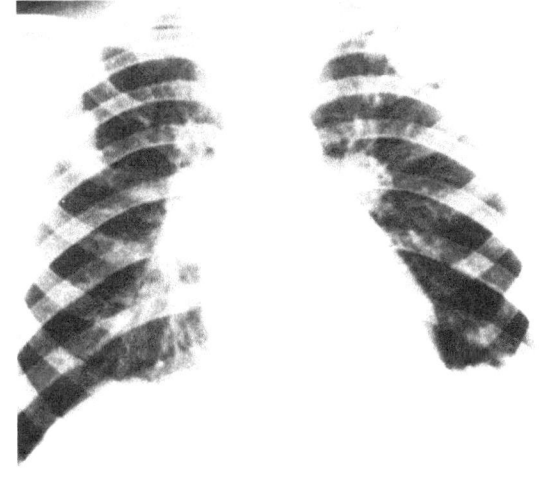

Fig. 9.14. Recurrent Wilms' tumour. LS supine. When examined through the right flank a large homogeneous mass displaces some dilated calyces in an infiltrated right kidney, which is now almost unrecognizable as such. Previously the left kidney tumour had been removed, but recurrence in the hitherto normal right kidney rapidly developed

Fig. 9.15. Multiple pulmonary metastases in Wilms' tumour. Several round deposits are seen in the periphery of the upper zones of both lungs. There is a further deposit in line with the right hilum which increases its density. A pleural effusion is present in the left base

the upper aspect of the diaphragm and in the left base behind the heart.

When a Wilms' tumour is present and a pleural effusion is found in the chest there is almost invariably extensive malignancy in the chest.

There are three possible ways in which to resolve the questions which may arise in respect of pulmonary metastases; they are tomography, fluoroscopy, and CT scanning of the lungs.

Traditionally classic tomography of the lungs in adult patients has been the method for detecting pulmonary metastases which may not be visible on ordinary chest radiographs. Standard antero-posterior projections with cuts at 1-cm intervals through the lungs have been carried out. Similar studies in children can be made, but in young children it is difficult to co-ordinate respiratory movement with the movement of the tomographic equipment consistently. In a supine child most of the blood flow passes through the posterior aspect of the lungs and the differences in radiolucency between posteriorly located metastases and the surrounding lung is less than that seen in anterior cuts. To enhance the prospects of seeing metastases on standard tomographic projections lateral sections through the lung may be taken; the child is placed lying first on one side and then on the other. Lateral tomographic cuts of the uppermost lung are then made for each lung.

Very high performance modern image intensifiers, with a manual control of KV for fluoroscopy, provide another way of looking for pulmonary metastases. The quality of image on modern intensifiers is quite remarkable. For this study the child lies on a horizontal radiographic table. Study of the lungs is then carried out with the child supine and prone. Subsequently the lungs are examined with oblique projections. By rotating a child carefully very steep oblique (nearly lateral) views of the lungs can be obtained. Again, advantage can be taken at fluoroscopy of the tendency for blood to flow into the most dependent part of the lung. Deposits near and at the margin of the lung can be seen along all but the mediastinal aspects. As the child breathes the pulmonary metastases move as the lung fills and empties; the TV image, being in shades of grey, enables the human eye to see the moving metastases, and pulmonary vessels can easily be differentiated from deposits. Because the child is breathing, rib shadows do not obscure deposits. Spot film devices can be used to record metastases (Fig. 9.16). Fluoroscopy of the chest is a quick and easy procedure to undertake once the observer has a little experience.

CT scanning has been adopted by some centres as a standard procedure in searching for pulmonary metastases. As with orthodox tomography and chest fluoroscopy the fact that the image of a deposit is enhanced when blood flow in the vicinity is low has to be taken into account. Accordingly it is essential to carry out sections through the lungs when the child is both supine and prone. Obviously CT scanners with a fast scan time are a great advantage in this type of work.

In planning treatment it is essential to know if any pulmonary metastasis has occurred; if it has, then the number and location of the deposits is important. When there is an isolated deposit, surgical resection can be contemplated.

9.2.1.3.4 Metastasis to Bone. It is strange but true that Wilms' tumour seldom metastasizes to bone. There are reports of bone deposits in the literature

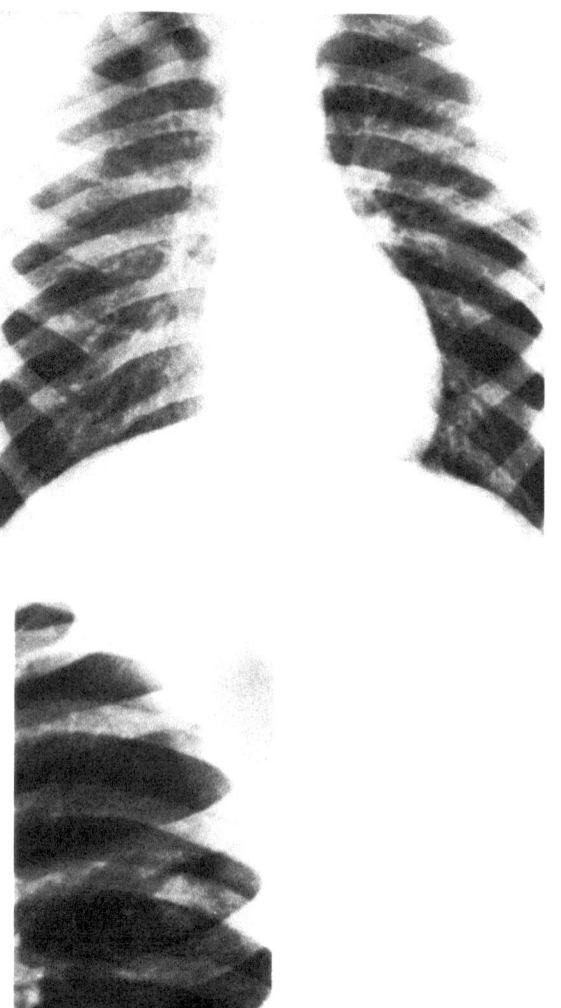

Fig. 9.16 a, b. Metastases to the lung in Wilms' tumour. What appears to be a solitary deposit is seen in the apex of the right lung on the AP chest radiograph (**a**). Fluoroscopy with a high-performance intensifier showed further deposits including that shown in the spot film (**b**) in the left lung

but this very fact emphasizes the rarity of the event. Bone metastases may be lytic, sclerotic or of mixed type on orthodox radiological examination. Often bone metastases are associated with high accumulation of 99 m-Tc polyphosphonate but this is not invariably so. Since bone metastasis is so very rare it would appear that, once the diagnosis of Wilms' tumour has been established, it is not necessary to search for bone metastases routinely either by radiology or isotope studies.

9.2.1.4 Staging of Wilms' Tumour

In essence this is a combined clinical operative and radiological exercise. The generally accepted staging is that along the lines given by Marsden and Steward who report as follows: [1]

Stage I. A well-encapsulated tumour which is entirely removed at operation. Spillage of the tumour does not take place at operation and there is no involvement of the para-aortic nodes at biopsy.

Stage II. There is extension of the tumour beyond the capsule either by:
1. Local infiltration or
2. Extension along the renal vein or
3. Involvement of the para-aortic glands

but where the surgeon believes total removal of macroscopic disease is possible.

Stage III. There is extension of the tumour beyond the capsule and:
1. Spillage of the tumour at operation or
2. Tumour is felt to have been left behind at the time of operation or
3. There are peritoneal metastases.

Stage IV. Spread to the liver, lungs, bones or brain is found at diagnosis.

Stage V. Tumours of both kidneys.

9.2.1.5 Follow-up Examination in Wilms' Tumour

For many years it has been known that Wilms' tumour is most likely to recur within the first 2 years after the initial diagnosis and treatment. It follows that the most intensive follow-up is required during this period if the best results are to be obtained. Wilms' tumour is therefore best investigated, treated and followed-up in centres which have the appropriate facilities and where the many disciplines required can co-ordinate effort.

When removal of the affected kidney has been accomplished repeat studies of the contralateral kidney should be carried out quite soon after operation and thereafter at about 6-monthly intervals for at least 2 years by IVU and more frequently by echography. Early identification and resection of a second tumour is then most likely to be possible.

Pulmonary metastasis is a common mode of spread. A careful initial evaluation of the lungs is essential and this can be repeated at 3-monthly intervals for the first year, then at 6-monthly intervals for 4 years thereafter. Treatment of multiple metastases may be necessary. Single isolated lesions in one lobe may be resected at thoracotomy.

Bone deposits in the radiographs of the thorax and abdomen and pelvis should always be sought for but general skeletal examination specifically for bone disease is not carried out.

Sonography can always be carried out to study the liver, the contralateral kidney, the bed of the tumour and retroperitoneal and retrocrural lymph nodes. Ultrasound studies can also be used with advantage to assess the size of any tumour which is being irradiated prior to operation so that the field size can be adjusted to that occupied by the tumour mass.

Radiation sequelae are potentially important but with skill and use of chemotherapy the problems can be minimized. For example, radiation pneumonitis is a complication which we have not encountered and children treated always appear to have had good lung growth.

Another complication is scoliosis; it may be simply good fortune, but this has not been a sequel, either early or late, to radiation therapy at the Hospital for Sick Children. There is no doubt that radiotherapy can and does inhibit growth and reduction in subcutaneous tissue and muscle mass may occur. Bone growth is also affected. From our experience it would seem that if the field of radiation to the tumour bed is such that less than one-half of each of the vertebral bodies in the field is affected no scoliosis, even at adolescence, develops. It would appear that vertebral bodies in the lumbar region on the side of the lesion may be reduced in height for about one-third of their width without spinal curvature developing.

Radiation ileitis and jejunitis is a rare complication as is symptomatic radiation nephritis [19] which can lead to renal atrophy in the unaffected remnant.

9.2.2 Mesoblastic Nephroma

This tumour is found in the very young (usually in the infant) and it is usually detected as an abdominal mass [20, 21, 22, 23]. Histologically the tumour is complex – such a lesion has variously been described as neonatal fibromatosis, fibroma, fibrosarcoma, leiomyosarcoma and leiomyomatous hamartoma. At investigation and at IVU (Fig. 9.17) the lesion is indistinguishable in its characteristics from Wilms' tumour which is found in the slightly older patient. However, the chest radiograph is invariably devoid of pulmonary deposits and there is no sign of any bony metastasis. Whilst Wilms' tumour is a malignant lesion mesoblastic nephroma is not. Provided that the tumour is completely excised at surgery the lesion is benign. However, if any mesoblastic nephroma element is left behind then local invasion of tissue can occur. In the very young patient who has a Wilms' tumour type of investigatory finding it is important to undertake surgical exploration and excision and avoid chemotherapy which can induce an unwelcome and unnecessary depression of bone marrow function.

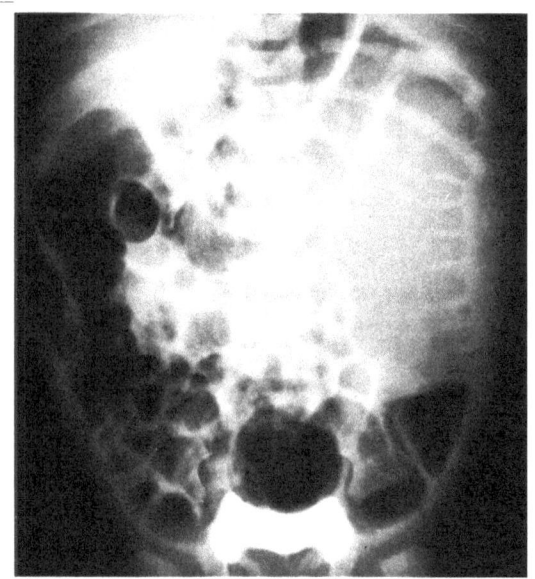

Fig. 9.17. Mesoblastic nephroma. The large mass in the left side contains, in its most lateral part, small pools of contrast medium at this IVU. The right kidney is normal. The patient's very young age makes the diagnosis of mesoblastic nephroma very probable indeed. Note the bladder ears – an insignificant phenomenon

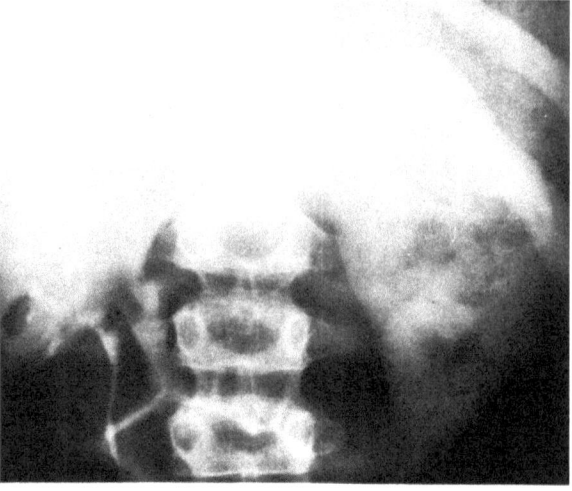

Fig. 9.18. Adenocarcinoma. At IVU the right kidney is normal but the large left kidney shows a dense nephrogram due to acute obstruction. However, the dense nephrogram is not uniform but irregular in density and the kidney is exceptionally large

9.2.3 Renal Carcinoma

These are exceptionally rare tumours in children but they do occur (Figs. 9.18 and 9.19) [24, 25]. They are of course malignant but if encapsulated and circumscribed they can be resected completely.

9.2.4 Other Tumours Affecting the Kidney

These tumours fall into two categories. The first is the very small residue of primary renal tumours such as angiosarcoma. The second category concerns lesions which affect the kidney as part of a more widespread disease process. Such lesions include leukaemia and lymphoma which may affect and involve the kidneys [26, 27].

Diffuse infiltration of both kidneys by these secondary leukaemic lesions produces kidneys which are large and the enlargement may be considerable. Symmetrical renal involvement produces symmetrical enlargement with a uniform distribution of the calyces within the renal contour at IVU (Fig. 9.20). There may on occasion be localized deposits which produce mass-like lesions, palpable at clinical examination and at investigation in the child with leukaemia (Fig. 9.21). Non-function of one kidney in the child with leukaemia can occur as a transient

phenomenon before treatment takes effect, presumably because of ureteric occlusion by the malignancy in the vicinity.

Children with non-Hodgkin's lymphoma may have an intrinsic renal mass lesion of the kidney (Fig. 9.22) but in this circumstance there is likely to be renal displacement associated with large para-aortic lymph nodes among other features (Fig. 9.23). Burkitt's lymphoma is also responsible for renal mass lesions and renal enlargement [28, 29]. In this condition the renal problem is but one feature of a more widespread symptom complex. Neuroblastoma *very rarely* invades the renal parenchyma (*see* Fig. 9.37).

▷

Fig 9.19 a–d. Papillary carcinoma. This 10-year-old girl had haematuria for 18 months. **a** The IVU shows a filling defect in the right renal pelvis. The preliminary film showed faint calcification in this region. **b** Ultrasound: (i) LS prone view of the right kidney shows the collecting cluster distended by a mass of similar echo amplitude to surrounding parenchyma but slightly more coarse. (ii) LS prone of the left kidney (for comparison). (iii) TS prone. Striking demonstration of the difference between the two kidneys. The right is large with the mass distending the collecting system. **c** DMSA isotope scan failed to show any significant abnormality. **d** CT scan demonstrated the mass to lie mainly in the lower portion of the renal pelvis. It appears to involve the renal substance. A nephroureterectomy was carried out. Histology revealed that the tumour was a well-differentiated papillary carcinoma which was multicentric in origin (i. e. from multiple minor calyces), lying in the renal pelvis

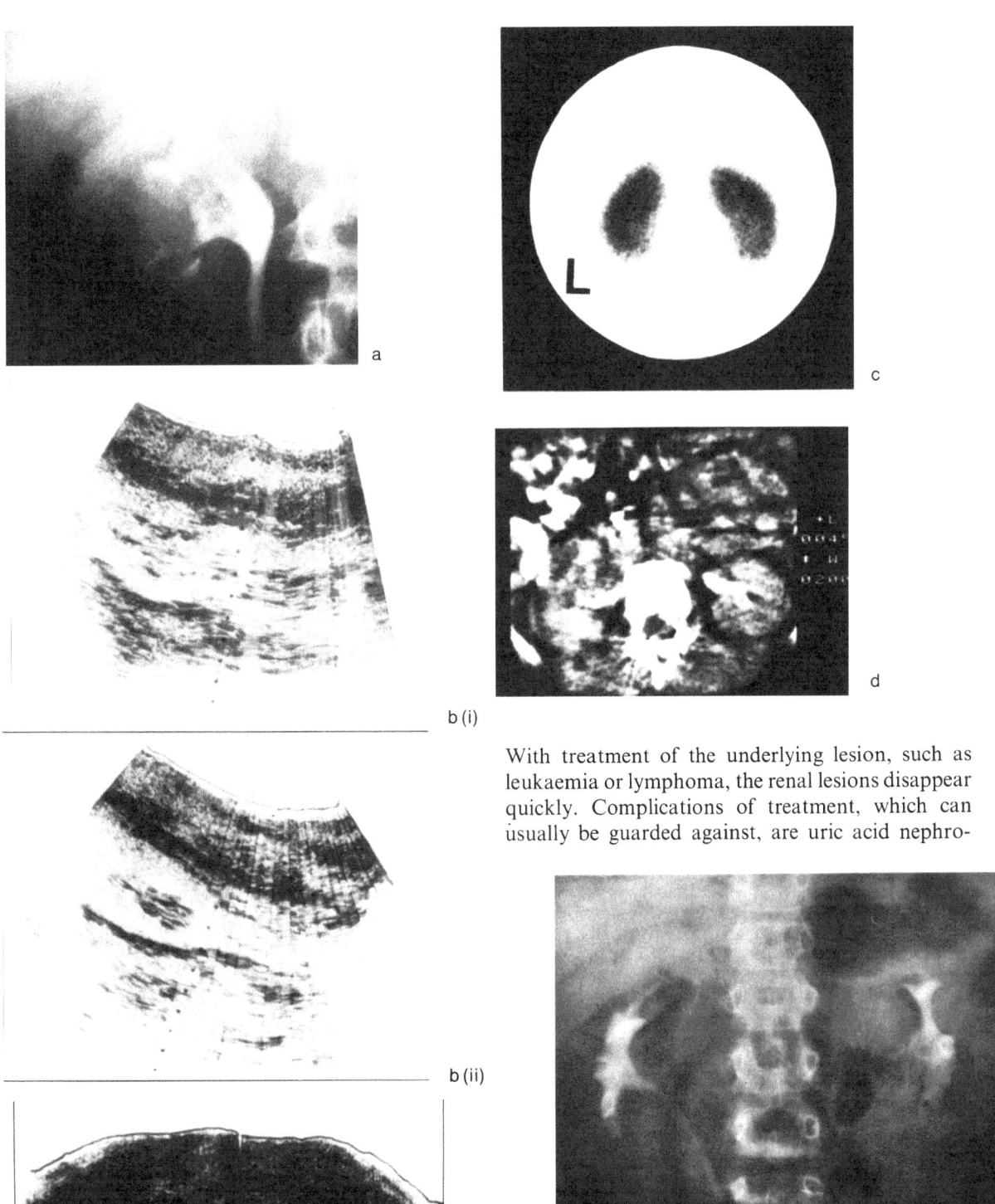

With treatment of the underlying lesion, such as leukaemia or lymphoma, the renal lesions disappear quickly. Complications of treatment, which can usually be guarded against, are uric acid nephro-

Fig. 9.20. Leukaemic infiltration. This boy's IVU shows considerable symmetrical increase in parenchymal thickness with no intrarenal distortion of the pelvicalyceal system, features of a diffuse renal lesion. However, the kidneys and proximal parts of the ureters are displaced laterally by retroperitoneal gland enlargement

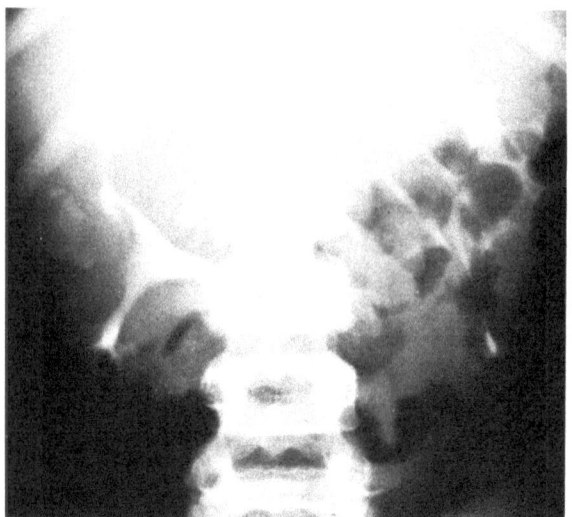

Fig. 9.21. Leukaemia. The IVU was carried out because the kidneys were large in this unwell boy. The IVU confirms bilateral renal enlargement with considerable distortion of the calyx system within the kidneys. Note the bone change in the iliac crest, which suggests the diagnosis despite the presence of a normal peripheral blood picture at this stage

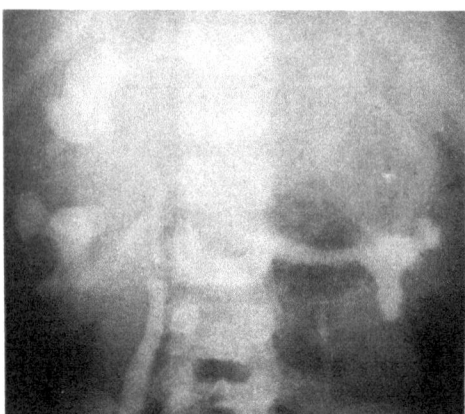

Fig. 9.22. Non-Hodgkin's lymphoma. At IVU the kidneys are large. The right is duplex and there is calyx dilatation with compression of the renal pelves. In the left kidney only the lower group of calyces opacifies and the left ureter is displaced laterally. This diffuse lesion affects the parenchyma of both kidneys to a varying degree with ureteric displacement and compression of the renal pelves

Fig. 9.23. See page 149.

pathy and renal colic caused by excessive uric acid being rapidly cleared through the kidneys. Opportunistic infection of the upper urinary tract by *Monilia* can cause obstruction in the ureter as well as invading the lower urinary tract.

9.2.5 Conclusion

The prognosis of malignant disease in childhood when it affects the kidneys is rather different from the situation in adult life. Clearly mesoblastic nephroma should carry a very good prognosis when treated by skilled surgeons in centres accustomed to such problems of childhood. Likewise, the prognosis in all but the very advanced cases of Wilms' tumour is excellent in terms of long-term survival and quality of life. Patients with leukaemia have a good chance of protracted remission and survival: the same cannot be said, however, for patients with non-Hodgkin's lymphoma. These observations simply underline the need to investigate renal mass lesions fully, reach a definitive diagnosis and institute the appropriate treatment.

9.3 Non-Neoplastic Renal Masses and Lesions Simulating Masses

Variations in tissue development can result in lesions which may present clinically as mass lesions or appear as mass lesions at IVU. Since the diagnosis is established after nephrectomy there is no need to elaborate unduly. These lesions include hamartoma (Fig. 9.24), angiomas, lymphangiomatous cysts (Fig. 9.25) and cystadenomas (Fig. 9.26).

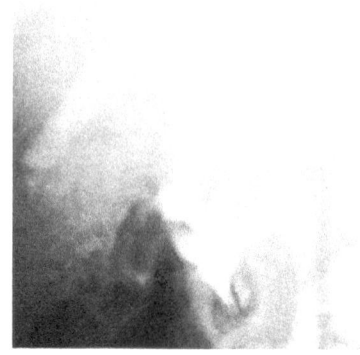

Fig. 9.24. Intrarenal hamartoma. This IVU was carried out because of haematuria. The mass lesion in the upper pole of the right kidney distorts the calyx system in the vicinity and extends into the pelvis. After nephrectomy the lesion was found to be a benign intrarenal hamartoma

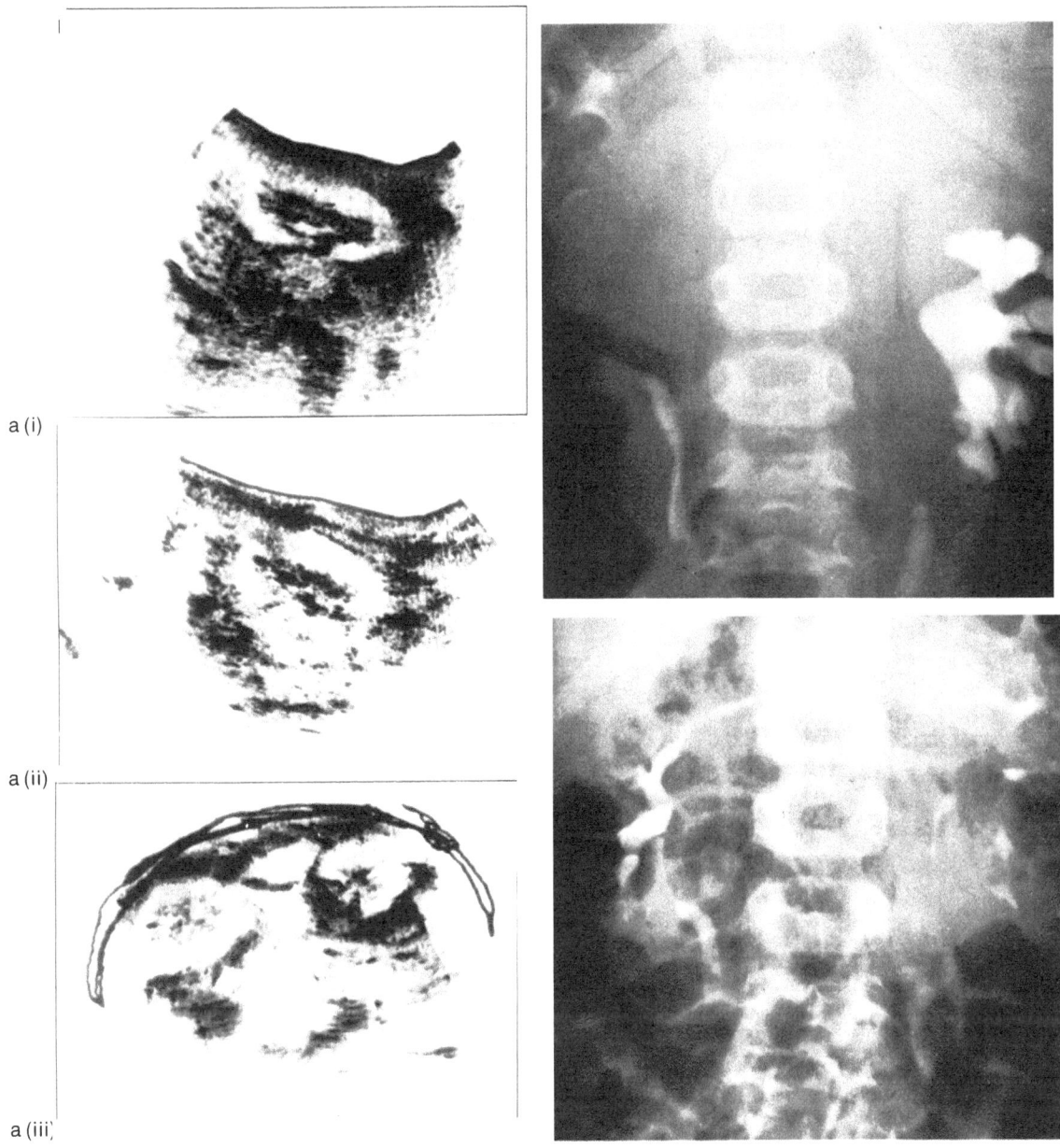

a (i)

a (ii)

a (iii)

Fig. 9.23 a Ultrasound: (i) LS prone, left kidney. The mass anterior to the kidney is a neuroblastoma (better seen in other views). Note the boundary between it and the kidney. (ii) LS prone. Follow-up examination weeks later shows breakdown of the boundary between the neuroblastoma and the kidney with disturbance of the collecting cluster better seen in the transverse plane. (iii) TS prone shows enlargement of the left kidney with a disturbed echo cluster. This suggested invasion of the kidney by the neuroblastoma. **b** IVU prior to treatment, showing displacement of the right kidney and hydronephrosis on the left. **c** IVU performed after the ultrasound shows the shrinkage of the tumour but infiltration of the left kidney

9.3.1 General Disease with Renal Masses

Mass lesions of the kidney occur in tuberous sclerosis and in hydatid disease.

9.3.1.1 Tuberous Sclerosis

In tuberous sclerosis a wide range of clinical features, including hypertension may be associated either with cystic (Chapter 6) or angiomyolipomatous changes (Fig. 9.27) in the kidneys [30]; these have characteristic features at IVU, angiography and echography.

9.3.1.2 Hydatid Disease

Hydatid disease (echinococcosis) is a disseminated parasitic disease which most commonly affects the

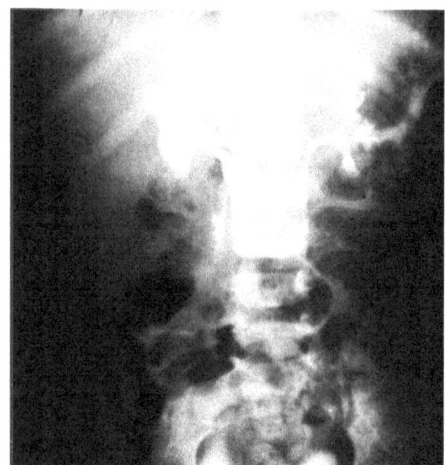

a

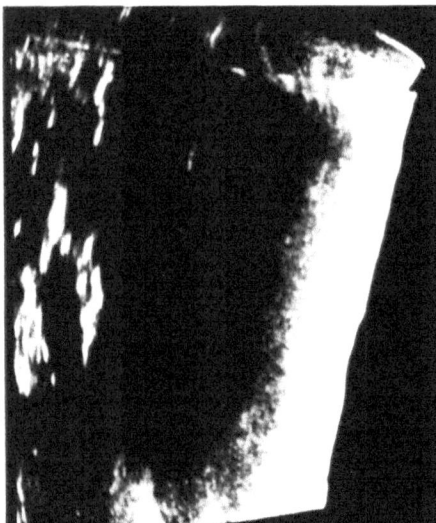

b

Fig. 9.25 a, b. Lymphangiomatous cyst. This child with a large right-sided abdominal mass demonstrates at IVU (**a**) compression of part of the right renal pelvis, with stretching of upper and lower pole calyces. A faintly opacified thin rim is present around the edge of the mass. The left kidney appears normal. The ultrasound study (**b**) demonstrates a large transonic cystic area. A few echoes are present within this area and this suggests that the cyst is not a "simple" one

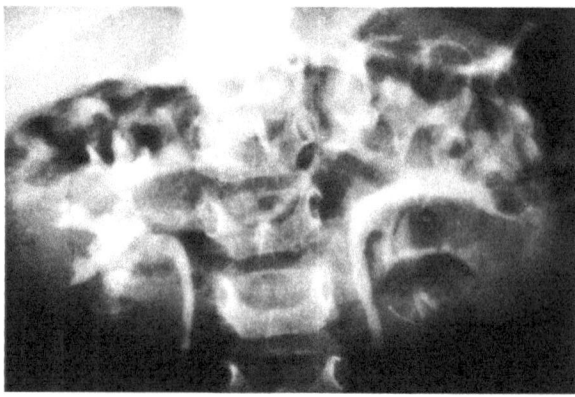

Fig. 9.26. Cystadenoma. The mass lesion in the lower pole of the left kidney causes stretching and distortion of the calyces in the vicinity. Cystadenoma was found and removed at operation

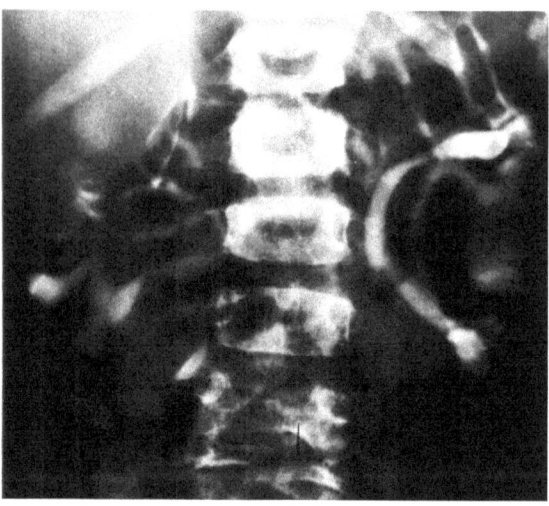

Fig. 9.27. Tuberous sclerosis. This child had the typical stigmata of the condition and was referred because of hypertension. The IVU shows changes typical for angio-myolipomata in tuberous sclerosis, with gross distortion of intrarenal anatomy in the large kidneys

lungs and liver; a concomitant kidney lesion occurs quite commonly, although seldom in isolation [31, 32]. The parasite produces a reaction in the host tissue around the hydatid cyst which has a double-layered capsular wall. Within the cyst lie many daughter cysts. Calcification in the wall of the cyst may be apparent in an IVU series. Sonography demonstrates echographic features which are complex but may be diagnostic [33]. Haemogglutination tests further substantiate the diagnosis prior to operation in the majority of children.

9.3.2 Obstruction in the Urinary Tract

Certain particular types of obstruction in the urinary tract can have features at IVU which suggest a tumour may be present. Among such lesions are hydrocalicosis, obstruction of one component of a duplex kidney [34] (Fig. 9.28) and obstruction of a kidney which is non-functioning at IVU. If pyonephrosis supervenes the kidney mass may be hard on palpation. However, as indicated in Chapters 3 and 5, studies by ultrasound, isotope scans and

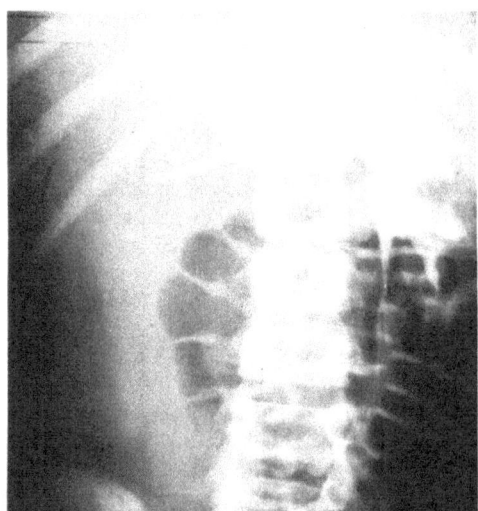

a

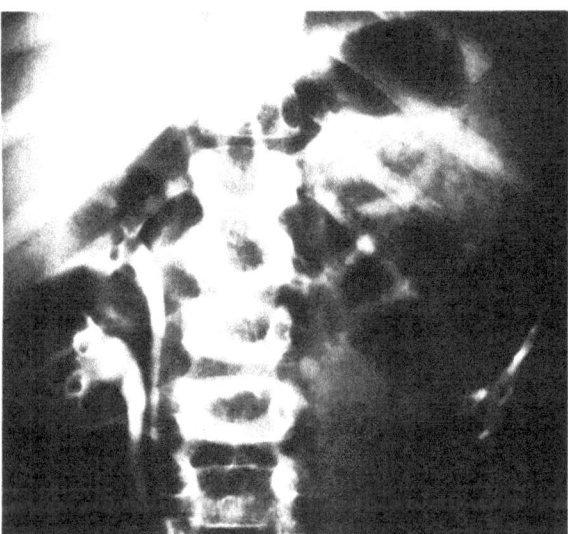

b

Fig. 9.28 a Duplication with hydronephrosis. Mass lesion in the right side is caused by a duplex kidney in which the lower component is grossly hydronephrotic and non-functioning because of pelvi-ureteric obstruction. The upper component continues to function well, but the overall impression at IVU might deceive and renal malignancy be considered, especially because there is an element of obstruction of the upper pole calyces.
b Left duplex kidney with hydronephrosis. There is a simple duplication of the right kidney at this IVU. It can reasonably be suspected that the left-sided mass lesion is caused by an obstruction and hydronephrosis of an upper renal component on the left side, despite the gross displacement of the unobstructed lower component

9.3.3.2 Adult-Type Polycystic Disease

Of the remaining types of cystic disease of the kidney only adult-type polycystic disease is likely to present occasional diagnostic difficulties [see Chapter 6]. These can arise if the lesion presents with haematuria and there is no clear-cut family background of the disease. The problems can be enhanced when, as sometimes happens, enlargement of one kidney is considerable and the other kidney is virtually normal in size (Fig. 9.29). Echography will demonstrate cysts in both kidneys; should a survey of the family by ultrasound study be carried out it may reveal lesions in other members of the family. Angiography can be helpful for it can show the bilateral nature of the problem but angiography or other investigatory measures may not always yield that element of confidence needed in diagnosis. Ultimately, exploration of the kidney and biopsy may be necessary and a deleterious nephrectomy must be avoided.

9.3.4 Ectopic Kidneys

Ectopic kidneys may simulate mass lesions in the abdomen and pelvis, especially if the kidney is large and single or if there is fused crossed ectopia (*see* Chapter 6). Rarely a kidney may extend through a posterior diaphragmatic defect to produce a "mass-like" feature in the chest posteriorly.

9.3.5 Pseudotumour: Cleft Kidney

This condition has been discussed in Chapter 6 under the title *Cleft kidney*. There is an infolding of the cortex producing an indentation of the renal contour and a short truncated minor calyx arising directly from the infundibulum of a middle – or

MCU should mean misdiagnoses are not made in this sector and an erroneous diagnosis of tumour is avoided.

9.3.3 Cystic Disease in the Kidney

9.3.3.1 Multicystic Disease

Multicystic disease of a large kidney with an atretic ureter in a young infant is unlikely to be mistaken for a non-functioning mesoblastic nephroma on clinical examination [35]. Dysplastic changes or obstruction in the contralateral kidney point, at IVU, to the likelihood of multicystic disease and sonograms show the cystic features of the lesion. Very rarely Wilms' tumour can have a predominantly cystic character.

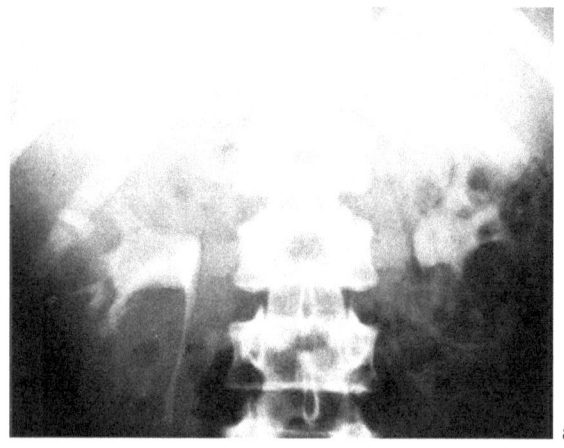

a

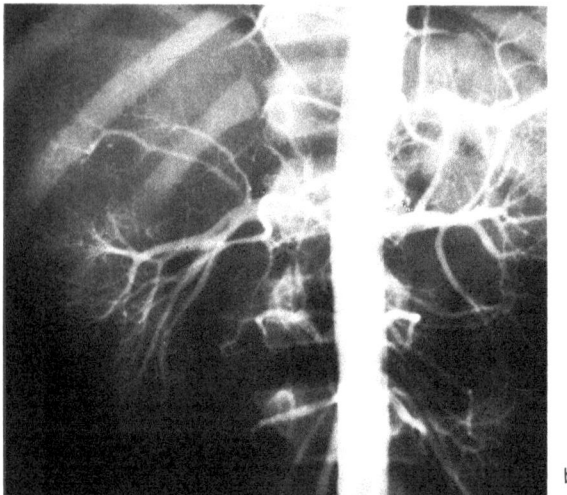

b

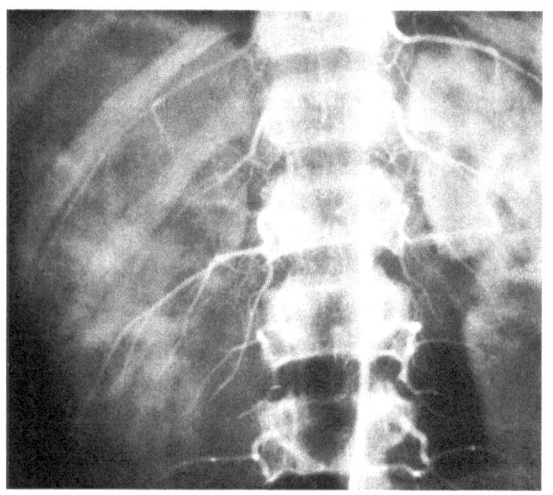

c

Fig. 9.29 a–c. Adult polycystic disease. **a** This boy had haematuria and IVU shows the right kidney is large with a smooth contour and calyces evenly distributed throughout the kidney. But the upper calyces are slightly irregular and compressed. No definite lesion shown in the left kidney. Differential diagnosis includes renal neoplasm, lymphoma, renal infection and cystic disease. **b** Ultrasonics study was inconclusive. The arterial phase of the aortogram shows a generally avascular upper pole. **c** Nephrographic phase of the angiogram demonstrates very extensive defects throughout the right kidney, but there are also defects in the left kidney. Ultrasonics study of the family was inconclusive and further limited studies were negative. Proof of diagnosis was essential and the biopsy indicated adult polycystic disease. From time to time children are encountered whose cystic disease enlarges one kidney predominantly

◁

kidney or pseudotumour and angiography is unnecessary [39]. If it has been seriously suggested the lesion is a malignancy then there must be a very high element of confidence about the findings from investigation.

9.3.6 Disappearing Calyces

For the unwary observer this phenomenon may present a problem [40]. A calyx, often in the mid part of a kidney, may not opacify with contrast medium at IVU. And so it might seem there is a mass lesion within the kidney in the vicinity of the non-opacified calyx. The measures outlined in respect of the cleft

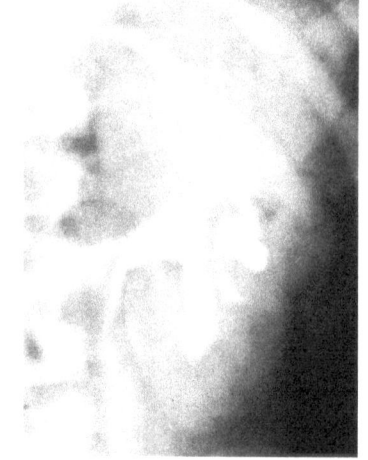

Fig. 9.30. Cleft kidney. This boy had a palpable solitary left kidney. The IVU shows the indentation of renal contour at the site of the cleft and the characteristic arrangement of calyces described in Chap. 6. Because of the particular circumstances of the case surgical exploration was carried out to confirm the diagnosis

upper-pole major calyx (Fig. 9.30). At IVU the nephrographic phase is uniform throughout the kidney, uptake of isotope at renal scan is either uniform or increased because of the local nephric tissue, and there is no disturbance of tissue echo texture on the sonogram [36, 37, 38]. These measures are sufficient to establish the diagnosis of cleft

kidney will show the normality of the renal parenchyma. Usually, if the IVU is carefully controlled,
one radiograph in a series will show the calyx
opacifying.

9.3.7 Renal Venous Thrombosis

When this condition affects one kidney in an infant
the kidney may be greatly enlarged in the acute
phase and there is invariably haematuria and non-
function at IVU. Sonography establishes the size of
the kidney, the uniform echogenic pattern in the
kidney parenchyma and the characteristic squashed
appearance of the central collecting system cluster.
Renal venous thrombosis may be bilateral and it is
discussed more fully in Chapter 8.

9.3.8 Renal Abscess Formation

In acute lesions the child has a high fever, polymorphonuclear leucocytosis and loin pain. The affected
kidney may be palpated. Septicaemia may be found
when the child has developed the lesion but bacteria
may not be present in the urine. Sometimes there is
haematuria. These clinical features in the acutely ill
child should suggest the possible diagnosis. As in all

septicaemic conditions other viscera may be affected, for example the heart by bacterial endocarditis.
At IVU localized renal abscess is usually confined to
the polar region of the kidney and this is enlarged
(Fig. 9.31) [41, 42, 43, 44]. The margin of the kidney
in the vicinity may be seen with undue clarity – the
clear rim sign. There may also be a localized increase
in the density of the nephrogram at the site of the
abscess. In the early stages the renal isotope scan can
be disappointing in defining the abscess; this is
because in the acute phase no cavity has developed,
and the "pre-abscess" stage only has been reached.
However the localized enlargement will be shown on
the sonogram and the echo pattern of the inflamed
zone is of lower amplitude than that of healthy renal
tissue (Fig. 9.32).

If the renal tissue becomes necrotic then an irregular
echolucent ring (produced by the oedematous parenchyma) surrounds an amorphous echo cluster which
represents the breaking down debris of the potential
abscess cavity. Once an abscess cavity has formed
then an outline of variable irregularity is noted and
within this the largely fluid content is transonic and
echofree. Debris tends to gravitate to the most
dependent part of the cavity and so as the patient is
rotated the debris (and its different echo pattern)
changes its relationship to a particular part of the
wall. At this stage the perinephric inflammatory

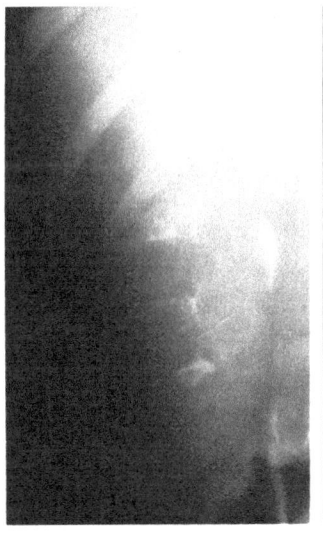 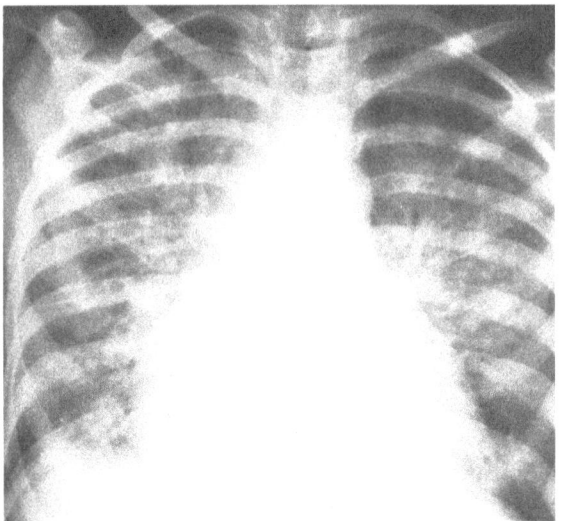

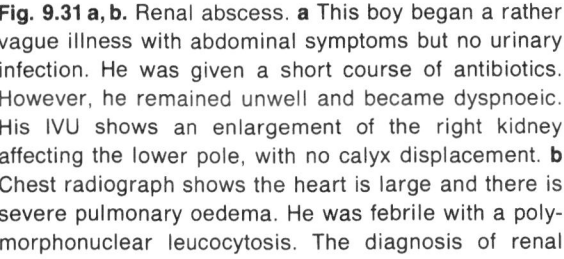

a, b

Fig. 9.31 a, b. Renal abscess. **a** This boy began a rather
vague illness with abdominal symptoms but no urinary
infection. He was given a short course of antibiotics.
However, he remained unwell and became dyspnoeic.
His IVU shows an enlargement of the right kidney
affecting the lower pole, with no calyx displacement. **b**
Chest radiograph shows the heart is large and there is
severe pulmonary oedema. He was febrile with a polymorphonuclear leucocytosis. The diagnosis of renal

abscess with bacterial endocarditis associated with myo-
pathy was made. No organism was isolated but intensive
treatment with antibiotics and for heart failure was
immediately started. He recovered quite rapidly and
repeat IVU some 2 weeks later showed the kidney length
had diminished by 3 cm and the definable mass in the
lower pole had disappeared. Several months later he had
fully recovered in all respects

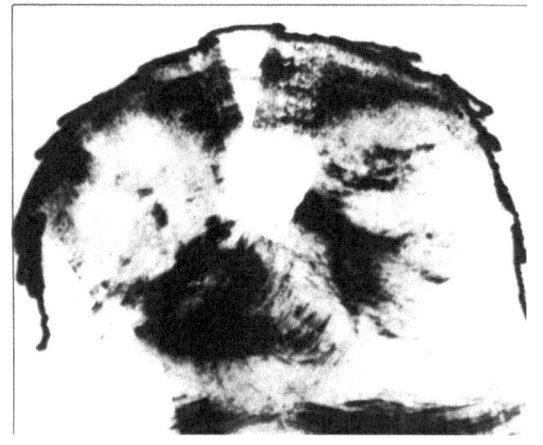

a

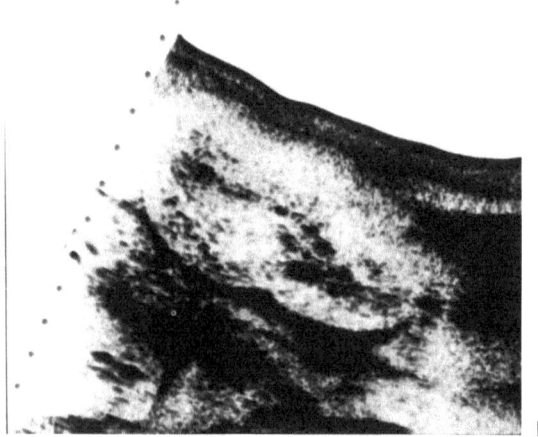

b

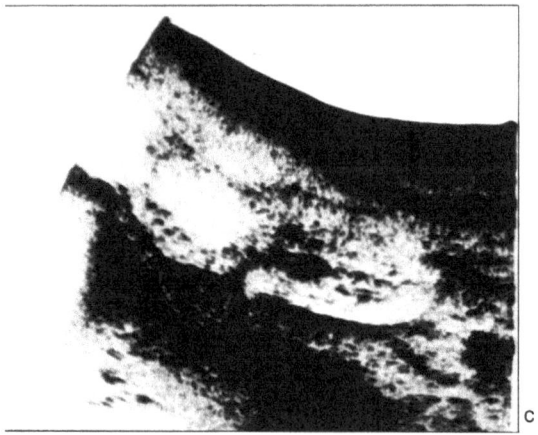

c

Fig. 9.32 a–c. Renal abscess. **a** TS prone. Scan shows a slightly large left kidney with areas of relatively lower echogenecity and some squashing of the collecting system. **b** LS prone. Left kidney shows a swollen cortex with an area suggesting abscess formation anteriorly. Probable diagnosis on this evidence: "pre-abscess" stage. **c** LS prone. After 1 week's antibiotic therapy the cortex is generally less swollen, but the anterior mass is even more echolucent. This is characteristic of a healing abscess
◁

organisms) rapidly brings the acute lesion under control. Scarring of varying degree may be a late sequel with at worst a thinned parenchyma containing a clubbed calyx. Small fibrotic scars show as a bright echo cluster within the parenchyma. Complete resolution of a lesion leaves no scarring at all. Not all renal abscesses are localized to one part of a kidney. Multiple small abscesses may be disseminated widely throughout the renal parenchyma. A kidney affected in this way is large and such renal infection may be unilateral or bilateral. Sometimes there may be surprisingly little systemic manifestation of infection in the child. At IVU the kidney may function surprisingly well. Although the infected kidney is large the overall symmetry of kidney structure is maintained because the abscesses are small and collectively they do not distort the calyx distribution within the renal contour. Such cases are rare, but it is important to be mindful of their existence so that a precipitate nephrectomy is avoided.

9.3.9 Perinephric Infection and Abscess

Perhaps the most common cause of perinephric abscess is underlying calculus disease in the kidney (*see* Chapter 5). Nevertheless, other causes of perinephric infection do occur, perhaps more commonly than is recognised. Appendicitis with abscess spreading to the perinephric space is one such case. Extension of renal abscess into the perinephric space is a more direct spread of infection (Fig. 9.33). A very rare cause is infection following renal biopsy in a nephrotic patient on a regime of therapy predisposing to infection. The classic staphylococcal primary perinephric abscess of former times is a rarity. If there is no calculus disease perinephric infection can potentially provide diagnostic problems.

IVU can show an increase in parenchymal thickness in the vicinity of the lesion with concomitant compression of calyces in the vicinity. Tomography at an early stage in the IVU will demonstrate an

change is usually sufficient to limit the normal respiratory excursion of the kidney.
An old abscess will have a well-defined margin and an echofree fluid content; calcification may develop in the wall and this is then highly echogenic and casts a shadow.
Clearly ultrasound study can provide the ideal way to check the progress of the lesion in a systematic way. Effective chemotherapy against the infecting organism (usually *E. coli,* but sometimes other

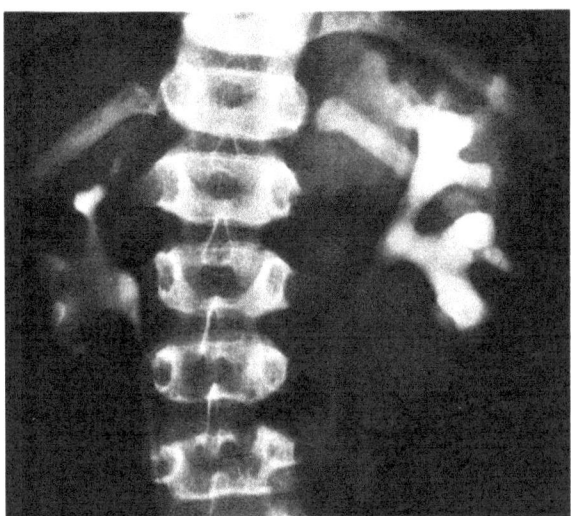

Fig. 9.33. Renal and peri-ureteric abscess. This 8-year-old had abdominal pain, anorexia fever and tenderness in the left flank. The IVU shows the left kidney is displaced laterally, the calyces are dilated. Below the small renal pelvis, the ureter is narrowed and no lower pole renal contour can be identified because of the abscess of the kidney and the extension into the vicinity of the ureter

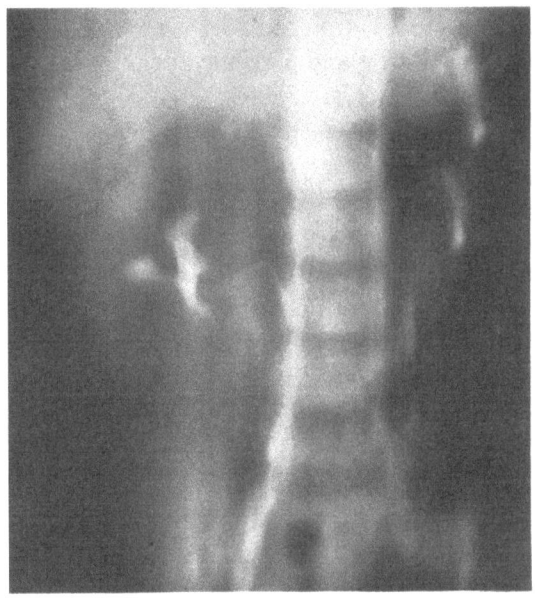

Fig. 9.34. Xanthogranulomatous pyelonephritis. This 3-year-old had right-sided abdominal pain, a mass on the right and pus cells in the urine. Nephrotomogram at IVU shows enlargement of the lower pole of the right kidney with distorted calyces. After nephrectomy histological examination confirmed the diagnosis

increase in the with of the perinephric space with rather dense opacification of the kidney cortex along the inner margin and the inflammatory tissue along the outer margin of the abscess.

Ultrasound study can be crucial in defining the spatial features and show the perinephric nature of the problem which characteristically has a reduced echo amplitude. A subcapsular haemorrhage may produce identical features at IVU and sonography.

9.3.10 Xanthogranulomatous Pyelonephritis

Commonly this is a feature of children who have calculus disease (Chapter 5) and a non-functioning kidney. However this is not invariably so (Fig. 9.34). The lesion can occasionally be found in children who have impaired immune responses. The clinical presentation in these circumstances may be acute and associated with urinary tract infection. In children xanthogranulomatous pyelonephritis is often localized or segmental.

At IVU a local mass lesion [45, 46, 47] may be suggested by the findings. The sonogram shows a bizarre echo complex and this might be thought to support the possibility of a tumour. However, small cystic spaces (due to obstructed calyces) and highly echogenic areas with acoustic shadows (caused by small amounts of calcium which may not be visible

on a radiograph) alert the ultrasonographer to the possibility of this diagnosis.

These findings, placed in the clinical context, should heighten the index of suspicion for this lesion. Angiography is of very limited help for there is, as so often is the case in renal mass lesions in children, no distinctive vascular pattern, although abnormal new vessels have been described.

Xanthogranulomatous pyelonephritis is the pathological term used to describe a condition whose precise causes lie well into the past and are often unknown and unknowable. In practical terms the lesion prior to excision is a mass lesion necessitating exploration and excision after its extent has been defined.

9.3.11 Trauma

When trauma has occurred a mass lesion in the vicinity of the kidney is not usually palpated. Intravenous urography and ultrasound studies are generally the first investigatory steps. Minor trauma can produce less severe degrees of damage such as subcapsular haematoma.

A late sequel of renal trauma may be a cyst within the kidney.

9.4 Extrinsic Malignant Masses Affecting the Kidney and Urinary Tract

9.4.1 Neuroblastoma

Neuroblastoma is a malignant tumour particularly associated with the sympathetic neural system and the adrenal medulla [1]. The tumour may develop primarily in the lower neck, thorax and abdomen. It is noted for its tendency to calcify and extend by direct spread so that an abdominal tumour mass traverses the diaphragm and invades the thorax. Metastasis is very common. Of radiological concern is the proclivity for bone metastases to develop; these may be lytic, sclerotic or of mixed form and they can be associated with periosteal new bone formation which may be the initial radiological finding. In the skull, suture widening can result from either raised intracranial pressure or direct erosion of suture margins. Liver enlargement follows the growth of deposits in the liver and direct invasion of a kidney may occur. Proptosis is a classic presenting feature of the disease and underlines the value of utilizing the contrast medium enhancement of a CT scan with a sequential radiograph of the abdomen to demonstrate any renal or ureteric displacement caused by the primary abdominal neuroblastoma.

Intravenous urogram series is often carried out as part of a study for an intra-abdominal mass lesion. Calcification in the tumour is quite commonly present. Neuroblastoma in the posterior abdominal wall displaces the intact kidney (Fig. 9.35). The primary displacement is lateral and because the tumour spreads across the retroperitoneal space both kidneys may be displaced (Fig. 9.36). There may be an element of rotation of either kidney and in addition displacement downward or less commonly upward. Upward extension of the tumour above the diaphragm into the thorax is common and is seen because of the wide paravertebral shadows.

When neuroblastoma arises in the adrenal there is an adrenal mass lesion which generally displaces the kidney downward and which may also rotate the kidney at IVU. Even in the presence of adrenal neuroblastoma the IVU may be normal [48], but echography will identify the lesion.

The urogram gives the diagnosis by inference drawn from the calcification which is so commonly present and the characteristic renal displacement. Extension into the paravertebral spaces alongside in the dorsal region may be seen on a chest radiograph. Since bone metastases are so very common with this tumour they must be carefully sought on all radiographs.

The tumour tends to invade the spinal canal. Erosion and reduction of the size of the pedicles can

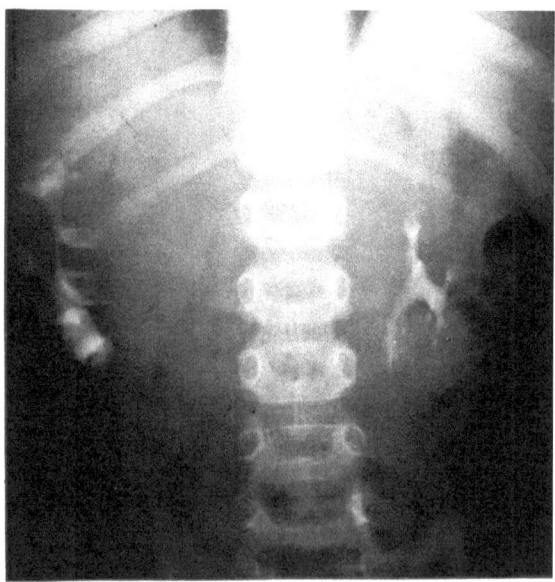

Fig. 9.35. Neuroblastoma. In this IVU the tumour displaces the right kidney, whose essential structure is intact. The left kidney is almost, but not quite, normally located. The differentiation from Wilms' tumour is clinched by the bilateral paravertebral shadows at D10-11 level

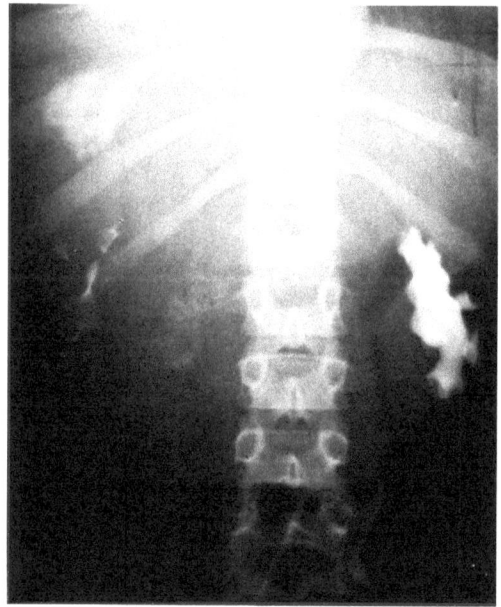

Fig. 9.36. Neuroblastoma. In this IVU the tumour contains areas of speckled calcification. The kidneys are intact structurally but grossly displaced laterally. The left kidney shows some obstruction of its collecting system and its ureter is displaced laterally. The right kidney is compressed by the tumour and its ureter too is displaced. Extension into the thorax is present because of the paravertebral shadow to the left of the dorsal spine

suggest this has occurred. On lateral and oblique views of the spine there may be an increase in the size of the exit foramina. These spinal features are all too often associated clinically with either paraparesis or frank paraplegia because of spinal cord compression. CT scan of the spine and its canal can confirm the problem.

Neuroblastoma in the posterior abdominal wall is a very echogenic tumour (Fig. 9.37, 9.38). Large deposits of calcium produce acoustic shadows. An IVU gives information about the extent of the lesion only by inferences drawn from displacement of the kidneys and bone changes. Sonograms define the degree of invasiveness of the lesion locally. Metastases to the liver and extension into the kidney can be kidney can be detected on sonograms. Prospects for resection of the lesion are determined by the extent of its localization and by the presence of metastases. Not all patients with retroperitoneal neuroblastoma have a tumour in the abdomen which is clinically recognisable. The first sign may be a secondary deposit in bone. In an isotope study of any patient suspected of bone disease it is always important to do an early blood pool phase. Neuroblastoma is noted for its ability to accumulate a bone-seeking isotope at this stage of the examination (Fig. 9.38). In this way the true cause of a bone lesion can be defined on occasion.

Nearly all children with neuroblastoma have elevated excretion of catecholamines or their derivatives and so this is an important screening test.

9.4.2 Hodgkin's Disease

Hodgkin's disease has an interesting epidemiology. Two peaks of incidence are found; the first is in the

▷

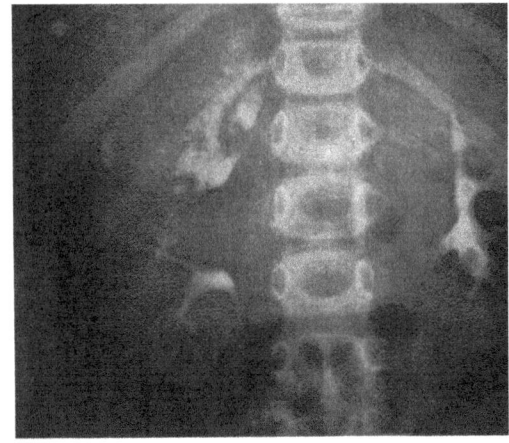

a

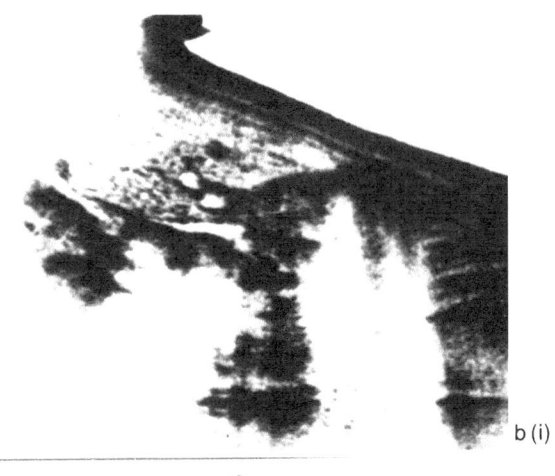

b (i)

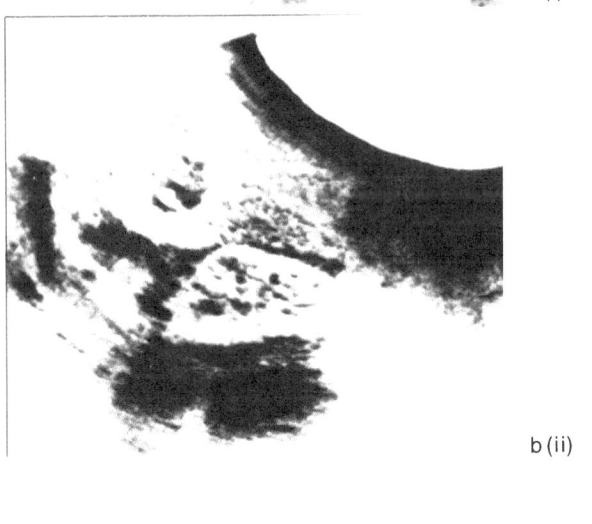

b (ii)

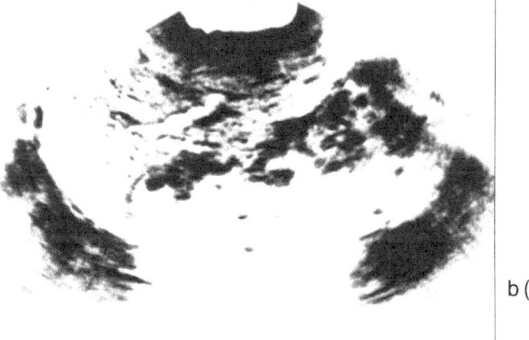

b (iii)

Fig. 9.37 a, b. Neuroblastoma. **a** This girl presented with headache and anorexia. The IVU shows extensive non-homogeneous calcification in the right side. The left kidney is normal in structure but slightly laterally placed. The right kidney is displaced downward and rotated by the right tumour originating in the right adrenal. Tumour spread is extensive and is responsible among the other features for the paravertebral shadow lying to the left of the spine in the thorax. **b** Ultrasound: (i) LS supine. The inferior vena cava is compressed from behind by a mass of highly echogenic character casting a dense acoustic shadow. (ii) LS supine through the right kidney. The acoustic density of the mass is again shown. Compare its shadow to that of the kidney. (iii) TS supine shows the echogenic tumour. The inference was that this was a lesion of the right adrenal gland containing calcium – a neuroblastoma in the clinical context

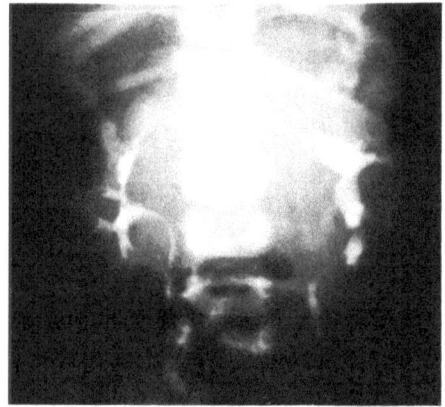

a

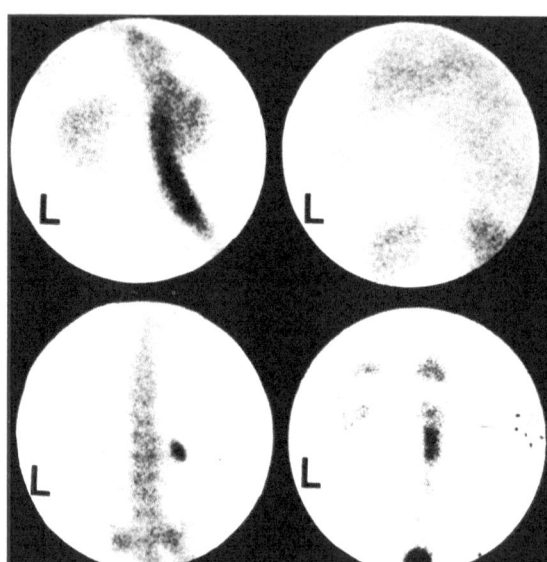

b

c

Fig. 9.38 a–c. Neuroblastoma. A 2-year-old boy who had diarrhoea for 4 days and progressive abdominal swelling for 1 week. He was found to have an abdominal mass on examination. IVU (**a**) shows a central abdominal mass extending to the left with compression of the left kidney and enlargement of this kidney. Note the calcification in the left suprarenal area. **b** Isotope scan: Tc99m polyphosphate. Images I and II: blood pool with deviated inferior vena cava and an avascular mass. Images III and IV show isotope within the tumour and a secondary deposit in the upper end of the right tibia respectively. **c** Ultrasound LS supine left flank. There is a large multilobulate mass squashing the left kidney

second half of childhood and adolescence and the second peak occurs in old people.

Staging of this disease is important for the prognosis is in part related to the stage found at presentation [49].

Stage I. Involvement of a single lymph node region (I) or a single extra lymphatic organ or site (IE).

Stage II. Involvement of two or more lymph node regions on the same side of the diaphragm (II) or localised involvement of extra-lymphatic organ or site and of one or more lymph node regions on the same side of the diaphragm (IIE).

Stage III. Involvement of lymph node regions on both sides of the diaphragm (III) which may also be accompanied by localised involvement of extra-lymphatic origin or site (IIIE) or involvement of the spleen (IIIS) or both (IIISE).

Stage IV. Diffuse or disseminated involvement of one or more extra-lymphatic organs or tissues with or without associated lymph node involvement.

From this description of the staging of this reticuloendothelial tumour it is clear that the kidney and urinary tract may be involved. Of all children with Hodgkin's disease the IVU is abnormal in about 30% [49]. Retroperitoneal lymph nodes are involved in about 30% of children (see Fig. 9.40). Retroperitoneal masses may be studied by several techniques, an IVU series including plain film studies, CT scanning, lymphography, ultrasonics and isotope techniques, but if the lesion is confined to structures below the diaphragm the diagnosis is made by histological examination of material obtained at surgery. Therefore, there should be a reasonable limit placed on investigatory routines.

Of all possible investigations lymphography is perhaps the most time consuming and it does not establish the diagnosis. At ultrasonography the finding of exceptionally echo-free tissue masses in the posterior abdominal wall can be very helpful in leading to the next diagnostic step (Fig. 9.41). Sonography can also show involvement of the kidney, liver and spleen. Intravenous urograms may give direct evidence of renal involvement and the course and displacement of the ureters can suggest the presence of large retroperitoneal nodes.

Obviously once the diagnosis is suspected and then established a complete investigatory protocol must be followed to stage the lesion accurately. Such a

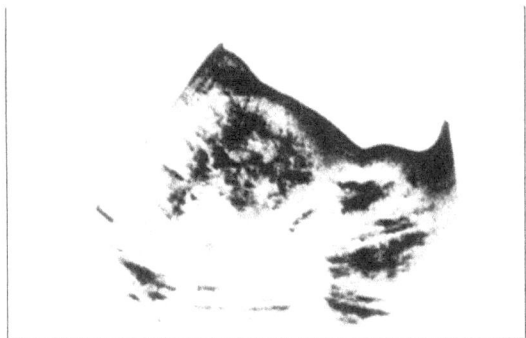

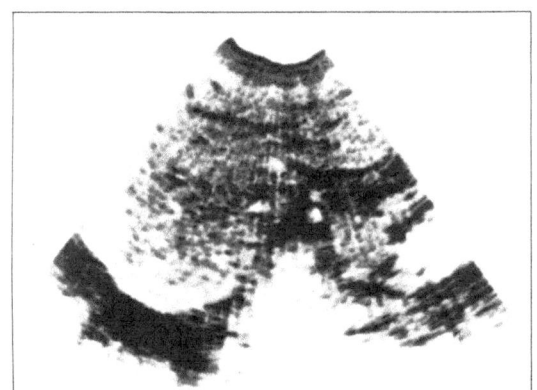

Fig. 9.39. a Age 3 -years: Large neuroblastoma. LS supine. The kidney is displaced inferiorly by a large mass containing many high-amplitude echoes with distal acoustic shadowing, suggesting a considerable degree of calcium deposition and therefore a possible neuroblastoma. This was confirmed histologically. b Age 4 years: small neuroblastoma. TS supine scan, upper abdomen. This boy presented with fever and a bone lesion. The IVU was normal with the exception of slight displacement of the upper pole of the left kidney. Ultrasound revealed a 2-cm solid mass in the position of the left adrenal. Diagnosis: neuroblastoma

protocol must include examining the chest and bones, quite apart from what may emerge from clinical findings.

9.4.3 Non Hodgkin's Lymphoma

In children non-Hodgkin's lymphoma tends to be more pervasive than Hodgkin's disease from the outset [49], with perhaps one exception; this is ileocoecal lymphosarcoma. Whilst the prognosis in Hodgkin's disease may be good the same cannot be said for non-Hodgkin's lymphoma in general.

Within this disease group lie what in former times were known as lymphosarcoma and reticulosarcoma. The initial presentation may, as in Hodgkin's disease, be with an abdominal mass and investigation routines are similar. Patients who present

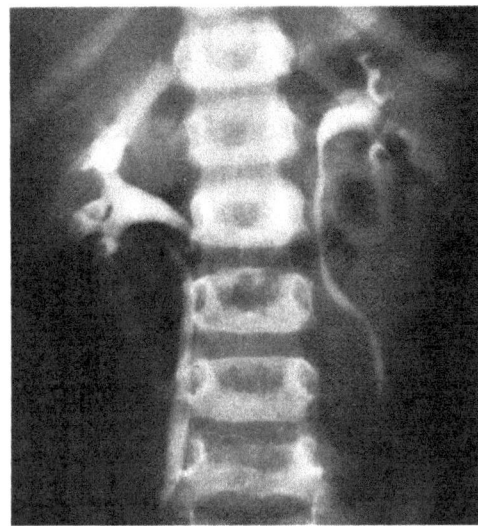

Fig. 9.40. Non-Hodgkin's lymphoma. The nodes in the paravertebral region have deviated the left ureter on this urogram. Sometimes in the reticuloses the ureter may be completely or partially obstructed. However, all the renal and ureteric features seen on IVU fail to display the situation cephalad, so such studies have distinct limitations when assessing lymphoma. Other modes of investigation are much more helpful in themselves and as an adjunct

with lymphoma in the ileum and caecum may have a lesion which occludes the lumen of the right ureter and so an obstructed or non-functioning kidney is present. Alternatively this mass may simply displace the right kidney cephalad.

9.4.4 Hepatoblastoma

This tumour is an important cause of a mass lesion in childhood. It may calcify. The important information needed is that which ensures the lesion is a primary liver lesion and not a metastasis from another primary source such as neuroblastoma.

Massive enlargement of the liver such as is found in hepatoblastoma may displace the kidney slightly upwards or downwards and this is shown on IVU. The large liver may also squash the kidney because of the size of the liver, and the kidney may be seen with great clarity on a radiograph because of the homogenous tissue which encompasses the kidney. However, ultrasonics study defines the intrinsic hepatic nature of the problem and excludes a primary retroperitoneal lesion such as neuroblastoma. Together, an IVU and sonography provide that information related to the liver lesion which is essential before surgical exploration can proceed. Scintigrams may define further the nature of the problem.

9.4.5 Teratomas

These tumours are most commonly found in infancy in the pelvic region. Provided the lesion can be removed in its entirety the prognosis is not unfavourable. An IVU is generally carried out to help define (by inference) the extent of the lesion and ultrasonics study gives additional information of a direct nature as in ovarian cysts and dermoids. Although teratomas commonly arise as sacrococcygeal tumours or ovarian tumours, this is not invariably so and lesions arising from the posterior abdominal wall should be anticipated (Fig. 9.42) [49].

9.5 Extrinsic Benign Masses Affecting the Kidney and Urinary Tract

9.5.1 Enlargement of Liver and Spleen

Gross enlargement of either the liver or spleen may displace the kidney on the side of the mass either upward or downward to a minor degree. When only one of these viscera is enlarged the kidney on that side may be squashed by the mass and appear to be increased in size on an intravenous urogram (Fig. 9.43). However the contour of such a kidney is smooth and the calyces are normally distributed within the kidney outline. Furthermore, echography will clearly show the nature of the problem and confirm the essential normality of the kidney (Fig. 9.43).

9.5.2 Neurofibromatosis

Large neurofibromatous masses may develop in the posterior abdominal wall and pelvis. These masses may (i) displace a kidney or ureter, (ii) narrow a

renal artery, (iii) be associated with abdominal aortic coarctation, (iv) have a concomitant phaeochromocytoma or other endocrinological problems, (v) extensively infiltrate the pelvis, narrowing and displacing the rectum forward from the sacrum and elevating the base of the bladder and narrowing the lower ends of the ureters [51].

These masses of neurofibromatous tissue may be the first and dominant clinical manifestation of this generalised disease.

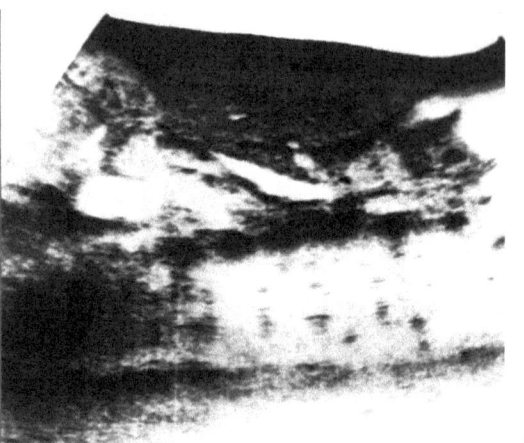
a

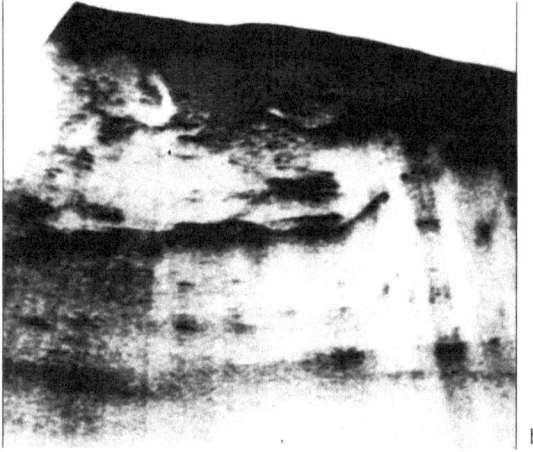
b

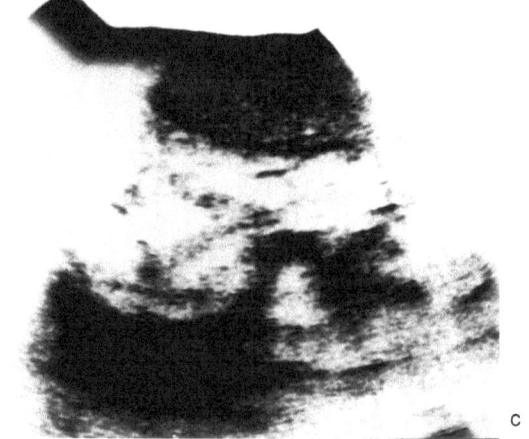
c

▷

Fig. 9.41 a–c. Retroperitoneal and mediastinal lymphomatous nodes. Age 4. **a** LS supine echogram. This child presented with fever, pleural effusion and an abdominal mass. The echogram shows the IVC displaced by a large relatively echolucent retroperitoneal mass extending into the mediastinum. **b** (Same case) LS supine through the aortic region. Note how the mass is echolucent despite the high sensitivity setting. This feature and the lobulated appeareance is characteristic of lymphoma. **c** (Same case) TS supine (30° tilt to the head). The large lower mediastinal mass is shown behind the left lobe of the liver. Such mediastinal enlargement is usually easily seen on a plain chest radiograph, but in this case the pleural effusions masked the shadows

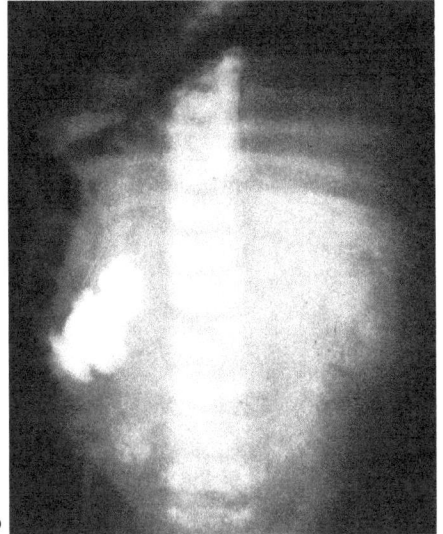
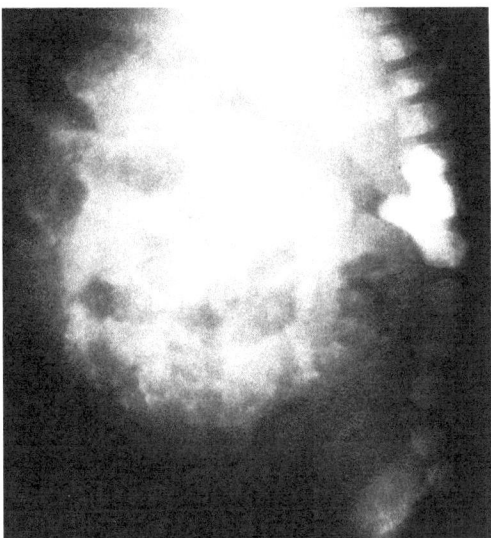

a, b

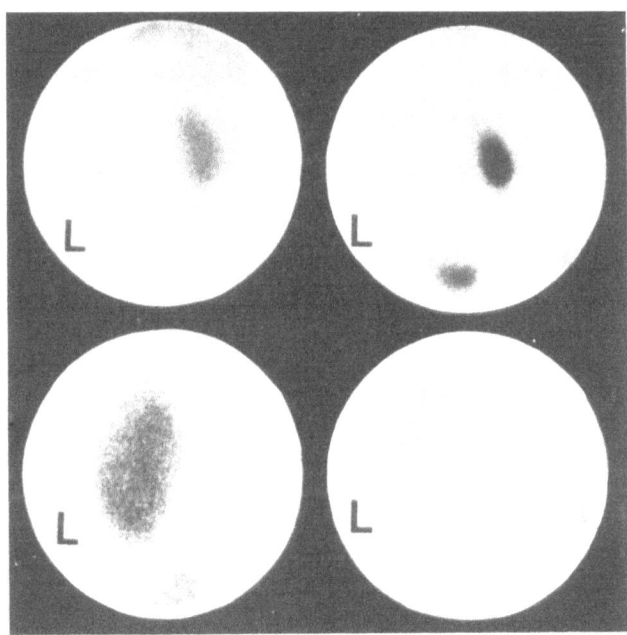

Fig. 9.42 a–c. Teratoma. This 18-month-old boy was found to have an abdominal mass. **a** The IVU at 2 h reveals a dilated collecting system on the right with malrotation of this kidney. Faint opacification of the left collecting system is visible. The calcification in the mass is well seen. **b** The lateral film reveals the anterior location of the mass containing calcification. **c** DTPA isotope scan shows prompt accumulation of isotope in the right kidney. The second image at 30 min shows hold-up of the isotope in the right renal pelvis. The third and fourth images were obtained at 3 h. These reveal isotope in a very dilated left renal pelvis. There is no extrarenal accumulation of isotope   c

9.5.3 Ganglioneuroma

This benign tumour has a similar derivation to that of neuroblastoma. Retroperitoneal ganglioneuroma causes displacement of posterior abdominal wall structures. Since it is truly benign total resection of the lesion may be feasible, but one of the main problems to look for is intraspinal extension (Fig. 9.44) as in neuroblastoma [52].

9.5.4 Parapelvic Cyst

These cystic lesions lie in the vicinity of the renal pelvis and produce an impression on the pelvis. They may be found incidentally on investigation of the urinary tract. Once discovered exploration and removal usually follows thereby establishing the diagnosis. Ultrasound can show the cystic nature of the lesion and may be used to guide aspiration needles for confirmatory diagnosis.

9.5.5 Hydrometrocolpos

When the lower genital tract in a femal infant or child is not canalized during development secretions accumulate because of the obstruction. A large cyst-like lesion then develops in the pelvis and this may obstruct the ureters which pass alongside the mass

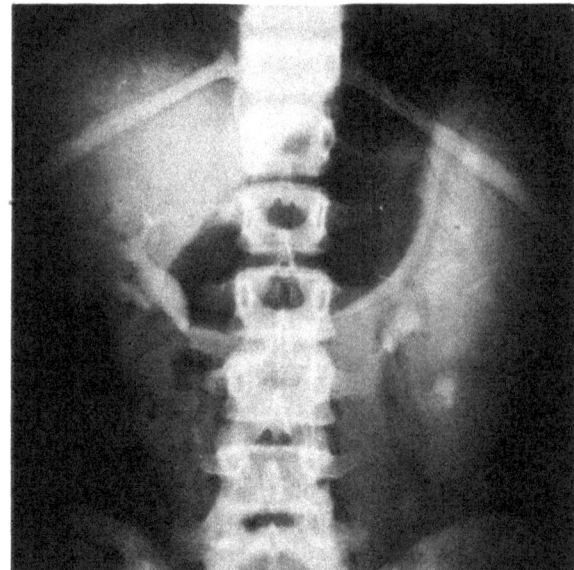

a

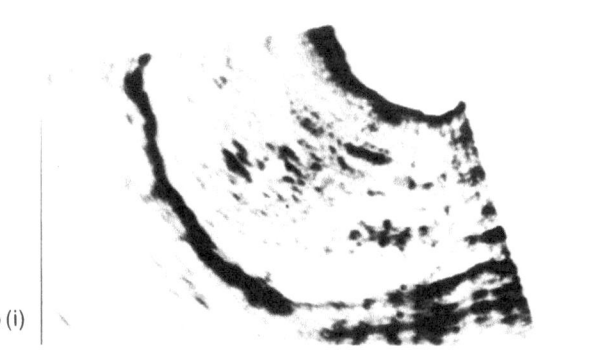

b (i)

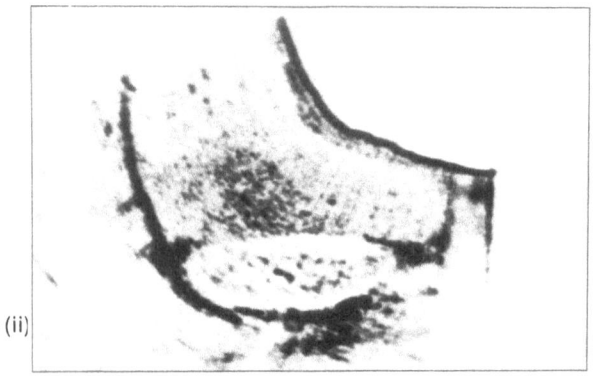

b (ii)

Fig. 9.43 a, b. The squashed kidney. **a** This child with gross splenic enlargement has a kidney which has been squashed with its contour enlarged and its calyces and pelvis compressed. Such changes can be seen at IVU in patients with gross splenic or liver enlargement from any cause. The kidney is not necessarily pathological because of its increase in size on AP projections **b** Ultrasound: (i) Squashed kidney. Age 5. LS supine through the right lobe of the liver, showing the normal kidney. (ii) [Same case as in (i)]. LS supine scan through the enlarged spleen and squashed left kidney

◁

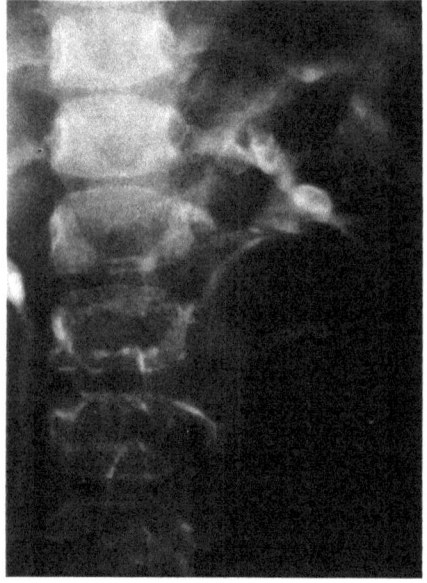

Fig. 9.44. Ganglioneuroma. The tumour has displaced and rotated the left kidney and the left ureter lies medially. Note the expansion of the spinal canal from D11 downwards and the marked thinning of the pedicles of the vertebral bodies associated with this lesion lying paravertebrally, in the exit foramina and intraspinally. Neurogenic tumours tend to invade the spinal canal

[53]. In the young infant this cystic mass lesion may participate in the whole-body opacification effect at IVU. Potentially, sonography should be diagnositc pre-operatively.

9.5.6 Large Ovarian Cysts and Dermoids

These lesions may present as large cystic masses. The dermoid may have the complex of tissue components so often associated with this lesion and these may be apparent at radiography. Ureteric displacement and extrinsic vesical compression may be a consequence of these lesions.

Echographically dermoids and teratomas are complex masses; however they may occasionally have features which suggest their true nature. They often contain pockets of fluid of variable size and number with well-defined margins around these fluid collections. Necrotic liquefied tumours and abscesses usually have poorly defined margins. Dermal elements within the mass manifest themselves either as high amplitude echo areas casting shadows (teeth) or as horizontal levels within cystic spaces which demonstrate gravitational shift (hair floating at the bottom). Cartilage and bone rests are highly echogenic and cast acoustic shadows.

Septae within cystic areas are often thickened. This feature often denotes malignancy in other cystic tumours but must not be misinterpreted as such when teratodermoids are present.

Large teratodermoids can fill the abdomen and be mistaken for ascites with matted bowel.

9.5.7 Pelvic Abscess

Abscess localisation to the pelvis, which is a small structure in young patients, may displace and compress ureters. Clinical evaluation suggests the likely diagnosis. Among others, two causes for such abscesses may be sought; the primary lesion may be appendicitis going on to abscess formation [54] and the second is the unfortunately traumatic use of a rectal thermometer.

9.6 Strategy in Investigation

If, on clinical assessment, a child has an abdominal mass which seems likely to be related to the posterior abdominal wall it is essential to take into account all the clinical facets when interpreting the findings from investigation. Age is important. The multicystic kidney, the mesoblastic nephroma and renal venous thrombosis occur especially in the very young infant. Wilms' tumour has a peak incidence between 2 and 7 years of age. Fever and anaemia are found both in Wilms' tumour and in sepsis, although a considerable polymorphonuclear leucocytosis should point to an infective problem. However, protracted infection (as in pyonephrosis or diffuse multiple renal abscess formation) may have only low-grade systemic effects. The duration of illness is of limited help; at times serious malignancy may be manifest for only a few days prior to clinical presentation or alternatively the history may be very much longer [55]. Careful evaluation of the family history may suggest a familial problem, as in cystic disease of various types. Certain conditions, for example echinococcosis, occur more commonly in some parts of the world. Urinalysis is mandatory but the immediate results are not always instantly helpful: haematuria may occur in Wilms' tumour, hydronephrosis and renal venous thrombosis; not all children with renal infection, even acute infection, have bacteria in the urine or urinary infection at the outset.

Chest radiographs may show pleural effusion, pulmonary metastases, direct upward extension into the thorax or concomitant supradiaphragmatic involvement in, forexample, lymphoma and leukaemia. Certain infective conditions, such as tuberculosis, echinococcosis and multifocal staphylococcal disease, may have both pulmonary and renal manifestations. In bacterial endocarditis (with or without an associated cardiomyopathy) blood culture may be difficult to interpret when antibiotics have been given in the very recent past.

In the vast majority of patients presenting for the first time the chest radiograph, echography and IVU [56] should make it possible to decide the following issues – namely whether the lesion is extrarenal, intrarenal or intrarenal with associated extrarenal problems. These issues may be viewed against the matrix presented in the context of this chapter. Once the anatomical location has been defined attention must be directed to the possibilities of the lesion being neoplastic (either malignant or benign), obstructive, inflammatory or infective, vascular, or an inherent abnormality of renal development.

Where the lesion is clearly intrarenal the most careful study of the contralateral kidney is imperative because prognosis is so very often determined by it. Clearly if the contralateral kidney is normal this is helpful, but not all such apparently normal kidneys are actually normal – for example Wilms' tumour and cystic disease may be cryptically bilateral. When the contralateral kidney is large and compensatory hypertrophy could be present this suggests a longstanding lesion in the affected kidney (such as severe hydronephrosis or pyonephrosis) may be present.

A presumptive diagnosis based on the investigatory findings taken in conjunction with the clinical context is then possible. In terms of management of the renal problem the decision as to an initially medical or surgical approach can then be made. When the decision favours a surgical course of action it is generally essential to determine whether total nephrectomy has to be undertaken or if partial nephrectomy will suffice. Not all patients with renal mass lesions require total nephrectomy. But it is imperative, if partial nephrectomy is contemplated, to know what functional value may be placed on any likely residual kidney remnant and for this assessment DMSA radioisotope studies are very helpful. Biopsy of renal mass lesions can have an important role in providing a tissue diagnosis in patients suspected of having advanced malignancy or adult-type polycystic disease.

In general the evidence is sufficiently clear cut to determine the course of action to be pursued expeditiously. Nevertheless, in uncommon or uncertain circumstances precipitate nephrectomy must be avoided and broadly two conditions, above others, present such uncertainties; these are certain variants of cystic disease and diffuse renal infection with multiple renal abscesses, and, in both renal function at IVU may be surprisingly and deceptively good.

References

1. Marsden, H. B., Steward, J. K.: Renal tumours. In: Recent results in cancer research. Vol. 13: Tumours in Children, 2nd ed. Marsden, H. B., Steward, J. K. (eds.), p. 327. Berlin, Heidelberg, New York: Springer 1976
2. Shashikumar, V. L., Somers, L. A., Pilling, G. P., Cresson, S. L.: Wilms' tumor in the horseshoe kidney. J. Pediatr. Surg. 9, 185 (1974)
3. Miller, R. W., Fraumeni, J. F., Manning, M. D.: Association of Wilms' tumour with aniridia hemitrypertrophy and other congenital malformations. N. Engl. J. Med. 270, 922 (1964)
4. Fraumeni, J. F., Geiser, C. F., Manning, M. D.: Wilms' tumor and congenital hemihypertrophy report of five new cases and review of literature. Pediatrics 40, 886 (1967)
5. Mankad, V. N., Gray, G. F., Miller, D. R.: Bilateral nephroblastomatosis and Klippel Trenaunay, syndrome. Cancer 33, 1462 (1974)
6. Cochran, W., Froggott, P.: Bilateral nephroblastoma in two sisters. J. Urol. 97, 216 (1967)
7. Sukarochana, K., Tolentino, N., Kiesenetter, W. B.: Wilms' tumour and hypertension. J. Pediatr. Surg. 7, 573 (1972)
8. Mitchell, J. D., Baxter, T. J., Blair-West, J. R., McCreddie, D. A.: Renin levels in nephroblastoma. Arch. Dis. Child. 45, 376 (1970)
9. Cope, J. R., Roylance, J., Gordon, I. R.: The radiological features of Wilms' tumour. Clin. Radiol. 23, 331 (1972)
10. Hunig, R., Kinser, J.: Ultrasonic diagnosis of Wilms' tumors. Am. J. Roentgenol. 117, 119 (1973)
11. Fay, R., Brosman, S., Williams, D. I.: Bilateral nephroblastoma. J. Urol. 110, 119 (1973)
12. Ragat, A. H., Vietti, T. J., Crist, W., Perez, C., McAllister, W.: Bilateral Wilms' tumour: a review. Cancer 30, 983 (1972)
13. Garrett, R. A., Donohue, J. P.: Bilateral Wilms' tumors. J. Urol. 120, 586 (1978)
14. Pagano, F., Pennelli, N.: Ureteral and vesical metastases in nephroblastoma. Br. J. Urol. 46, 409 (1974)
15. Anselmi, G., Suarez, J. A., Machado, I., Moleiro, R., Blancho, P.: Wilms' tumour propagated through the inferior vena cava into the right heart cavities. Br. Heart J. 32, 575 (1970)
16. McDonald, P., Hiller, H. G.: Angiography in abdominal tumours in childhood with particular reference to neuroblastoma and Wilms' tumour. Clin. Radiol. 19, 1 (1968)
17. Follin, J.: Angiography in Wilms' tumor. Acta Radiol. [Diagn.] (Stockh.) 8, 201 (1968)
18. Clark, R. E., Moss, A. D., Lorimier, A. A. de, Palubinskas, A. J.: Arteriography of Wilms' tumor. Am. J. Roentgenol. 113, 476 (1971)
19. Arneil, G. C., Harris, F., Emmanuel, I. G., Young D. G., Flatman, G. E., Zachary, R. B.: Nephritis in two children after irradiation and chemotherapy for nephroblastoma. Lancet 1974 I, 960
20. Bolande, R. P., Brough, A. J., Izart, R. J.: Congenital mesoblastic nephroma of infancy. Pediatrics 40, 272 (1967)
21. Keeling, J. W., Hilton, C.: Neonatal renal tumours. Br. J. Urol. 46, 157 (1974)
22. Berdon, W. E., Wigger, H. J., Baker, D. H.: Fetal renal hamartoma – a benign tumour to be distinguished from Wilms' tumour. Am. J. Roentgenol. 118, 18 (1973)
23. Favara, B. B., Johnson, W.: Renal tumors in neonatal period. Cancer 22, 845 (1968)
24. Cassady, J. R. Carcinoma of kidney in children. Radiology 112, 691 (1974)
25. Fisher, R. G.: Renal adenocarcinomain adolescence and childhood: emphasis on angiographic findings. J. Urol. 118, 83 (1977)
26. Benz, G., Brandeis, W. E., Willich, E.: Radiological aspects of leukaemia in childhood; an analysis of 89 children. Pediatr. Radiol. 4, 201 (1976)
27. Jaffe, N., Teft, M.: Unsuspected lymphosarcoma of kidneys diagnosed as bilateral Wilms' tumour. J. Urol. 110, 593 (1973)
28. Dunnick, N. R., Cunningham, J. J.: Burkitt's lymphoma involving the kidney. J. Urol. 112, 394 (1974)
29. Lamm, D. L., Kaplan, G. W.: Urological manifestations of Burkitt's lymphoma. J. Urol. 112, 402 (1974)
30. McCullogh, D. L., Scott, R., Seybold, H. M.: Renal angiomyolipoma (hamartoma), review of literature and report of 7 cases. J. Urol. 105, 32 (1971)
31. Gharbi, H. A., Ben Cheikh, M., Hamza, R., Jeddi, M., Hamza, B., Jedidi, H., Bendridi, M. F.: Les localisations rares del'hydatidose chez l'enfant. Ann. Radiol. (Paris) 20, 151 (1977)
32. Saidi, F.: Surgery of hydatid disease, p. 322. London, Philadelphia, Toronto: Saunders 1976
33. Babcock, D. S., Kaufman, L., Cosnow, I.: Ultrasound diagnosis of hydatid disease (echinococcosis) in two cases. Am. J. Roentgenol. 131, 895 (1978)
34. Nusbacher, N., Bryk, D.: Hydronephrosis of the lower pole of the duplex kidney: another pseudotumour. Am. J. Roentgenol. 130, 967 (1978)
35. Eklöf, O.: Radiological aspects of benign renal mass lesions in infancy and early childhood. Pediatr. Radiol. 1, 53 (1973)
36. Parker, J. A., Lebowitz, R., Mascatello, V., Treves, S.: Magnification renal scintigraphy in the differen-

tial diagnosis of septa of Bertin. Pediatr. Radiol. **4**, 157 (1976)

37. Pollack, H. M., Edell, S., Morales, J. O.: Radionucleide imaging in renal pseudotumor. Radiology **111**, 639 (1974)

38. Flynn, V. J., Gittes, R. F.: Benign cortical rest: "pseudotumor of the kidney". J. Urol. **108**, 54 (1972)

39. Lima, A. C. De, Iker, M., Burros, H. M., Keenan, G. R.: Renal pseudotumor: importance of selective arteriogram. Urology **5**, 572 (1975)

40. Friedland, G. W., Filly, R.: Appearing and disappearing calyces. Pediatr. Radiol. **1**, 237 (1973)

41. Moenne-Lecloz, J. P., Bomsel, F., Gatti, J. M., Prot, D.: Renal abscess in children. Pediatr. Radiol. **7**, 150 (1978)

42. Lebowitz, R. L., Fellows, K. E., Colodney, A. H.: Renal parenchymal infection in children. Radiol. Clin. North Am. **15**, 37 (1977)

43. Simonovits, D. A., Reyes, H. M.: Renal abscess mimicking a Wilms' tumour. J. Pediatr. Surg. **11**, 269 (1976)

44. Segura, J. W., Panayotis, P.: Localised renal parenchymal infection in children. J. Urol. **109**, 1029 (1970)

45. Shanser, J. D., Herzog, K. A., Palubinskas, A. J.: Xanthogranulomatous pyelonephritis in childhood. Pediatr. Radiol. **3**, 12 (1975)

46. Gravier, L., Vargas, M. A.: Xanthogranulomatous pyelonephritis in childhood. Am. J. Dis. Child. **123**, 156 (1972)

47. Fahr, K., Oppermann, M. C., Schärer, K., Greinacher, I.: Xanthogranulomatous pyelonephritis in childhood: report of three cases and review of literature. Pediatr. Radiol. **8**, 10 (1979)

48. Haller, J. O., Berdon, W. E., Baker, D. H., Kassner, E. G.: Left adrenal neuroblastoma with normal appearing urogram. Am. J. Roentgenol. **129**, 1051 (1977)

49. Marsden, H. B., Steward, J. K.: Tumours of the sympathetic system. In: Recent results in cancer research, Vol. 13: Tumours in Children, 2nd ed. Marsden, H. B., Steward, J. K., (eds.), p. 194. Berlin, Heidelberg, New York: Springer 1976

50. deleted in production

51. Daneman, A., Gralton-Smith, P.: Neurofibromatosis involving the lower urinary tract in children: a report of three cases and a review of the literature. Pediatr. Radiol. **4**, 161 (1976)

52. Fagan, J., Swischuk, L. E.: Dumbell neuroblastoma or ganglioneuroma of the spinal canal. Am. J. Roentgenol. **120**, 451 (1974)

53. Young, L. W., O'Connell, D. J.: Hydrometrocolpos. Am. J. Dis. Child. **131**, 457 (1977)

54. Cooke, T. G.: Appendiceal abscess causing urinary obstruction. J. Urol. **10**, 212 (1969)

55. Rogers, P. C., Wood, B. J., Smith, D. F., Teasdale, J. M.: Slow growth of an untreated Wilms' tumour in the adolescent. Arch. Dis. Child. **53**, 822 (1978)

56. Micsky, L.: Optimal diagnosis of renal masses in children by combining and correlating sonography and radiography. Am. J. Roentgenol. **120**, 438 (1974)

10 Adrenal and Gonadal Lesions

10.1 Introduction

Neither the adrenals nor the gonads are part of the kidney or urinary tract. And yet their relationships to each other and the kidney are close, both medically and in terms of investigations. Two lesions which affect the adrenal, neuroblastoma and phaeochromocytoma, are dealt with in other sections (Chapter 9 and Chapter 11 respectively). Neuroblastoma commonly presents as a mass lesion, which may be already very extensive at the time of diagnosis. Phaeochromocytoma primarily, but not invariably, manifests its presence in the clinical feature of hypertension. Neither phaeochromocytoma nor neuroblastoma have the adrenal gland as their only site of origin.

One adrenal tumour, manifesting its presence with systemic hypertension, is Conn's syndrome with hyperaldosteronism. The diagnosis is established in the first instance by biochemical analysis.

In the newborn the adrenal is large and ordinarily it rapidly involutes after birth. During these early weeks of life it seems peculiarly vulnerable to haemorrhage in circumstances when the infant is under severe stress, as in the respiratory distress syndrome.

The endocrinological role of the normal adrenal gland can be pathologically altered, as in congenital adrenal hyperplasia. Cushing's syndrome may be a consequence of either bilateral hyperplasia or tumour; in children it is sometimes associated with elements of virilization in addition to the classic increased glucocorticoid output. In childhood, tumours of either the gonad or the adrenal may produce virilization or feminization as the primary presentation. Precocious puberty represents another feature of endocrinological disturbance. The biochemical investigation and evaluation of all these problems is complex and outside the scope of this text. The primary concern here is with the localization of the underlying lesion.

10.2 Tactics in Investigation of the Adrenal

10.2.1 Clinical Information

A close dialogue with the clinician is essential. The results of complex biochemical analyses can be interpreted in conjunction with the imaging studies. In this way a synthesis may be achieved and from this the diagnosis of the causative lesion and the next step in management follow.

10.2.2 Plain Radiographs

Plain films of the abdomen may show whether calcium has been deposited in the adrenal region. The character of the calcium may suggest the presence of a benign or malignant lesion.

10.2.3 Ultrasonography

Ultrasound may show whether enlargement is unilateral, as with a tumour, or bilateral as in hyperplasia. When ultrasound is available it is not essential to undertake an IVU, whose interpretation can be difficult. Additionally the femal genital pelvic organs can also be examined.

10.2.4 Scintigraphy

Isotope scanning is a protracted investigation because accumulation of the labelled substrate (for instance 17-substituted iodocholesterol) is a gradual process.
The information from such a study is functional and shows whether uptake is bilateral and symmetrical, indicating hyperplasia, or unilateral with poor uptake on the contralateral side indicating the presence of a tumour with suppression of the normal side.

10.2.5 Angiography

Modern imaging methods have made angiography of the adrenal, at least in children, almost superfluous. Its potential hazard is no longer justified. Perhaps there is still a place for venous sampling, especially in the ectopically situated adrenal tumour.

10.2.6 Retroperitoneal Gas Insufflation

Pneumography either by the presacral or direct retroperitoneal route is no longer necessary.

10.2.7 Computerized Tomography

The place of CT scanning of the paediatric adrenal gland would seem to be limited. It may be particularly useful in those cases of Cushing's syndrome in which adequate echograms are unobtainable because of the thickness of adipose tissue, a feature which specifically emphasises organ boundaries as shown by CT.

10.3 Adrenal Haemorrhage and Abscess

Adrenal haemorrhage is a particular feature of the infant or child who, classically, is subject to serious stress leading to a shock state. In the perinatal period the stress of delivery, apnoeic attacks and respiratory distress and sepsis provide the background for adrenal haemorrhage. However, it may be found in neonates who do not have such a

dramatic history. It is more common on the right. This is probably an effect of the difference in venous drainage. Among older children the classic adrenal haemorrhage is associated with meningococcal septicaemia. The reaction of the adrenal to a shock state is that of hyperactivity and haemorrhage is a collateral event. Because of the stresses which may be associated with delivery and the sudden requirement for the newborn to survive independently, young infants are among the most commonly affected by adrenal haemorrhage.

10.3.1 Adrenal Haemorrhage

The large adrenal of the neonate increases in size as the haemorrhage within it develops [1, 2, 3]. Bleeding may extend from the adrenal into the peritoneal cavity, which fills with heavily blood-stained fluid. Once the infant enters a recovery phase the gland shrinks and it often starts to calcify within 2–3 weeks (Figs. 10.2 and 10.3). Such calcification tends to persist and it may be discovered as an incidental finding on chest or abdominal radiographs taken later in life, for example chest radiographs taken in the assessment of congenital heart disease. Perhaps surprisingly, overall adrenal function in the long term seems unimpaired by the acute catastrophe.
When considering the possibility of adrenal haemorrhage the clinical context must be to the fore. The adrenal mass may be palpable clinically. Traditionally an IVU series has established the diagnosis. The enlarged adrenal displaces the kidney downward and may rotate it slightly as well. Following the relatively large volume of contrast medium

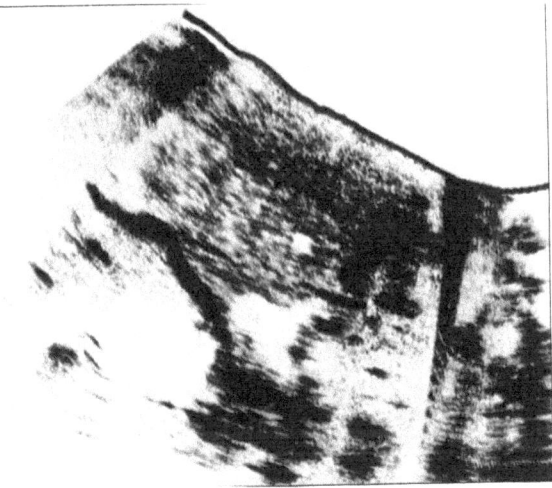

Fig. 10.1. Age 3 weeks. LS supine, showing a clearly visible slightly enlarged right adrenal gland

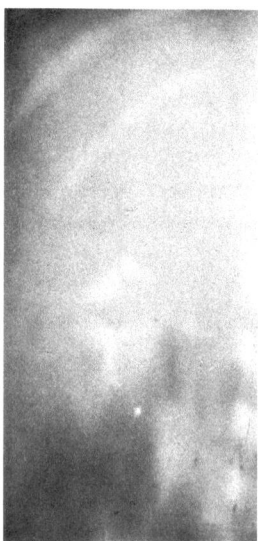
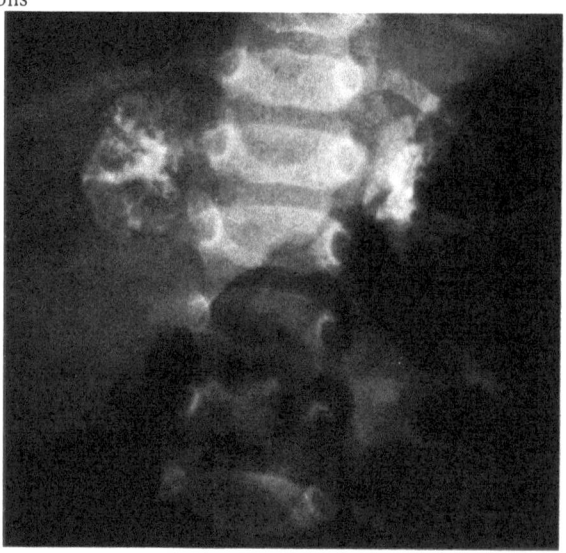

a, b

Fig. 10.2 a, b. Adrenal haemorrhage. **a** Rim along margin of haemorrhagic adrenal in a neonate on tomography at IVU. **b** Infant now aged 4 months with densely calcified adrenal glands as a late sequel to haemorrhage

injected for this study the adrenal may show a denser thin marginal rim with a relatively transradiant central zone on the radiograph: the *precise* reason for this pheomenon is related to the whole body opacification effect in some way or other, but this is not a constant finding in an adrenal which is the site of haemorrhage. Subsequent radiographs, often taken because of a respiratory problem, can show the development of calcification.

Adrenal haemorrhage may be accompanied by acute damage to the kidney and brain (Chapter 8). If haemorrhage occurs into the peritoneal cavity then, on radiographs taken with the infant in the supine position, the abdomen appears featureless except for the gas-containing loops of gut which lie centrally in the field. The gas seen in the gut may extend from the stomach only into the most proximal part of the small intestine: because of the shock state the infant ceases to swallow air and peristaltic activity is in abeyance.

10.3.2 Adrenal Abscess

Infants who suffer a shock in the perinatal period often are infected also. It might therefore be anticipated that infection of a haemorrhagic adrenal would be a quite common event but this is not so [4, 5]. Most infants with uncomplicated haemorrhage present with clinical features suggesting the lesion in the first 2 weeks or so, but when adrenal abscess has developed this lesion usually is delayed in its presentation until a later date (Fig. 10.4). As in adrenal

haemorrhage, the kidney is displaced downward by the adrenal mass and the abscess cavity in the adrenal may show as a thick dense rim surrounding a radiolucent centre at IVU.

When an abscess is present clinical signs of infection are also present and drainage of the lesion is carried out. If haemorrhage only has occurred it is the practice in some centres to drain the lesion but in others conservative measures are preferred.

In both adrenal abscess and adrenal haemorrhage intravenous urography may be completely replaced as a method of investigation by ultrasound exam-

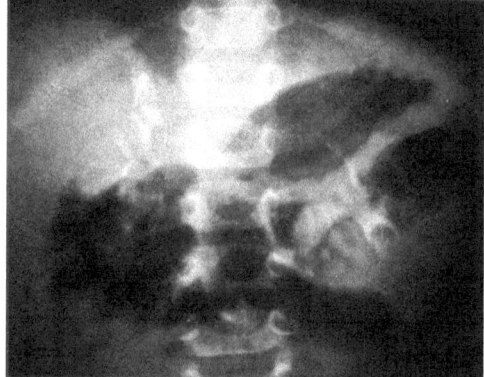

Fig. 10.3. Adrenal haemorrhage with renal vein thrombosis. This infant had an episode of intravascular coagulation resulting in right renal vein thrombosis and haemorrhage of the right adrenal gland. This IVU taken several months later demonstrates right adrenal gland calcification and atrophy of the right kidney. There is compensatory hypertrophy of the normal left kidney

ination. Intravenous urography and CT scanning are far from ideal methods of investigation in these critically ill infants. Radioisotope studies take too long to provide the answer at a time when it may be most critical.

10.4 Congenital Adrenal Hyperplasia (Adrenogenital Syndrome)

In essence, this condition is two-fold in its effect: there is a diminished production of cortisol by the adrenals and this insufficiency gives rise to the electrolyte problems encountered in the infant; there is an over-production of androgens which begins in foetal life.

Radiological examination may be sought to exclude lesions in the urinary tract and to help ensure that the lesion is truly bilateral hyperplasia rather than a tumour – but there is usually clear-cut evidence from other sources to suggest this anyhow. At IVU the adrenal glands in patients with congenital adrenal hyperplasia may show as a faint blush during the early nephrographic phase. Echograms show enlarged, relatively echolucent adrenals. In the neonatal period allowance must be made for the normal enlarged state of the adrenal.

Virilization occurs. In females the enlarged clitoris and the fused labial folds necessitate plastic surgical procedures. In male infants the virilizing effect may be delayed. In both sexes there is a tendency to accelerated skeletal maturation and, since the disorder is treated medically by steroids, patients with this disorder accumulate radiological records of skeletal maturation.

10.5 Cushing's Syndrome

This syndrome [7, 8, 9] may have as its cause either adrenal hyperplasia (Figs. 10.4 and 10.5) or an adrenal tumour. Tumour is the commoner lesion (Figs. 10.6 and 10.7). The clinical features of obesity, hypertension, osteoporosis, retarded skeletal maturation are familiar to all; sometimes signs of virilization may also be present.

The nature of the adrenal lesion can be established simply by ultrasound and intravenous urography in most patients. A tumour of one adrenal is accompanied by a small adrenal gland on the other side. If ultrasound is not available it can be helpful to carry

out tomography of the region during the nephrographic phase of the IVU and both antero-posterior and lateral tomograms can be helpful if there is difficulty in producing good direct radiographs of the regions. Sometimes the tumour lesion can extend forward over the anterior aspect of the kidney and lateral tomograms will elucidate such a feature. Displacement of the kidney on the side of a tumour may be minimal. When hyperplasia is present the adrenal glands are of equal size and no tumour is found.

A careful dialogue between the radiologist and paediatrician and paediatric surgeon must be initiated in all patients who have endocrinologically hyperactive adrenal lesions. Biochemical analysis with supression tests can usually differentiate between adrenal hyperplasia and tumour. This alerts the radiologist to the particular objective of investigation. If IVU results are unsatisfactory then sonography, isotope studies and CT scans should be sufficient to provide the essential information.

Adrenal tumours are frequently encapsulated and they can be resected completely. However, they may be locally invasive and ultimately metastasize. One complication of Cushing's syndrome, which has been mentioned in Chapter 5, is calculus formation in the urinary tract.

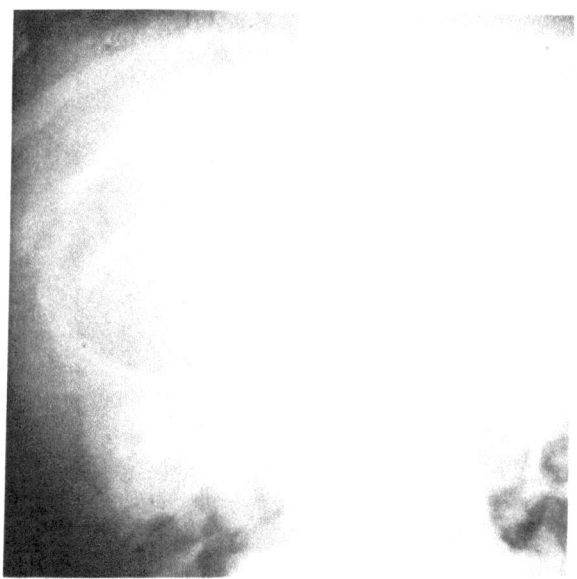

Fig. 10.4. Adrenal haemorrhage and abscess. IVU in a young infant shows the kidneys are displaced downward and rotated by the large haemorrhagic adrenal glands in an infant who had septicaemia. The adrenal is well seen on the right where it shows a central zone of increased transradiancy with a denser marginal rim opacified positively by contrast medium

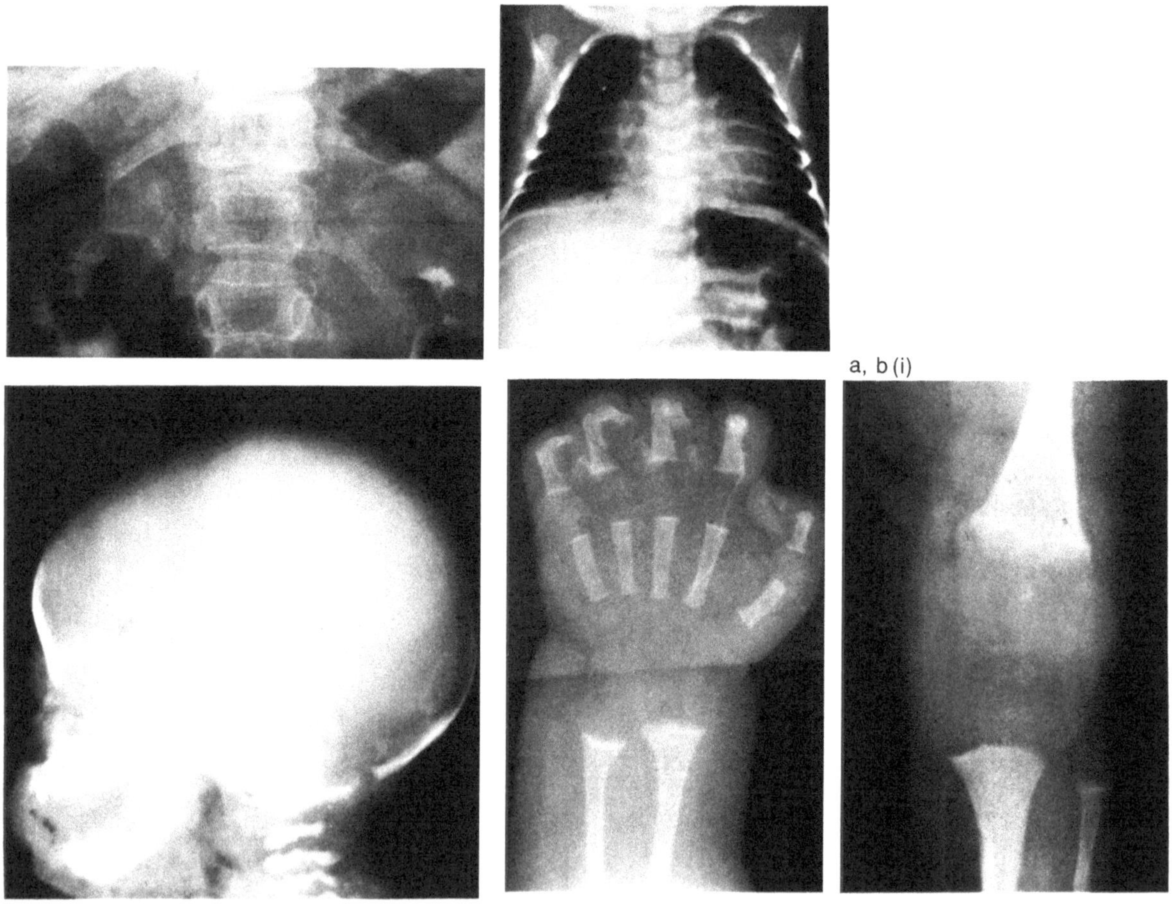

a, b (i)

Fig. 10.5. (Legend see page 171)   b (ii)   b (iii)   b (iv)

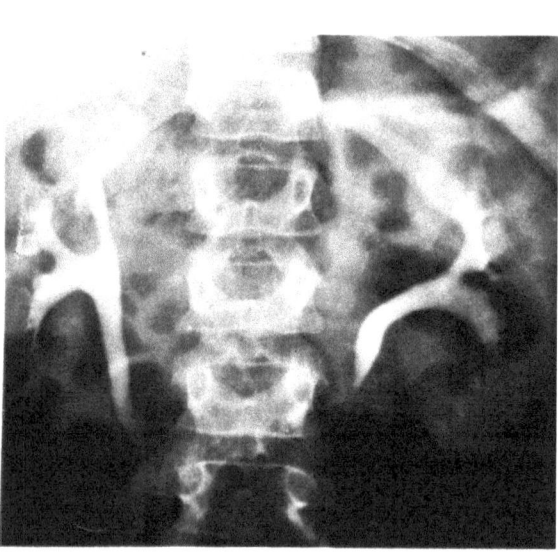

Fig. 10.6. Cushings's syndrome with left adrenal tumour. At IVU the right kidney is normally located, but the left kidney is displaced downward and slightly laterally by the left adrenal adenoma. The right kidney is normally positioned and the right adrenal is not large

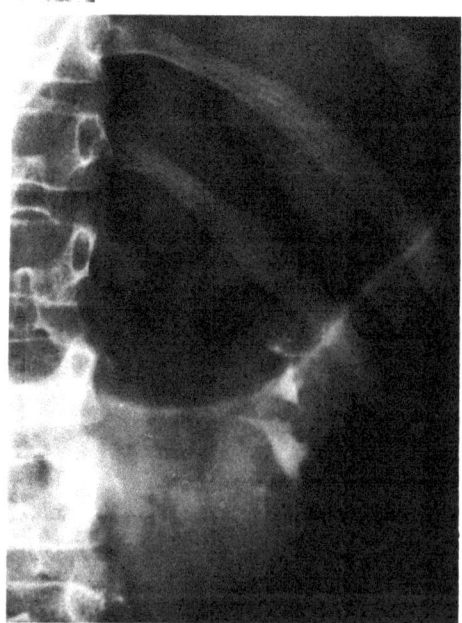

Fig. 10.7. Cushings's syndrome caused by left adrenal tumour. The adrenal adenoma is not calcified and lies above and slightly to the front of the left kidney. At IVU the tumour has displaced the left kidney downward

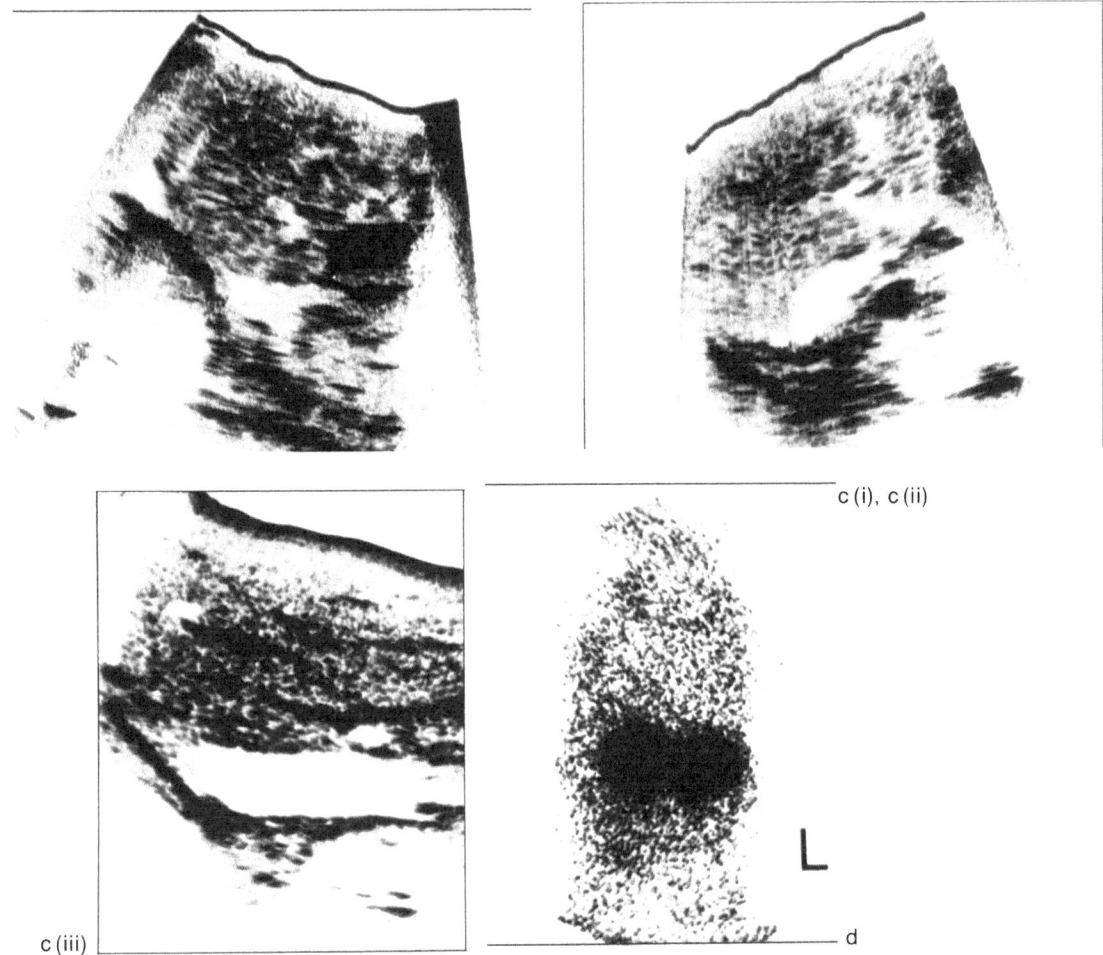

c (i), c (ii)

c (iii)

d

Fig. 10.5 a–d. Cushing's syndrome: methods of imaging in hyperplasia. **a** In this child at IVU both adrenal glands are seen. They are rather large and of equal size, synonymous with bilateral hyperplasia, confirmed by biochemical assay and isotope scan. **b** (i) Chest radiograph of a 4-week-old girl showing undermineralized gracile ribs. (ii) Skull radiograph showing poorly ossified bone and wide fontanelles. (iii) Left hand with very poorly mineralized and underdeveloped bones. (iv) Left knee, also showing poor development and undermineralization, delay in bone age (bone maturity 32 weeks). Note also the thick fat line and diminished muscle shadow **c** (i) LS supine echogram through the right liver a large echolucent adrenal capping the right kidney. (ii) TS supine echogram shows the enlarged right adrenal under the liver. The left adrenal could not be demonstrated with such clarity but was thought to be enlarged. (iii) Age 10 years. Normal right adrenal (for comparison). Tilted LS supine echogram through the left lobe of the liver and IVC showing the upper pole of the right kidney capped by the normal right adrenal. The adrenal medulla can be discerned within the more echolucent adrenal cortex. **d** Adrenal isotope scan using ^{75}Se-methionine iodocholesterol. Bilateral adrenal hyperplasia clearly demonstrated in the infant

10.6 Virilizing and Feminizing Tumours of the Adrenal Gland or Gonad

10.6.1 The Clinical Problem

Preoccupation with sex can start at an early age and it can be very serious if there are clinical signs that boys are feminizing or girls virilizing, or if puberty is precocious. Intensive hormonal assays invariably ensue.

10.6.2 Virilization

Virilization in boys has different consequences from girls but certain lesions are common to both sexes [10]. Advanced skeletal maturation is often present.

Adrenal adenoma [10] occurs as a cause of virilization more commonly in girls than boys, and it is benign (Fig. 10.8).

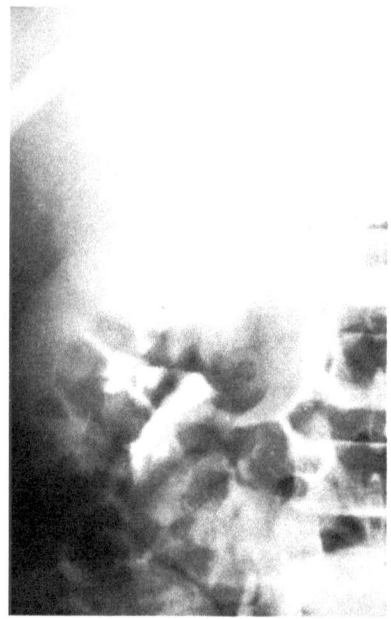

Fig. 10.8. Virilizing right adrenal adenoma in a boy. IVU shows the slightly calcified tumour lying above the right kidney. The right kidney is displaced downward and slightly rotated by the adenoma

Adrenal carcinoma [10] is a rare cause of virilization in either sex (Fig. 10.9).

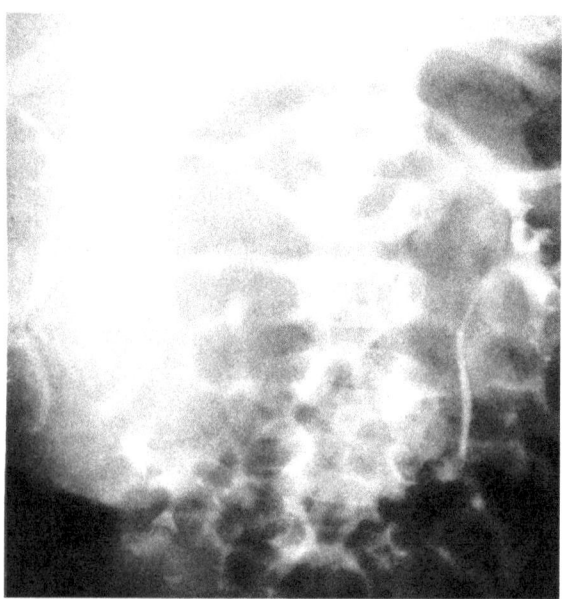

Fig. 10.9 Virilizing right adrenal carcinoma in a young girl. IVU shows a normally positioned left kidney, but the right kidney is displaced downward and rotated. The right adrenal tumour which is extensively calcified has caused this displacement

Gonadoblastoma [11, 12] in dysgenetic gonadal structures (ovary or testis) is a malignant lesion metastasizing to liver and lung. It is sometimes associated with virilization.

Androblastoma [13] (arrhenoblastoma) occurs in the ovaries of girls. The tumour may be benign or malignant and virilization may occur.

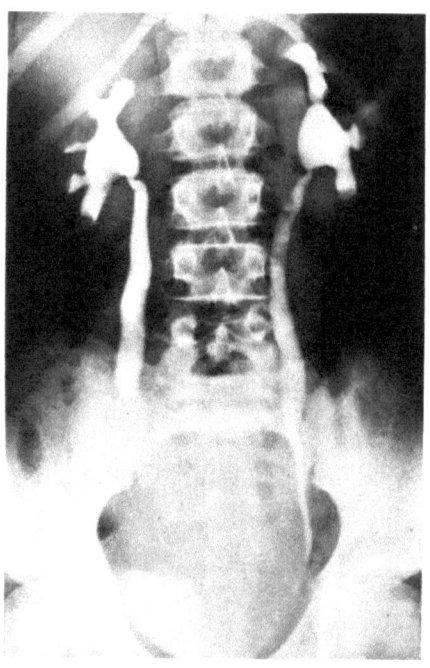

Fig. 10.10. Ovarian dysgerminoma. IVU shows the mass lesion in the pelvis, which compresses the bladder from above. Both ureters are compressed by the lesion at the pelvic brim, producing obstruction and upper tract dilatation, which is greater on the right side

10.6.3 Feminization

Feminization is associated with gynaecomastia in boys, but in girls it must be differentiated from precocious puberty.

Adrenal carcinoma [10] may cause feminization and this malignant lesion metastasizes to either the lungs or liver. Boys are more commonly affected than girls.

Adrenal adenoma [10] is a rare benign lesion causing feminization.

Sertoli cell tumour of testis [14] in males may be malignant and associated with feminization.

10.6.4 Precocious Puberty

Granulosa-Theca cell tumour [15] in the ovary of a girl is almost invariably a benign lesion and it causes precocious puberty.

Other lesions which cause precocious puberty include fibrous dysplasia and neurofibromatosis.

10.6.5 Role of Investigation

Obviously ultrasonics study, as in the adult patient, can be expected to identify a mass (if of sufficient size) in the ovary. In boys examination of the descended testis will indicate the lesion's site, should one be present, in the testis. These gonadal problems having been evaluated it may be, and very often is, important to study the adrenal glands. Since the lesion is commonly a tumour the question as to which adrenal is affected dominates the investigation. Ultrasonics and IVU and isotope scans will all identify the size of the affected adrenal gland in most instances, either directly or by inference. The main consideration is to decide whether there is hyperplasia (bilateral) or a tumour. Computerized tomographic study has a role also in this context. One thing is certain – there is now no place for any perirenal air insufflation studies and it is difficult to see how angiography can usefully add anything to the information derived from other modes of study.

10.7 Other Gonadal Lesions

Testicular lesions in the descended testis are clinically evident. Excluding such problems as mumps orchitis (rarely seen before puberty) and epidydimitis (which may be associated with maldevelopments of the urinary tract), the lesions of most concern are rare but significant; they include orchioblastoma [16], embryonic sarcoma (rhabdomyosarcoma), teratomas, seminomas [17], and lymphomas and leukaemia. In investigation the principal concern is to determine the extent of the lesion and spread to other sites such as para-aortic glands, lungs, liver and bone. The ways in which this is carried forward in principle can be found in Chapter 9.

After the sacrococcygeal location, the ovary is one of the commonest sites for teratomas (and der-

moids) to arise [18]. Teratomas, according to pathological study, are more commonly cystic than solid and frequently present as mass lesions palpable in the abdomen or pelvis. There may be associated abdominal pain of a continuing nature, or acute pain with vomiting when torsion of the tumour occurs. As with other pelvic lesions ultrasonics study should be able to localise the cause of the clinical problem and ectopic calcium in one form or another may be seen on plain radiographs of the pelvis and erect films may show a fat-water level.

Gonadoblastoma [11, 12] in a dysgenetic ovary or a testis has been discussed above, since it commonly occurs in phenotopic females who show signs of virilization.

Dysgerminomas [18] of the ovary, along with other ovarian lesions, may present with abdominal pain (which may be acute because of torsion) or a mass lesion. Precocious puberty may be present. However, in the paediatric age range these tumours, which follow a fairly benign course, are unlikely to present problems in diagnosis (Fig. 10.10).

Cystic ovarian benign tumours may, classically, present as large abdominal cystic mass lesions in childhood [19]. Again findings at investigation may determine what procedures may be necessary at subsequent laparotomy.

Finally there is a very tiny minority of congenital rest tumours including adrenal rest tumours, meso-metanephric rest tumours, and Brenner tumours which are extremely rarely found in childhood. Their adrenal, renal and ovarian connotations perhaps provide the aetiological raison d'etre for including lesions of the adrenal and gonad in this volume [20].

10.8 Conclusion

When the findings from (i) biochemical analyses and (ii) imaging are interpreted the conclusion about the underlying nature of the lesion will be obvious and the next step in management will logically follow. Although tumours may have a malignant type of appearance on histological examination, this is not necessarily reflected in the clinical course when complete excision of the local tumour produces a cure. Chest radiographs will show whether there are metastases but these are rare, as is a significantly elevated blood pressure. Echography provides a simple means of assessing the liver, and any possible lesions within it.

References

1. Black, J., Williams, D. I.: Natural history of adrenal haemorrhage in the newborn. Arch. Dis. Child. **48,** 183 (1973)
2. Eklöf, O., Grotte, G., Jonalf, H., Löhr, G., Ringertz, H.: Perinatal haemorrhage necrosis of the adrenal gland: a clinical and radiological evaluation of 24 consecutive cases. Pediatr. Radiol. **4,** 31 (1975)
3. Dickerman, J. D., Tampas, J. P.: Adrenal haemorrhage in the newborn. Clin. Pediatr. Phila. **16,** 314 (1977)
4. Stevenson, J., MacGregor, A. M., Connelly, P.: Calcification of the adrenal glands in young children. Arch. Dis. Child. **36,** 316–320 (1960)
5. Carty, A., Stanlex, P.: Bilateral adrenal abscesses in a neonate. Pediatr. Radiol. **1,** 63 (1973)
6. Favara, B. E., Akers, D. R., Franciosi, R. A.: Adrenal abscess in a neonate. J. Pediatr. **77,** 682 (1970)
7. Raiti, S., Grant, D. B., Williams, D. I., Newns, G. M.: Cushing's syndrome in childhood. Arch. Dis. Child. **47,** 597 (1972)
8. Gilbert, M. B., Cleveland, W. W.: Cushing's syndrome in infancy. Pediatrics **46,** 217 (1970)
9. Somers, S. C.: Adrenal glands. In: Pathology, 7th ed. Anderson, W. A. D. Kissane, J. M. (eds.), Vol. 2, p. 1658. St. Louis: Mosby 1977
10. Gyepes, M. T., Lindstrom, R. L., Merten, D., Goller, D., Lachman, R., Lippe, B.: Hormonally active adrenal adenomas and carcinomas in children. Ann. Radiol. (Paris) **20,** 123 (1977)
11. Scully, R. E.: Gonadoblastoma: a review of 74 cases. Cancer **25,** 1340 (1970)
12. Krause, F. T.: Ovary. In: Pathology, 7th ed. Anderson, W. A. D., Kissane, J. M. (eds.), Vol. 2, p. 1734. St. Louis: Mosby 1977
13. Teilum, G.: Acta Endocrinol. (Kbh.) **4,** 43 (1950)
14. Brown, N. J., Langley, F. A.: Teratomas and other genital tumours. In: Recent results in cancer research, Vol. 13: Tumours in children, 2nd ed. Marsden, H. B., Steward, J. K. (eds.), p. 397. Berlin, Heidelberg, New York: Springer 1976
15. Brown, N. J., Langley, F. A.: Teratomas and other genital tumours. In: Recent results in cancer research, Vol. 13: Tumours in Children, 2nd ed. Marsden, H. B., Steward, J. K. (eds.), p. 384. Berlin, Heidelberg, New York: Springer 1976
16. Brown, N. J., Langley, F. A.: Teratomas and other genital tumours. In: Recent results in cancer research, Vol. 13: Tumours in children, 2nd ed. Marsden, H. B., Steward, J. K. (eds.), p. 390. Berlin, Heidelberg, New York: Springer 1976
17. Brown, N. J., Langley, F. A.: Teratomas and other genital tumours. In: Recent results in cancer research, Vol. 13: Tumours in children, 2nd ed. Marsden, H. B., Steward, J. K. (eds.), p. 396. Berlin, Heidelberg, New York: Springer 1976
18. Breen, J. F., Neubecher, R. D.: Ovarian malignancy in children with special reference to the germ cell tumors. Ann. N. Y. Acad. Sci. **142,** 658 (1967)
19. Brown, N. J., Langley, F. A.: Teratomas and other genital tumours. In: Recent results in cancer research, Vol. 13: Tumours in children, 2nd ed. Marsden, H. B., Steward, J. K. (eds.), p. **000**. Berlin, Heidelberg, New York: Springer 1976
20. General References: Chapter 1

11 Systemic Hypertension

11.1 Introduction

Systemic arterial hypertension is a feature of a very wide range of diseases. Very often hypertension can be anticipated from what is already known about the infant or child's clinical background. For example, hypertension is a feature of such overt endocrinological conditions as Cushing's disease or other adrenal lesions. A wide variety of renal diseases whose presence is already known may be associated with hypertension; such diseases include nephritis and nephrotic syndromes, cystic disease of the kidneys, antecedant renal injury with damage to the parenchyma or renal vascular pedicle, obstructive renal atrophy and Wilms' tumour. Surgical operations on a kidney may precipitate an acute hypertensive episode. Hypertension may be a continuing feature of patients who have had a successful repair of coarctation of the aorta; such patients tend to have had the surgical correction in their childhood years and hypertension may reflect the fact that the carotid sinus baroreceptors have become set at a higher level (speculative) but such mild hypertension does not necessarily indicate underlying renovascular problems.

11.2 Clinical Presentation

There is a group of infants and more especially children in whom hypertension is responsible for the dominant clinical features and yet the underlying cause is not immediately apparent [1, 2, 3].

In young patients hypertension can present an immediate threat to life in four ways: the onset of severe pulmonary oedema; the development of acute hypertensive encephalopathy with fits, papilloedema and maybe blindness; bleeding from a berry aneurysm into the subarachnoid space; and, critically severe hypertension with diastolic pressures of 120–130 mm Hg. In the forefront are clinical features which may suggest a primary neurological disorder and so it is important always to measure the blood pressure carefully and accurately in children with such problems.

Less dramatic but significant clinical symptoms may develop. Transient facial nerve palsy may be the first sign. This may be a consequence of oedema or haemorrhage affecting the facial nerve as it passes through the long bony canal from the brain stem to the facial muscles but this is conjectural. Headache, irritability, unsteadiness of gait or acute incidents during the course of minor operations for, say, dental care with anaesthesia, may alert the perceptive clinician to the possibility of severe hypertension being present. Episodes of sweating, tachycardia, dizziness and anxiety, which are so often seen in adults with phaeochromocytoma, seldom occur in children with this lesion, for their hypertension is usually fixed and not periodic. Episodic hypertension, although rare in children, is seen in hypertension which is renal in origin or with phaeochromocytomas.

A chest radiograph is useful, for it shows the heart size and signs of pulmonary oedema if this is present. It is always wise to bring the hypertension under control by drug therapy before pursuing invasive investigation which may exacerbate the problems of hypertension.

11.3 Causes of Hypertension

11.3.1 Non-Congenital Coarctation

11.3.1.1 Coarctation due to a non-specific arteritis may narrow the descending aorta or abdominal aorta. There may be narrowing of renal arteries also when the abdominal aorta is affected.

It was thought that this lesion was found only in those living in Far Eastern and Middle Eastern countries, but recent work suggests it occurs more widely throughout the world [4, 5].

11.3.1.2 Neurofibromatosis may narrow the abdominal aorta and produce hypertension (Fig. 11.1 a and b). The hypertensive symptoms may be the first manifestation of the disease. Vascular disease may be widespread affecting arteries in other locations [6, 7, 8].

11.3.1.3 Chronic granulomatous disease may have an associated protracted mediastinitis which narrows the origins of the great arteries passing to the thoracic inlet. In such circumstances the hypertension may not be detectable in the arms (Fig. 11.2).

Comment. Careful clinical examination will show the disparity between arterial pressure measurement in the upper limbs and lower limbs. Since the disease process is slow to develop, the dramatic differences between the upper-limb and lower-limb pulses seen in congenital paraductal coarctation in the young infant may not be so apparent. Nevertheless, shrewd clinical assessment should lead to the suspicion of arterial narrowing which falls into this category. Very rarely indeed, hypertension may be caused by congenital coarctation of the abdominal aorta [9]. Further evaluation and confirmation is by cardiac catheterization (including manometric studies and

▷

Fig. 11.1 a, b. Four-year-old child with dyspnoea on exertion and hypertension in the upper limbs. No femoral pulses were palpable. Café au lait spots indicative of neurofibromatosis developed subsequently. **a** In this descending angiogram the aorta narrows below the origin of the coeliac axis. The aorta is completely interrupted immediately below the origin of the right renal artery and above the left renal artery. There is extensive filling of the collateral channels associated with the gut. **b** Later phase of angiogram shows the aorta distal to the interruption has filled via the collateral channels. Immediately below the site of interruption in the aortic lumen the left renal artery is seen. At IVU the left kidney was smaller than the right but both kidneys appeared structurally normal in other respects

angiography). Skilled surgical procedures can correct some of these problems; since the kidneys are, in general, protected from developing hypertensive nephrosclerosis it is worthwhile making all reasonable efforts, both investigatory and therapeutic.

11.3.2 Renal Parenchymal Lesions

Within this group lie conditions which cause a small kidney to be present. If both kidneys are small the

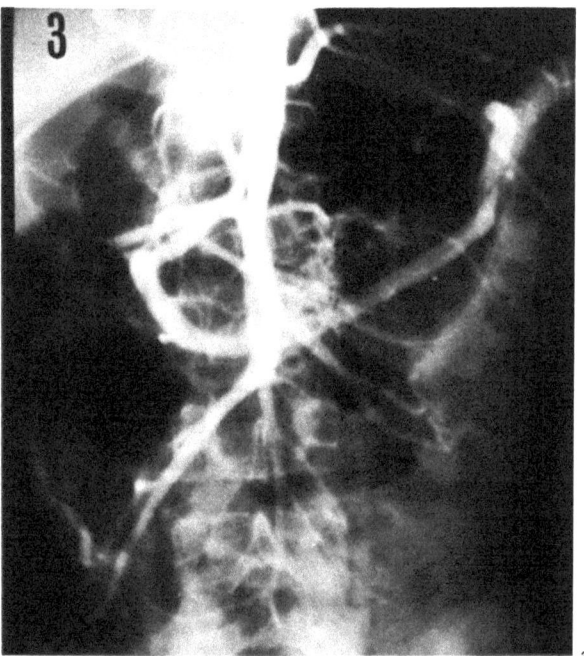

a

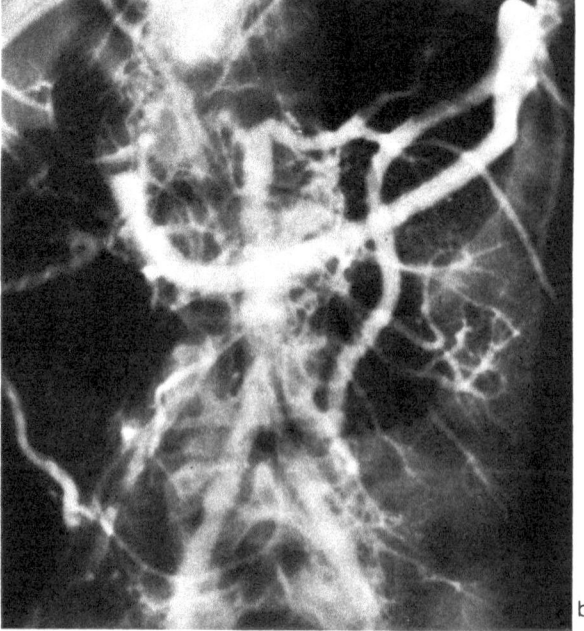

b

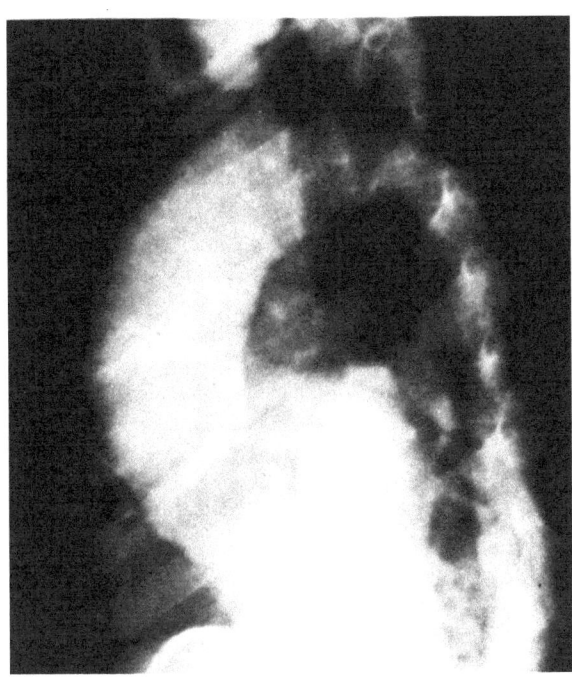

Fig. 11.2. Angiogram in a patient with left ventricular failure and severe hypertension. This girl was known to have chronic granulomatous disease and had long-standing infective mediastinitis. The descending thoracic aorta is narrow and all origins of arteries arising from the aortic arch are narrowed.
Patients with non-specifc arteritis may have similar narrowing of the descending aorta; the problem can be palliated by a conduit from the left ventricular apex to the lower part of the thoracic aorta

prospects for radical surgical correction are in general poor. However, if only one kidney is affected or the major part of one kidney remains undamaged by the pathological process, then surgical cure can be anticipated; in such circumstances it is worthwhile taking every step to define the extent of the problem because a balance has to be struck between loss of parenchyma which has some renal function and the possible relief of hypertension.
Parenchymal lesions within this category are detailed as follows:

11.3.2.1 Chronic nephritis (Chapter 9) can represent an end stage of a variety of types of acute nephritis which run a protracted course. The kidneys are equally affected by the disease process, there is usually a significant proteinuria and the initial episode of kidney damage may not have been a definable episode in the child's life.

11.3.2.2 Obstructive Atrophy (Chapter 3). If the lesion has affected one kidney only, then the other kidney will generally show marked compensatory hypertrophy. Unfortunately in children the common causes of obstructive atrophy so often affect both kidneys.

11.3.2.3 Renal Venous Thrombosis (Chapter 9). Renal venous thrombosis which affects one kidney may result in compensatory hypertrophy of the un-affected kidney and very marked shrinkage and growth failure in the affected kidney.

11.3.2.4 Atrophic Chronic Pyelonephritic Scarring (Chapter 4). This end stage of renal disease is increasingly associated with hypertension as the years go by with about 10%-15% of patients showing hypertension by the time they reach early adulthood [9, 10, 11]. As has been indicated previously (Chapter 4) the acute episode leading to kidney damage may not have been definable at the time it occurred and hypertension may be the first clinical feature at presentation.
The consequences of the acute episode may be bilateral and features of incipient renal failure may be present as well as hypertension. In such circumstances renal clearance studies highlight this problem. However, the renal lesion may affect solely or predominantly one kidney and this kidney is small; the contralateral kidney will then have undergone compensatory hypertrophy of its undamaged segments and so it is large. The possibility of hypertensive nephrosclerosis must always be borne in mind and when this has been present for a protracted period there may be no enlargement of the contralateral kidney.

11.3.2.5 Segmental renal hypoplasia (Ask Upmark Kidney) (Chapter 6) is one of a range of developmental renal lesions which is especially associated with systemic arterial hypertension [13, 14, 15]. The lesion may be impossible to differentiate from chronic pyelonephritic scarring on purely radiological grounds (Fig. 11.3). The condition seems to vary in its incidence among the different clinics and the reason for this may reflect the interpretation by their nephropathologists for pathological study is essential to establish the diagnosis.
The extent of the parenchymal problem must be defined for the same reasons as the scarring in chronic pyelonephritis.

11.3.2.6 Dysmorphic Kidney. Developmental anomalies with concomitant renal anomalies may cause severe hypertension (Fig. 11.4).

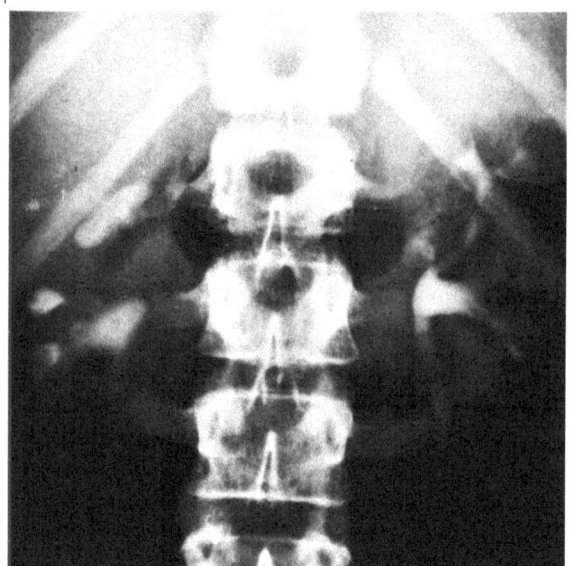

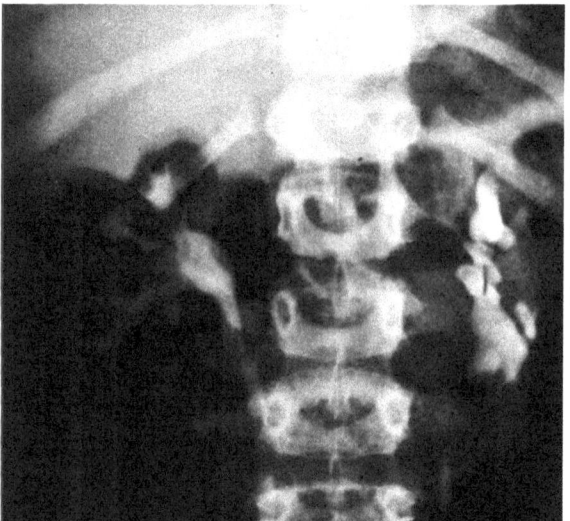

Fig. 11.3. This 10-year-old girl had serious headaches with hypertension. One identifiable urinary tract infection had occurred 5 years previously and IVU at that time had shown a small right kidney. Repeat IVU shows the left kidney is rather hypertrophied and structurally normal, but the right kidney is small with dilated calyces and reduced parenchymal thickness. Plasma renin levels were elevated. Careful study of the right kidney after nephrectomy showed extensive segmental renal hypoplasia (Ask-Upmark kidney)

11.3.2.7 Haemolytic Uraemic Syndrome (Chapter 8). This is dealt with in more detail in Chapter 8. Suffice it to say that hypertension develops in many of the affected children during the acute phase. Subsequently in the survivors hypertension may continue to be a dominant clinical problem In the haemolytic uraemic syndrome, after recovery from the acute phase, the IVU shows essentially normal structure, but at necrospy the widespread patchy infarction caused by vascular occlusion is seen.

11.3.2.8 Haemangiopericytoma. This is a tumour of the juxtaglomerular apparatus [16, 17, 18]. It secretes excessive quantities of renin and so in the course of investigation of hypertension renal vein renin assays may be expected to highlight the possible presence of the lesion. Angiographic studies can show the tumour's pathological circulation.

Comment. Sonography can be used to estimate renal size and the presence of focal parenchymal loss. If both kidneys are small (chronic nephritis, bilateral chronic atrophic pyelonephritis, bilateral extensive segmental hypoplasia), the prospects for a successful outcome to surgical intervention are poor. However,

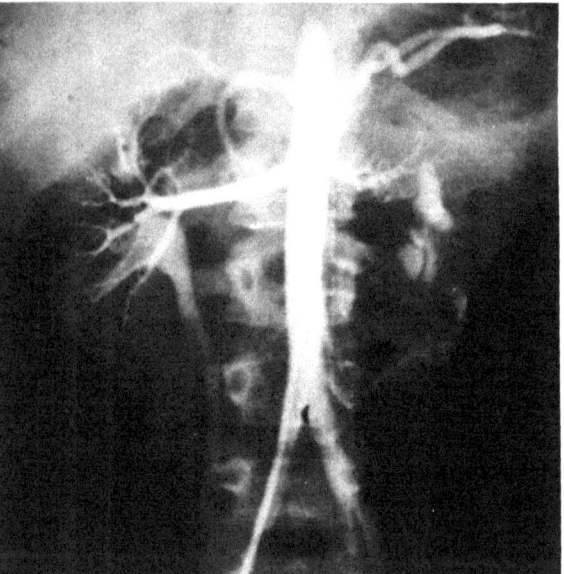

Fig. 11.4 a, b. This 5-year-old had headache and vomiting and was severely hypertensive. **a** IVU shows a normal right kidney with a rotated and misshapen left kidney with dilated calyces. **b** Aortogram shows the normal right renal artery, but on the left side two small renal arteries are seen, one supplying the upper pole and one the lower pole. There were at nephrectomy two more tiny arteries found supplying the middle part of the left kidney

when one kidney is large and the other small – it may be very small – then there is a reasonable prospect for successful surgical intervention. MCU will often show continuing vesico-ureteric reflux in patients who have chronic atrophic pyelonephritis. This procedure may provide the best chance of easily defining the clubbed calyces crowded together in an atrophic pyelonephritic kidney. IVU may show good clearance of contrast medium through both kidneys and it can define the kidney size, abnormalities of renal contour and calyx deformities; very severely damaged kidneys may be "non-functioning" at IVU.

If resection of damaged kidney or kidney segments is to be undertaken, then in principle it is rational to estimate the total renal function and that fraction of function which would remain after resection by studying "areas of interest" in a radioisotope renal scan. Static scans using DMSA should help delineate the undamaged sectors of kidney and dynamic DTPA scans will make it possible to assess renal function in the individual kidneys. It is helpful to utilize all the information about kidney structure which accrues from the IVU radiographs when undertaking this exercise. Co-ordinating the views of nephrologist, urologist and radiologist is essential.

Angiography has a rather uncertain role in this group of renal diseases associated with hypertension. Distortions and alterations in renal arterial anatomy are seen within areas already known to be damaged from information derived from the previous studies. The major role of angiography lies in selective renal arteriography to ensure the normality of the contralateral kidney if surgery is contemplated. Selective and super-selective renal vein renin levels should also be obtained to ensure that the apparently normal kidney is not the "driving source" for hypertension.

11.3.3 Renal Arterial Disease

Broadly, renal arterial disease falls into two categories: (A) arterial lesions lying outside the kidney itself; and (B) arterial lesions lying deep in the renal parenchyma. In Group A the abnormality may be amenable to surgical correction, but in Group B the prospects for such a correction are non-existent or at best extremely poor in bilateral lesions.

11.3.3.1 Group A. Arterial Lesions Outside the Kidney

11.3.3.1.1 Fibromuscular Hyperplasia (Fig. 11.5).
This is a generic word describing a variety of findings whose pathology has been correlated with radiological features by McCormack and co-workers [19]. In children fibromuscular hyperplasia [20] is probably the principal cause of isolated renal artery stenosis and hypertension. Internal fibrotic narrowing [21] may be associated with arterial dilatation distally, but the "chain of beads" appearance due to break up of elastic tissue in the arterial wall is rarely seen in children. The aorta in the vicinity of the renal arteries may be narrow (Fig. 11.6) and there may be stenosis of many other arteries including those

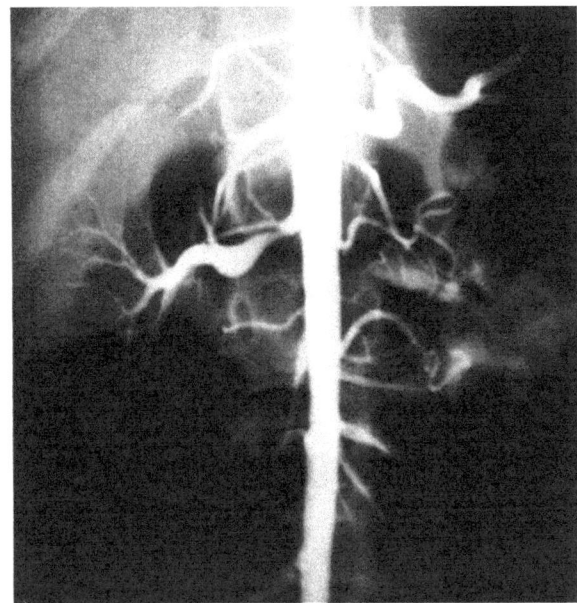

Fig. 11.5. Eleven-year-old girl with severe headache and subarachnoid haemorrhage due to berry aneurysm of the right middle cerebral artery. Angiogram shows the right renal artery is stenosed, just beyond its origin from the aorta; distal to the renal artery stenosis there is dilatation. The left renal aretry is very severely narrowed near its origin, but distal to the stenosis the artery is dilated

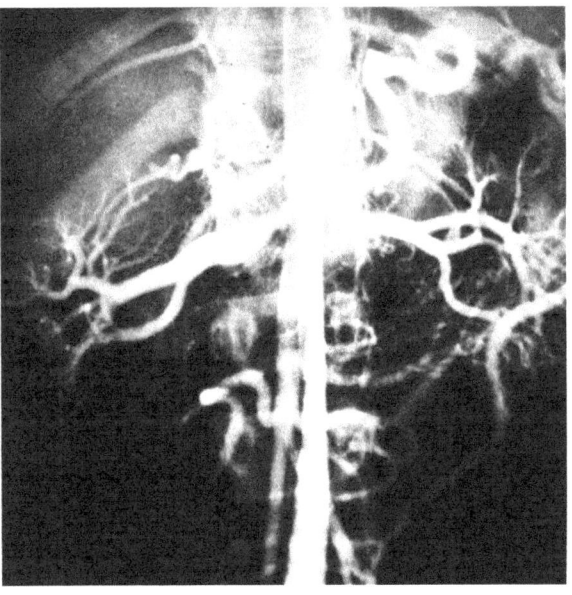

Fig. 11.6. Coarctation of the abdominal aorta has produced narrowing at the level where the renal arteries arise. The origins of the renal arteries are also narrowed. No filling of any hepatic artery branches. Diagnosis presumed to be fibromuscular hyperplasia

arising from the abdominal aorta as well as the carotid and vertebral arteries.

11.3.3.1.2 Neurofibromatosis.
Hypertension may be the first manifestation of neurofibromatosis, but as with fibromuscular hyperplasia arteries other than the renal arteries may be affected; coarctation may also be present [6, 7, 8]. The narrowing of the renal arteries may be due to intimal proliferation or extrinsic compression by sheets of neurofibromatous tissue in the posterior abdominal wall. Intrarenal arterial abnormalities may also be seen either alone or in conjunction with main renal artery narrowing (Fig. 11.7).

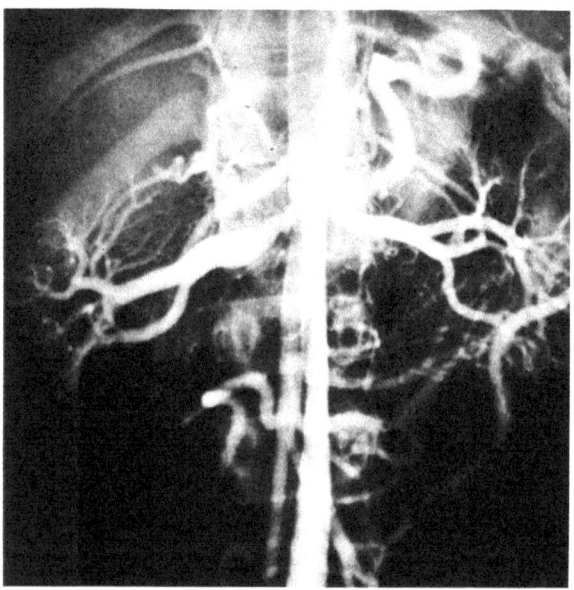

Fig. 11.7. Child neurofibromatosis associated among other things with a small left pedicle of L4. Aortogram showed no aortic or main renal artery anomaly. The selective left renal arteriogram shows stenoses in the arteries supplying part of the lower pole of the left kidney. Selective renal vein renin assays showed high values only in the samples from the left lower renal pole

11.3.3.1.3 Other Causes of Renal Artery Stenosis.
These include idiopathic hypercalcaemia [22], the rubella syndrome [23] and errors in lipid metabolism [24] which lead to premature atherosclerosis and sometimes arterial calcification.

Comment. When renal arterial stenosis is unilateral the kidney on the side of the lesion is smaller than it would otherwise be. Normally the left kidney is larger than the right so the significance of this generalisation can be uncertain. A murmur audible at clinical examination may be found at the back of the child or in the abdomen. The stenosis has functional effects which can sometimes (though very

rarely) be seen at IVU; the affected kidney shows a slower development of a nephrographic phase, a greater concentration of contrast medium within its calyces and a slower clearing of this contrast medium at diuresis (the Amplatz phenomenon) [25]. The same physiological changes may affect a dynamic isotope study, where the change can be quantified, with a slower accumulation of counts in the affected kidney and longer persistence of counts. Such isotope studies are theoretically helpful, for they can show the difference between the kidneys and the possibility of hypertensive nephrosclerotic change being present in the unprotected kidney. But here lies but one difficulty in interpreting with certainty the isotope study in isolation.
The definitive demonstration of the site of stenosis is given by aortography and selective renal arteriography.

*11.3.3.2 Group B. Arterial Lesions
Within Renal Parenchyma*

Arterial lesions lying in the parenchyma may be a consequence of coexistent parenchymal damage. For example, chronic pyelonephritic scarred kidney segments show a diminished number of narrowed arteries with few branches in the scarred segment. However, there are arterial lesions which have their origin primarily within the blood vessel [19, 20].

11.3.3.2.1 Fibromuscular Hyperplasia.
Fibromuscular hyperplasia may solely narrow renal arteries towards the periphery of the arterial circulation [26] (Figs. 11.8 and 11.9).

11.3.3.2.2 Polyarteritis Nodosa.
Although this condition has generalised features affecting other viscera, the kidney may be affected by nephritic changes and systemic hypertension may dominate the clinical picture. Angiography can demonstrate stenoses of arteries lying within the kidney and also small aneurysms. In the classic type the arterial lesions are multiple and affect both kidneys. In the microscopic form the abnormalities are not seen in the major vessels but only at the 4th-5th intrarenal arterial level.

11.3.3.2.3 Other Arterial Lesions.
Rare congenital anomalies of intrarenal arteries may result in fewer arteries with an abnormal branching pattern in the kidney [27]. Arterio-venous fistulae may occur [28].

11.3.3.2.4 Tuberous Sclerosis with angiomyolipoma may have a distorted arterial pattern with pools of

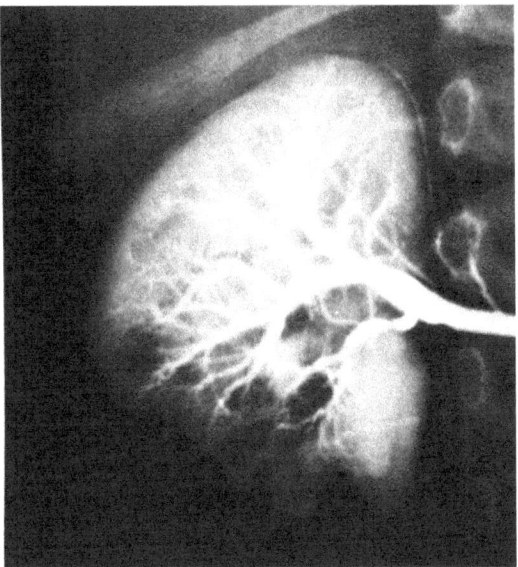

Fig. 11.8. Fibromuscular hyperplasia has narrowed the second division artery supplying to the lower part of the right kidney in this hypertensive child. Selective angiography is helpful in clearly delineating this type of lesion. High renal vein renin levels were found in the blood leaving the lower part of the right kidney

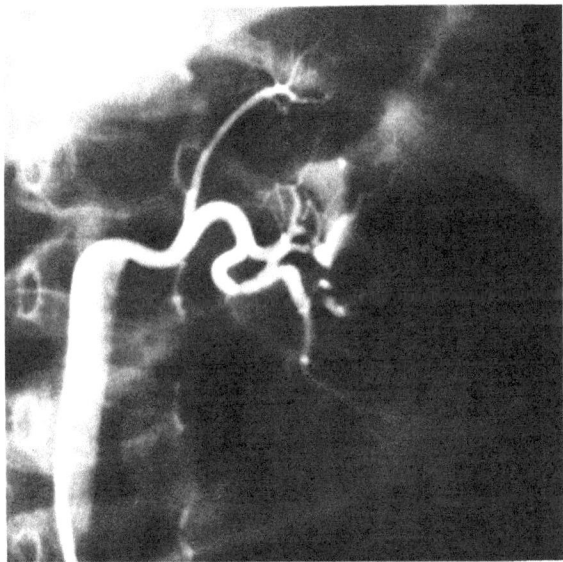

Fig. 11.9. Selective renal arteriogram showing severe stenosis and slight distal arterial dilatation of one artery supplying the mid-part of the left kidney. Diagnosis: presumed fibromuscular hypoplasia

opacified blood being seen at angiography; the nature of the hypertensive problem is not difficult to define in these circumstances and IVU alone may suffice as the definitive investigation when the lesion is bilateral, as it usually is.

11.3.3.2.5 Renal Trauma is an event which may damage the main renal artery or parenchymal arteries leaving a zone of relatively reduced vascularity.

11.3.3.2.6 Duplex Kidneys have a double drainage, but rarely may not be duplex in respect of their vascular supply so that resection of part of a duplex kidney may lead to under-perfusion of part of the remnant.

11.3.4 Phaeochromocytoma

Usually the phaeochromocytoma is a solitary benign tumour. Occasionally a second tumour coexists and may be revealed during the initial study of the child or may be found after a resection of one tumour and clinical relapse. Familial occurrence of this tumour has been reported [29].
The phaeochromocytoma may be located in the adrenal gland [30] (Fig. 11.10), renal hilum [31] (Fig. 11.11), the organ of Zuckerkandl, the mediastinum, [32] or the urinary bladder [33]. Hypertension associated with phaeochromocytoma in children is very commonly fixed and does not show the periodic character seen in adult life. The tumour secretes noradrenalin and adrenalin and screening tests include assays of catecholamines, VMA and metabolites, and the phentolamine test, all of which can support the diagnosis.

Comment. Angiography will, in most circumstances, demonstrate the phaeochromocytoma [34]. The tumour has an arterial supply and late in the angiographic study contrast medium often enters venous pools in the periphery of the tumour. Before searching for a possible phaeochromocytoma by angiography or IVU it is essential to establish the probability of the tumour by bioassay and pharmacological testing and then control hypertension by the appropriate drug therapy. This should be continued up to the time when the tumour is surgically removed.
A phaeochromocytoma lying within the adrenal distorts the anatomy of this gland and this can be demonstrated by iodo-cholesterol radioisotope studies. Echography is a simple, safe and non-invasive method of studying the adrenal and the various other locations in which phaeochromocytomas may be found; and so, echography may provide the fastest way of identifying the tumour.
After surgical removal the blood pressure falls dramatically and the fall may be difficult to control. Recurrence of hypertension should suggest a second tumour is present.

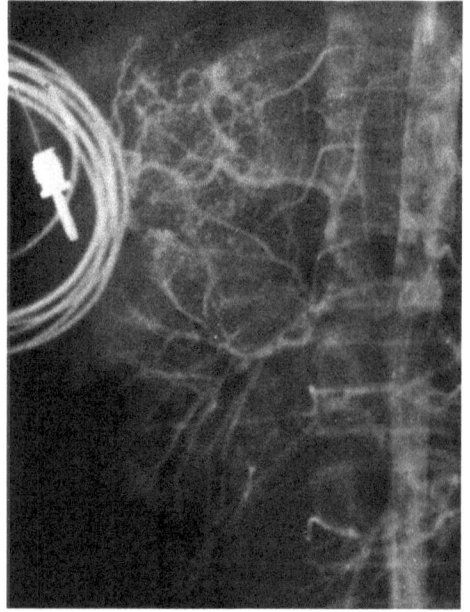

a

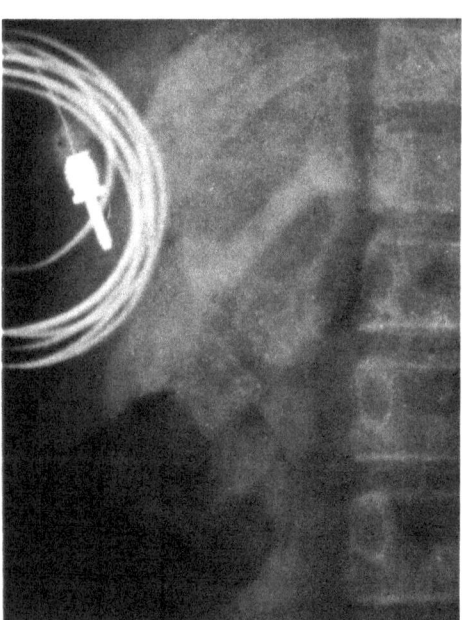

b

11.4 Conclusion: Tactics in Investigation

In adult life essential hypertension is common and even if hypertension is secondary to a renal or arterial lesion it is often doubted whether a radical approach to investigation or operative intervention is helpful. Rather, the increasing tendency is simply to treat the elevated blood pressure by an appropriate range of drugs. Such is not the case with children who are hypertensive for they have a variety of conditions, some of which may be amenable to surgical intervention. Perhaps there is one exception

◁ **Fig. 11.10. a** Phaeochromocytoma of the right adrenal showing, during the arterial phase, the pathological circulation to the tumour lying above the right kidney. **b** During the later phase the angiogram shows the dense periphery of the tumour containing contrast medium, whereas the central relatively avascular zone shows increased transradiancy. This ring-like effect was also visible during the nephrographic phase of the preceding urogram. Note the spare ECG lead: monitoring by ECG is imperative

to this concept; the child who has a pyelonephritic scar may have hypertension which resolves as scar formation progresses to its end-point and so drug therapy can be used to control hypertension as the process evolves.

In phaeochromocytoma there is an output of catecholamines which raises the blood pressure. Coarctation is associated with hypertension proximal to the site of aortic narrowing and the precise mechanism of the hypertension is uncertain and probably multifaceted. If aortic narrowing affects the site of origin of the renal arteries a by-pass graft from above the coarctation site to below may exacerbate hypertension.

Renovascular hypertension is the generic term which encompasses those causes of hypertension which relate to the kidney and its arterial supply. The concept of renovascular hypertension derives from the classic work of Goldblatt who experimentally produced hypertension by narrowing the artery to one kidney. In these circumstances the endocrinological function of the kidney is changed and increased amounts of renin are produced. This has led to the development of sophisticated techniques for renin assays in hypertensive children [35]. Hypertension is seldom a clinical problem in Wilms' tumour although increased renin output has been recorded [36, 37]. A rare renal tumour, the haemangiopericytoma, has a high renin output and this produces hypertension.

More generally, renin levels in the plasma of the general circulation and in the plasma in the blood of each of the renal veins can be assayed in order to find out the significance of a lesion which affects either the arterial supply to a kidney or a parenchymal lesion within the kidney. Such renin assays are especially important when surgical intervention is contemplated.

In children who have hypertension the objective of investigations is first to determine the cause and then decide if the lesion is amenable to surgical correction.

Renal parenchymal lesions are amongst the commonest of causes and so investigation of the kidneys

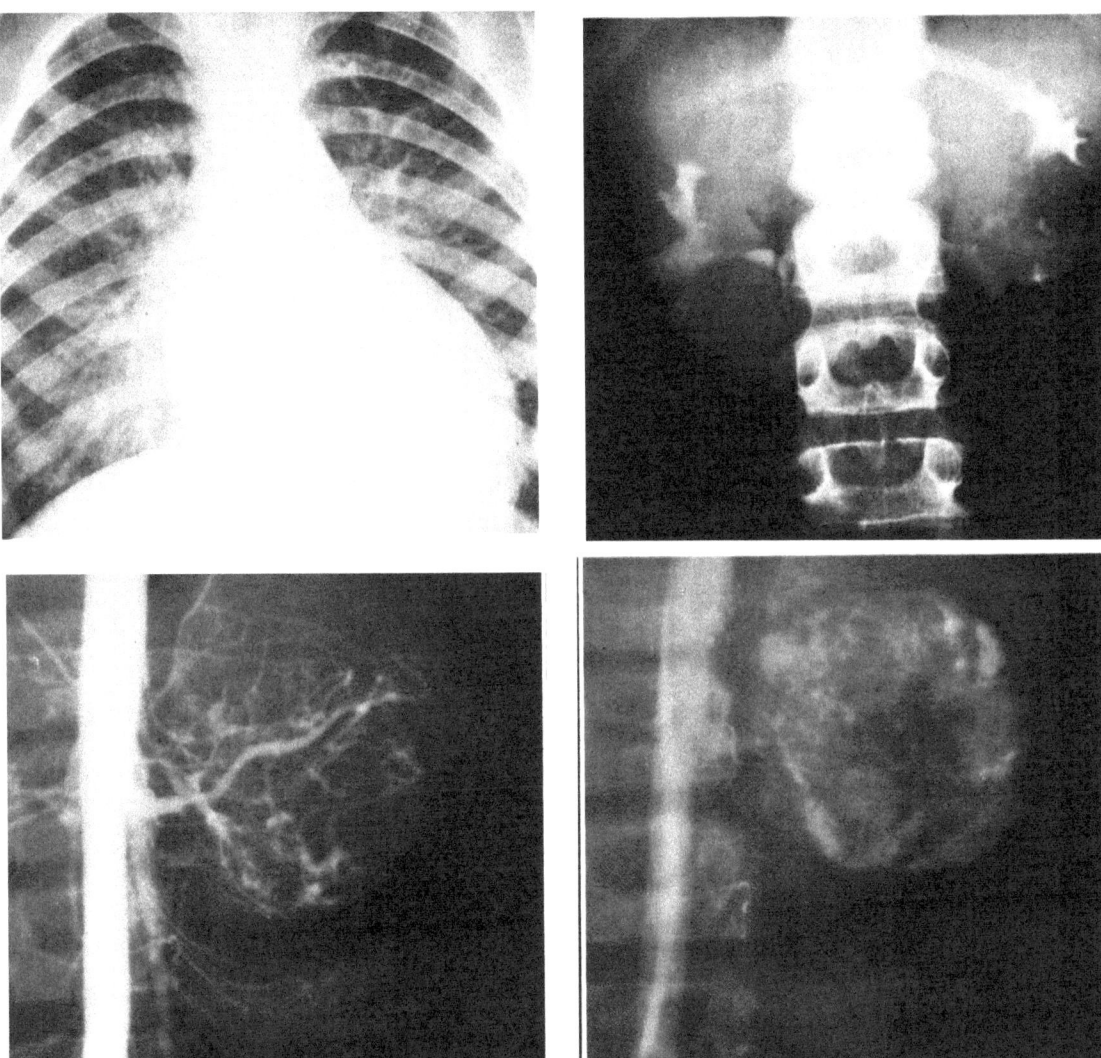

Fig. 11.11. a Chest radiograph in an 11-year-old boy with dyspnoea at rest. The heart is large and there is pulmonary oedema because of left ventricular failure due to sustained hypertension associated with phaeochromocytome. Medical measures to control blood pressure and cardiac failure are imperative before proceeding to investigation. Although this patient had phaeochromocytoma, this type of chest radiograph is more commonly seen in children with parenchymal renal disease, hypertension and an element of renal failure **b** IVU shows the normal right kidney and no opacification of the renal pelvis of the rather small left kidney. **c** Aortogram shows the left renal artery feeds the phaeochromocytoma and the supply to the tumour also steals the blood supply to the left kidney. Thus, there are two components to the hypertensive problem, namely that due to the tumour and that due to the renovascular problem. **d** Late phase of angiogram, showing dense opacification of the venous pools around the periphery of the tumour. Not all phaeochromocytoma have this degree of vascularization

is directed at ascertaining if the renal lesion is generalized, as in the various forms of nephritis, or localized in the form of, say, atrophic pyelonephritic scarring, segmental renal hypoplasia or a late sequel to renal venous thrombosis. The fact that lesions are localized may be shown by IVU, sonography and DMSA scans. When only one kidney is clearly affected the next point is to establish what is the contribution to renal function that the damaged kidney makes; dynamic DTPA scan and DMSA scan assessments yield this information. It is around the results of such evaluations that the decision about surgical excision revolves.

In children who have a combination of hypertension and impending renal failure, renal function is severely impaired. IVU and isotope scans are of limited value because neither can image the kidney satisfactorily. Ultrasound studies establish the size of such kidneys. Since reflux nephropathy and atrophic renal scarring are a common cause for this combination of clinical problems an MCU will often give detail of the calyx structure and, by inference, kidney structure and size.

When it is clear that hypertension is not (in the ordinary sense) endocrinologically based, then the possibility of abnormalities of renal vascular supply arises and it is here that angiography has a cardinal role and renal vein renin assays have great importance in evaluating the significance of the findings. Biochemical and pharmacological studies should be able to determine whether a phaeochromocytoma is present. The purpose of further investigation is then to elucidate where it is and, if more than one lesion is present, to define it as well. From IVU the presence of a sizeable tumour should be inferred. Ultrasound imaging of the adrenal is both desirable and feasible; it is important because not all phaeochromocytomas are vascular. Phaeochromocytomas are not common in children, but at the present state of the art it proves difficult to persuade clinicians not to have some angiographic evidence before embarking on surgery.

The hypertension of hyperaldosteronism due to Conn's tumour is usually suspected on the basis of the biochemical features of the lesion [37, 38]. Radioisotope studies of the adrenal will localize the side which is the site of the lesion [39].

Given these perspectives, it is clear that the approach to the problem of hypertension in children requires the integration of findings from clinical observation, biochemical analyses and assays and imaging techniques. This integration provides the basis on which rational judgements about management can be made.

References

1. Still, J. L., Cottom, D.: Severe hypertension in children. Arch. Dis. Child. **42,** 34 (1967)
2. Loggie, J. M. H.: Systemic hypertension in children and adolescents. Pediatr. Clin. North Am. **18,** 1273 (1971)
3. Lawson, J. D.: Diagnosis and management of renovascular hypertension in children. Arch. Surg. **112,** 1307 (1977)
4. Danara, J. J., Wong, O. H., Thomas, M. A.: Primary arteritis of aorta causing renal artery stenosis and hypertension. Br. Heart J. **25,** 153 (1963)
5. Golding, R. L., Perri, G., Cremin, B. J.: The arteriographic manifestations of Takayasu's arteritis in children. Pediatr. Radiol. **5,** 224 (1977)
6. Bruneton, J. N.: Hypertension artérielle et rein en fer à cheval au cours d'une maladie de von Recklinghausen. J. Radiol. Electrol. Med. Nucl. **59,** 149 (1978)
7. Klecker, R. L., Roth, J. B.: Visceral neurofibromatosis and hypertension in childhood. Pediatrics **52,** 417 (1974)
8. Halpern, M., Currarino, G.: Vascular lesions causing hypertension in neurofibromatosis. N. Engl. J. Med. **273,** 248 (1965)
9. Fisher, E. R., Corcoran, A. C.: Congenital coarctation of the abdominal aorta with resultant renal hypertension. Arch. Intern. Med. **89,** 943 (1952)
10. Poutasse, E. F.: Malignant hypertension in children secondary to chronic pyelonephritis: laboratory and radiological indications for partial or total nephrectomy. J. Urol. **119,** 264 (1978)
11. Heale, W. F.: Hypertension and reflux nephropathy. Aust. Paediatr. J. **13,** 56 (1977)
12. Wallace, D. M. A., Rothwell, D. L., Williams, D. I.: The long-term follow-up of surgically treated vesicoureteric reflux. Br. J. Urol. **50,** 479 (1978)
13. Habib, R., Courtecuisse, V., Ehrenspenger, J., Royer, P.: Hypoplasia segmentaire du rein avec hypertension artérielle chez l'enfant. Ann. Paediatr. (Basel) **41,** 954 (1965)
14. Ljungquist, A., Lagergren, C.: The Ask-Upmark kidney; a congenital renal anomaly studied by micro angiography and histology. Acta Pathol. Microbiol. Scand. [A] **56,** 277 (1962)
15. Benz, G., Willich, E., Scharer, K.: Segmental renal hypoplasia in childhood. Pediatr. Radiol. **5,** 86 (1976)
16. Robertson, P. W., Klidjian, A., Harding, L. K., Walters, G.: Hypertension due to a renin-secreting renal tumor. Am. J. Med. **43,** 963 (1967)
17. Davidson, J. K.: Renin-secreting juxta glomerular-cell tumour. Br. J. Radiol. **47,** 594 (1974)
18. Lee, M. R.: Renin secreting kidney tumours. Lancet *1971 II,* 254
19. McCormack, L. J., Poutasse, F. E., Meaney, T. F., Noto, J. J., Dunstan, H. P.: A patholo-arteriographic correlation of renal arterial disease. Am. Heart J. **72,** 188 (1966)
20. Eklund, L., Gerlock, J., Wolin, J., Smith, C.: Roentgenologic appearance of fibromuscular dysplasia. Acta Radiol. [Diagn.] (Stockh.) **19,** 433 (1978)
21. Schmidt, D. M., Rambo, O. N.: Segmental intimal hyperplasia of the abdominal aorta and renal arteries producing hypertension in an infant. Am. J. Clin. Pathol. **44,** 546 (1965)
22. Black, J. A., Bonham Carter, R. E.: Association between aortic stenosis and facies of severe infantile hypercalcaemia. Lancet *1963 II,* 745
23. Menser, M. A., Dorman, D. C., Reye, R. D. K., Reid, B. R.: Renal artery stenosis in the rubelly syndrome. Lancet *1966 I,* 790
24. Boggs, J. D., Usia, D. Y., Mais, R. F., Bigler, J. A.: The genetic mechanism of idiopathic hyperlipemia. N. Engl. J. Med. **257,** 1101 (1957)
25. Amplate, K.: Two radiographic tests for the assessment of renovascular hypertension. Radiology **79,** 807 (1962)
26. Bennett, S. P.: Juvenile hypertension caused by overproduction of renin within a renal segment. J. Pediatr. **84,** 689 (1974)

27. Chrispin, A. R., Scatcliff, J. H.: Systemic hypertension in childhood. Pediatr. Radiol. **1,** 75 (1973)

28. Long, L., Javid, H., Julian, O. C.: Arteriovenous fistula of renal vessels: report of a case believed to be congenital. Ann. Surg. **160,** 239 (1964)

29. Cone, T. E., Allen, M. S., Pearson, H. A.: Pheochromocytoma in children: a report of three familial cases in two unrelated families. Pediatrics **19,** 44 (1957)

30. Robinson, M. J., Kert, M., Stocks, J.: Phaeochromocytoma in childhood: report of 3 cases. Arch. Dis. Child. **48,** 137 (1973)

31. Weidman, P., Siegerthaler, W., Zeigler, W. H., Sulser, H., Endres, P., Werning, C.: Hypertension associated with tumor adjacent to renal arteries. Am. J. Med. **47,** 528 (1969)

32. McNeill, A. D., Groden, B. M., Neville, A. M.: Intrathoracic phaeochromocytoma. Br. J. Surg. **57,** 457 (1970)

33. Leestma, J. E., Price, E. B.: Paraganglioma of the urinary bladder. Cancer **28,** 1063 (1971)

34. Lanner, L. O., Rosencrantz, M.: Arteriographic appearances of phaeochromocytomas. Acta Radiol. [Diagn.] (Stockh.) **10,** 35 (1970)

35. Stockigt, J. R., Collins, R. D., Noakes, C. A., Schambelar, M., Biglieri, E. G.: Renal vein renin in various forms of renal hypertension. Lancet *1972 I,* 1194

36. Mitchell, J. D., Baxter, T. J., Blair-West, J. R., McCreddie, D. A.: Renin levels in nephroblastoma. Arch. Dis. Child. **45,** 376 (1970)

37. Slaton, P. E., Biglieri, E. F.: Hypertension and hyperaldosteronism of renal and adrenal origin. Am. J. Med. **38,** 324 (1965)

38. Cavell, B., Sandegard, E., Hökfelt, B.: Primary aldosteronism due to an adrenal adenoma in a 3 year old. Acta Paediatr. Scand. **53,** 205 (1964)

39. Conn, J. W., Beier Waltes, E. H., Liebermann, L. M., Ansari, A. N., Cohen, E. L., Bookstein, J. J., Herwig, K. R.: Primary aldosteronism: pre-operative tumor visualization by scintillation scanning. Endocrinology **89,** 713–716 (1971)

12 Bone Changes in Chronic Renal Failure

12.1 Introduction

Renal osteodystrophy may be defined as abnormal bone metabolism associated with renal disease. The basic defect is a failure to absorb calcium normally from the gut because of abnormal vitamin D metabolism. This may result in secondary hyperparathyroidism. The abnormal bone metabolism results in a disturbance of bone structure.

Because bone is a dynamic structure, responding to different stimuli in varying degrees, it follows that an understanding of the changes which occur can only be appreciated by considering the different responses of the different components of bone [1]. The response of cortical bone to altered metabolism is different from the response of cancellous bone. Likewise, in the growing child, the bone changes caused by abnormal metabolism vary according to the site predominantly affected; the epiphyseal plate, the metaphysis or the diaphysis. The range of appearances seen on radiographs in patients with renal osteodystrophy is shown in Figs. 12.1 to 12.9.

12.2 Cortical Bone

12.2.1 General Radiological Changes

Radiological changes in cortical bone [2] in patients with chronic renal failure are:
(i) A characteristic spiculated appearance along the cortical margin

(ii) Longitudinal striations in the core of cortical bone
(iii) endosteal cortical thinning

These three features are the result of secondary hyperparathyroidism which causes an accelerated remodelling rate at the periosteal, endosteal and Haversian surfaces.

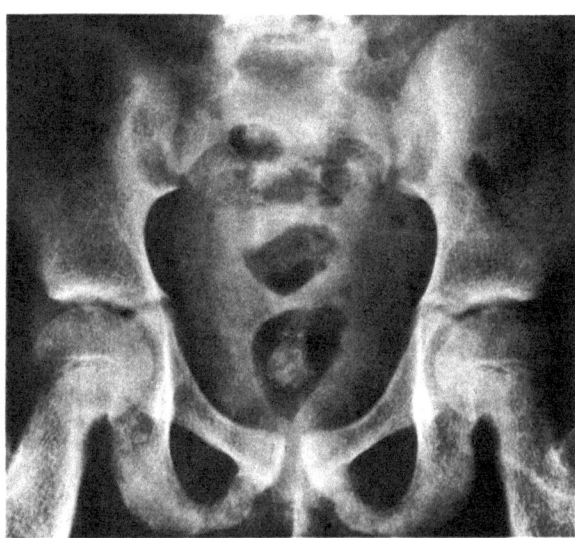

Fig. 12.1. Cortical bone lesions of the sacro-iliac joints and femoral necks. This child, with chronic renal failure due to juvenile nephronophthisis, demonstrates cortical changes of renal osteodystrophy in the pelvis. The sacroiliac joints are wide and indistinct. Both femoral necks show subperiosteal bone resorption along the upper and lower borders, giving rise to the "rotting stump" appearance

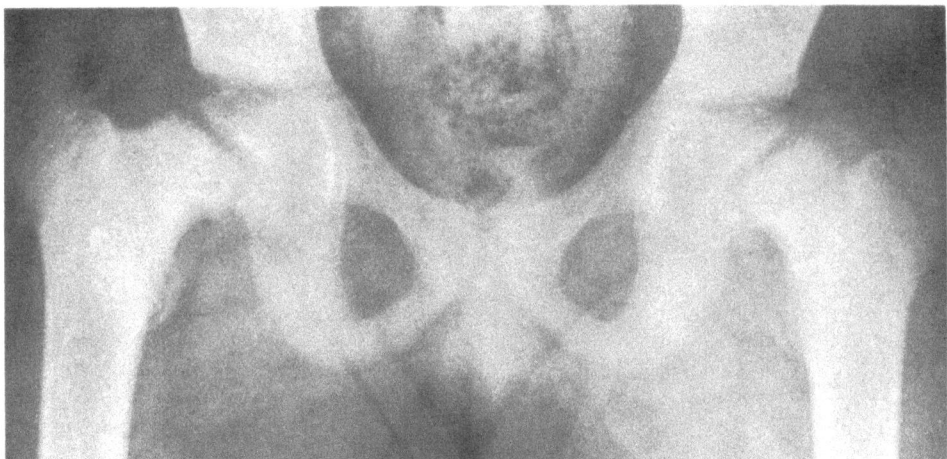

Fig. 12.2. Slip of both upper femoral epiphyses. Radiographs of the hips of this child with chronic renal failure demonstrate bilaterally symmetrical upper femoral epiphyseal slip. Poorly mineralized bone is present in the metaphyses. There is osteosclerosis and the trabecular pattern is coarse

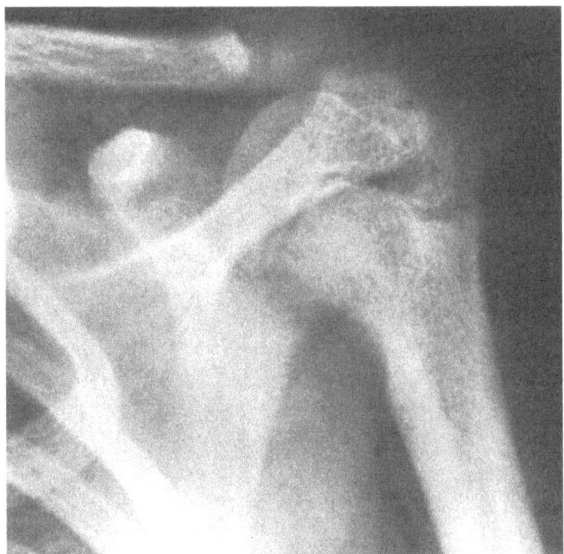

Fig. 12.3. Cortical bone resorption at the acromioclavicular joint. This child with end-stage renal failure illustrates cortical bone resorption of the upper medial humeral shaft and at the acromioclavicular joint with erosion of the distal end of the clavicle. The changes were bilaterally symmetrical

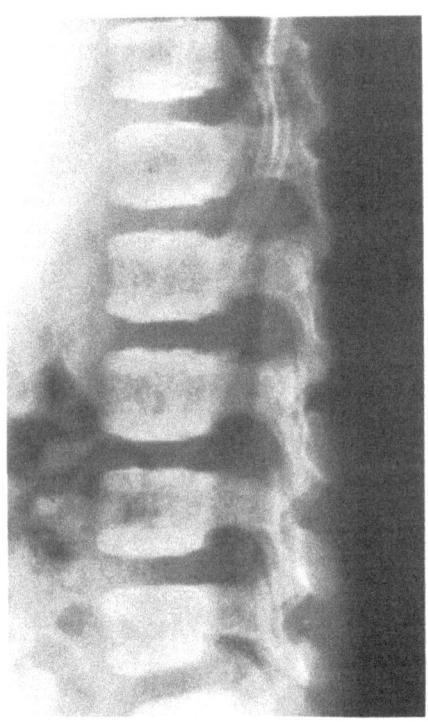

Fig. 12.4. Spinal changes in renal osteodystrophy. This child with chronic renal failure demonstrates changes of renal osteodystrophy in the cancellous bone of the spine. Increased cancellous bone mass is apparent beneath the vertebral end plates and gives rise to a "rugger-jersey" appearance

The spiculated appearance is caused by resorption of the outer circumferential lamellae, and replacement by fibrous tissue or loose woven bone. There is no loss of bone tissue, simply a replacement of well-mineralized by poorly mineralized bone. This explains why appropriate therapy usually results in a rapid restoration of the normal bone contours. Occasionally the bone resorption is truly subperiosteal and the cortical margin may be left intact.

Periosteal reactions of this sort occur in less than 10% of children with chronic renal failure and appear to be unrelated to peritoneal or haemodialysis, or to renal transplantation. These children may have bone pain.

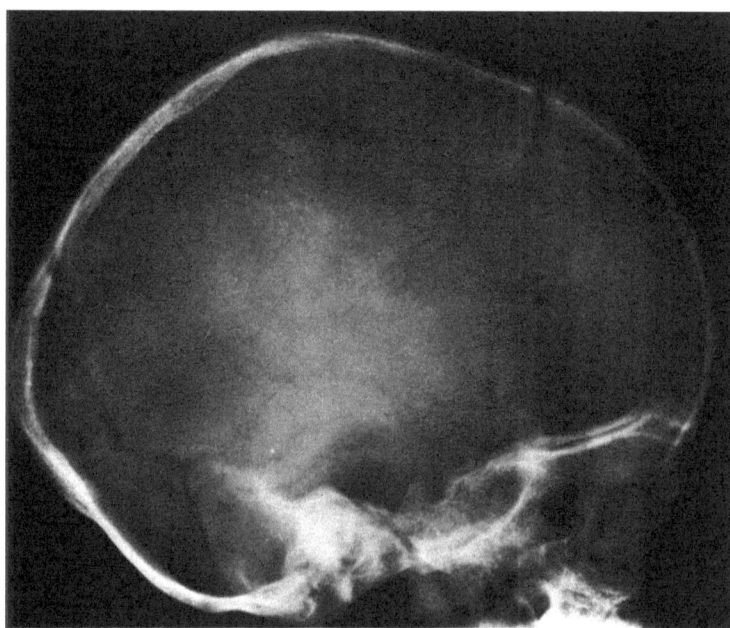

Fig. 12.5. Cancellous changes in the skull.
The lateral radiograph of the skull in this child with chronic renal failure demonstrates loss of definition between the inner and outer tables. There is a "ground glass" density of the skull vault. The skull base is dense

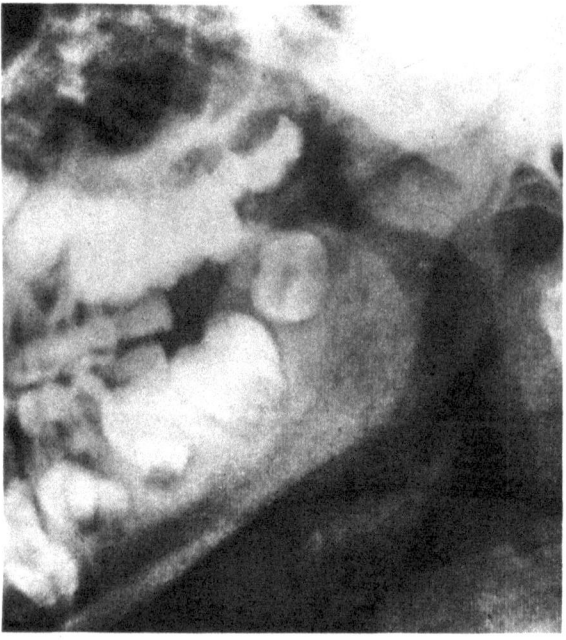

Fig. 12.6. Loss of lamina dura around the alveolar margins

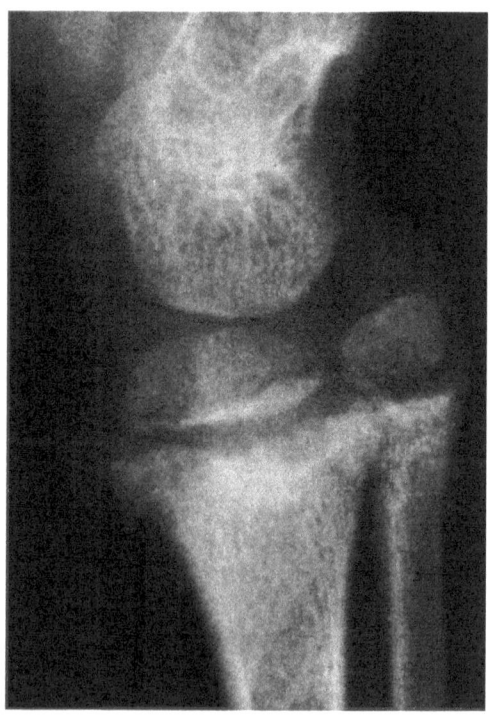

Fig. 12.7. Knee radiograph showing coarse trabecular pattern, disordered ossification in the metaphyses, and endosteal and some subperiosteal calcification deficiency

In the core of cortical bone increased osteoclastic activity is present in renal failure. When the resorption cavities are filled with poorly mineralized bone, or even fibrous tissue, longitudinal striations become apparent.

An increased rate of remodelling by secondary hyperparathyroidism induces bone loss at the endosteal surface, leading to cortical thinning.

12.2.2 Sites of Bone Resorption

Cortical bone resorption is seen in two sites. Firstly in areas where the rate of skeletal remodelling is high

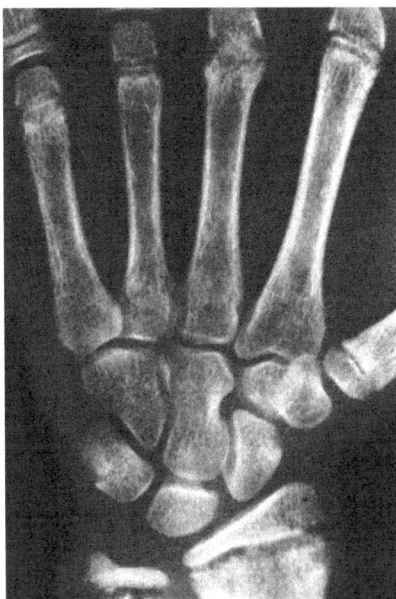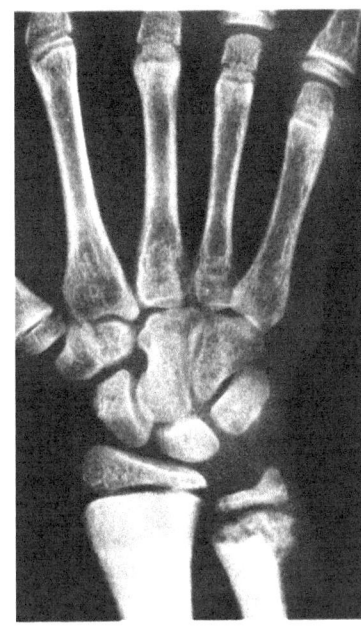

a, b

Fig. 12.8 a, b. Slip of the distal ulnar epiphysis: condition bilateral and symmetrical. **a** The wrist shows features of renal osteodystrophy. The distal ulnar epiphysis has slipped in an ulnar direction. There is a wedge-shaped defect of bone resorption of the ulnar metaphysis. The cortical margin is indistinct along the distal radius and ulna and there is osteosclerosis. **b** One year later, radiograph of other hand shows there is a wedge-shaped metaphyseal resorption defect of the distal ulnar metaphysis. This has resulted in further ulnar slip of the distal ulnar epiphysis. The epiphyseal growth plate of the radius is narrow and even following therapy there is still a metaphyseal zone of poorly mineralized bone. An osteoclastic resorption defect is also present on the ulnar side of the radial metaphysis. The diaphyses show coarsening of the trabecular pattern

in the normal child; and secondly at sites constantly subjected to mechanical stress.

The commoner areas of cortical bone resorption are:
(i) At the sites of tendinous and ligamentous insertions at the medial proximal tibiae and humeri, and at the bases of the phalanges.
(ii) At tight articulations, that is, at sites subject to excessive shearing forces, such as the acromioclavicular joints, the sterno-clavicular joints, the symphysis pubis, the tempero-mandibular joints and the sacroiliac joints. Radiologically the appearance suggests enlargement of the joint space but the apparent enlargement is caused by replacement of the well-mineralized lamellar bone, by poorly mineralized woven bone and fibrous tissue in the subchondral region.
(iii) At the lamina dura of alveolar bone.
(iv) At the outer circumference of the metaphyses of long bones.
In normal children bone modelling at the metaphyses is initiated by a collar of osteoclasts, which affects the reduction in the diameter of the epiphysis to the diameter of the diaphysis. Under the influence of excess parathormone there is an increase in osteoclastic activity. In advanced cases there is a circumferential metaphyseal defect under

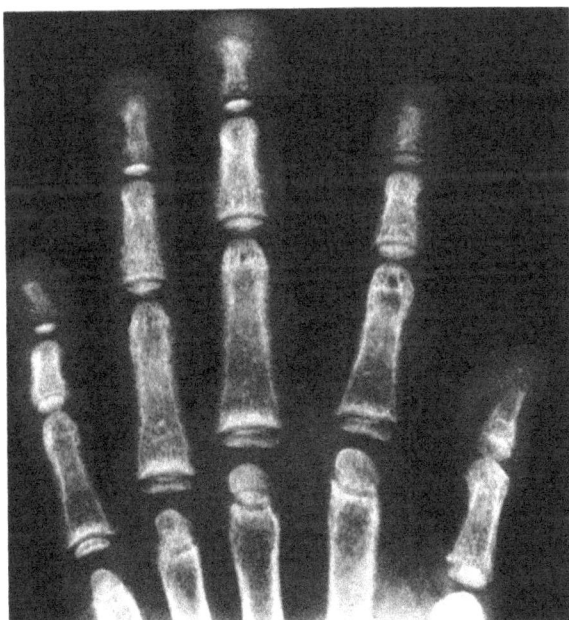

Fig. 12.9. Cortical bone resorption in the phalanges. Cortical resorption defects are present at the bases of the phalanges on the radial and ulnar aspects. Subperiosteal resorption is present along the shafts of the middle phalanges, particularly on the radial sides. "Pseudo-clubbing" is apparent in the terminal phalanges

the growth plate, and the entire epiphysis may slip sideways under the influence of shearing forces [3]. In this situation metaphyseal fractures may also occur.

12.3 Cancellous Bone

12.3.1 General Radiological Changes

Radiological changes in cancellous bone in patients with chronic renal failure are:
(i) An increase in the number and diameter of trabeculae in the metaphyses
(ii) Osteosclerosis
The increase in the amount of cancellous bone formed is a result of stimulation of osteoblastic activity by the excess bone resorption stimulated by parathormone. Transformation of metaphyseal spongiosa into diaphyseal spongiosa by loss of trabeculae, is disturbed. Dense metaphyseal spongiosa is encountered further down in the diaphysis. The increased cancellous bone mass becomes apparent after the mineral content of the increased bone matrix mass has been raised by therapy.

12.3.2 Sites of Cancellous Bone Lesions

Bones in which cancellous rather than cortical bone is present are the skull, pelvis, scapulae, vertebrae and metaphyses of long bones. These bones show an increase in bone mass and the overall effect is to produce sclerosis [4].

12.4 Diaphyseal Lesion

In addition to the cortical bone changes which have been described, children with chronic renal failure exhibit patchy rarefaction of the spongiosa of the diaphyses. The coarse trabecular pattern indicates the relative resistance of osteoid to osteoclastic resorption.

12.5 Epiphyseal Lesion

The epiphyseal growth plates of the long bones are characteristically narrow in children with chronic renal failure. Beneath the growth plate, with its disordered columns of cartilage cells, the primary spongiosa is both poorly mineralized and disorganized: the absence of radiographically detectable calcium gives the impression of widening and thickening of the growth plate.

12.6 General Considerations

In normal children, bone is a dynamic tissue constantly changing in response to various stimuli, either metabolic and hormonal or mechanical. Not only do the factors controlling bone development vary from time to time, but also the response of an individual child to specific stimuli may vary.

Similarly, children with chronic renal failure will demonstrate varying degrees and varying patterns of bone disease. For example, one child may show severe cortical bone changes at many sites, with bone resorption causing a spiculated appearance, and with longitudinal cortical striations, and the same child may have no radiological evidence of cancellous bone lesions. Another child may show only the osteosclerosis of cancellous bone.

The radiological bone changes may be affected by therapy. An immediate response may be seen in areas where there is poorly mineralized bone or fibrous tissue; that is, beneath the epiphyses and at sites of bone resorption. In this situation the template of the bone becomes clearer as bone mineralization proceeds. In contrast other bone changes appear to be unrelated to either vitamin D therapy or dialysis; for example the osteosclerosis of cancellous bone. Renal transplantation will, however, improve all the bone changes directly attributable to the chronic renal failure. However, renal transplants may induce other bone changes. Ischaemic necrosis may occur, and most frequently involves the hips, the knees and the humeral heads.

Whilst one child with chronic renal failure may have generalized osteoporosis, representing endosteal bone resorption, as the only bone change, and another may have only osteosclerosis, most children demonstrate a combination of bone lesions.

In general the bone changes are not a reflection of the severity of the underlying renal disease nor of its duration. (On average renal failure is present for at least 2 years before bone changes are apparent.) However certain radiological features can only be seen in severe renal failure of long standing. These are shortening and bowing of the long bones and also a retarded bone age.

12.7 Clinical Presentation

The child with chronic renal failure rarely presents for the first time as a result of the secondary bone disease. Occasionally the patient may present with shortness of stature and bowed long bones. In some children bone pain is incapacitating. This appears to be unrelated to the severity of the bone changes. Also the sites of bone pain appear to be unrelated to the sites of major radiological change.

Children in whom osteoporosis is a feature may present as a result of impaction fractures. The osteoporosis may be a manifestation of endosteal bone resorption, but other factors such as the general debility of the patient, or the bone pain, may be contributory.

Slipped epiphyses with or without the adjacent metaphyseal fractures may be the first indication of bone disease associated with chronic renal failure.

More commonly the children present with some other manifestation of renal disease. In practice the evolution of bone changes and their response to therapy can be monitored conveniently by means of comparable A. P. views of one hand and one knee, taken at regular intervals, and also if the clinical condition of the child changes.

12.8 Conclusion

The whole of this chapter has been taken up with the findings in renal osteodystrophy [5]: This aspect of renal disease has very specific connotations in management. As treatment for bone lesions proceeds continuing radiological surveillance is required. It is important to evaluate progress of bone lesions in zones where bone change is especially dynamic and where changes are easily accessible to radiographic study. In most young children the knee and the hand radiograph provide the information needed to monitor progress.

References

1. Mehls, O., Ritz, E., Krempien, B., Willich, E., Bommer, J., Schärer, K.: Roentgenological signs in the skeleton of uremic children. Pediatr. Radiol. **1**, 183 (1973)
2. Meema, H. E., Oreopoulos, D. G., Meema, S.: A roentgenologic study of cortical bone resorption in chronic renal failure. Radiology **126**, 67 (1978)
3. Goldman, A. B.: Slipped capital femoral epiphyses complicating renal osteodystrophy. Radiology **126**, 333 (1978)
4. Kaye, M., Pritchard, J. E., Halpenny, G. W., Light, W.: Bone disease in chronic renal failure with particular reference to osteosclerosis. Medicine (Baltimore) **39**, 157 (1964)
5. Chan, J. C. M.: Renal osteodystrophy in children. Clin. Pediatr. (Phila.) **15**, 996 (1976)
6. Mehls, O., Ritz, E., Krempian, B., Gilli, G., Link, K., Willich, E., Schärer, K.: Slipped epiphysis in renal osteodystrophy. Arch. Dis. Childh. **50**, 545 (1975)

13

Full Circle: An Epilogue

Within the broad perspectives discussed in the Preface to this book the concept of *revolution* was introduced; that is the radical change in circumstances, attitudes and conditions which new methods of investigation have brought. Chapter 1 is concerned with the clinical context and here the concept of *revolution* is used in a different sense, the circular movement of thought around the specific clinical phenomena which lead to investigation. All this is rational and as it should be.

As the mind circumambulates problems an analysis of them develops. Within any particular circle lie various diagnostic possibilities. An analysis of any particular case suggests there may be pre-eminence of one particular possibility, over and against all others. This may be clear-cut at an early stage because the evidence is overwhelming. Very often this is not so; the reason is simply that the evidence is incomplete and in a sense it always is. It follows that the pre-eminence of one particular diagnostic possibility is judged on the basis of a plenitude of factors in its favour and a paucity of factors against it. Other diagnostic possibilities decline in significance be

cause, whilst there may be some factors in their favour, there is no lack of factors against them. Judgements, therefore, are made by weighing and weighting the evidence.

Diagnosis is reached by a process of deduction based on clinical features and findings derived from investigation. Then follows an inductive process in which the various options for clinical management are considered; and this leads to clinical action. Thus, clinical action is determined by clinical features and investigatory findings. The importance of this is the reason for the recapitulation of investigatory findings and their possible causes which now follows. Within each circle lies the generic group in which specific entities lie. The circle implies no sense of hierarchy nor do the lists of specific entities. When considering the individual child's problem this concept is important because diagnosis is established by methods which concern degrees of confidence rather than by probabilities which, put crudely, simply state the obvious, namely that common things occur commonly!

13.1 Large Kidneys

When renal enlargement affects both kidneys the features may be considered in the following way:

Bilateral Renal Enlargement

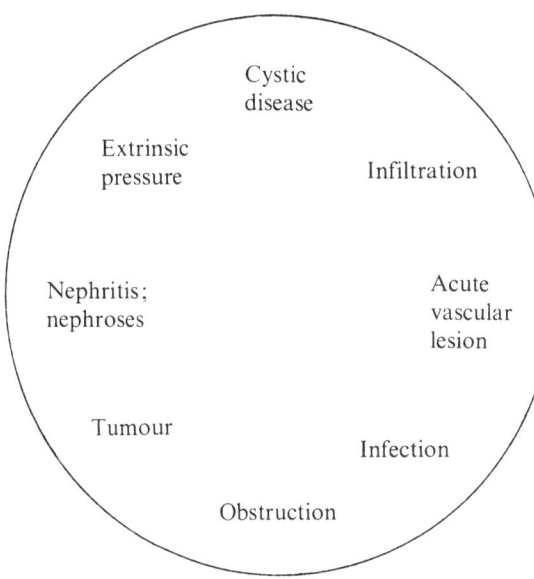

1. *Types of cystic disease*
   Infantile polycystic
   Juvenile polycystic
   Tubular ectasia
   Adult polycystic
   Tuberous sclerosis

2. *Infiltrations*
   Leukaemia
   Lymphoma
   Amyloid
   Glycogen storage disease

3. *Acute vascular lesions*
   bilateral renal venous thrombosis
       acute tubular necrosis
   severe haemolytic uraemic syndrome

4. *Infections*
   acute pyelonephritis
   multiple, diffuse abscess formation
   bilateral localized renal abscesses (may be with
       perinephric abscess)
   septicaemia
   infectious mononucleosis
   bilateral echinococcosis

5. *Obstruction*
   Causes given in Chapter 3

6. *Tumour*
   Nephroblastomatosis
   Bilateral Wilms' tumour in
       Aniridia and Beckwith-Weidemann syndrome

7. *Nephritis; nephrosis*
   All causes of acute nephritis which may lead to
   nephrosis, which may also develop
       directly from other causes

8. *Extrinsic pressure*
   Kidneys may appear large because they are
   "squashed" by gross enlargement of both liver
   and spleen

Renal enlargement may be one feature of a generalized visceromegaly, as in gigantism, and it is found in the Lawrence Seip syndrome.

13.2 Enlargement of one Kidney

Hemihypertrophy may be associated with unilateral renal enlargement: the connection is usually obvious.
Other causes may be considered in this way.

Unilateral Renal Enlargement

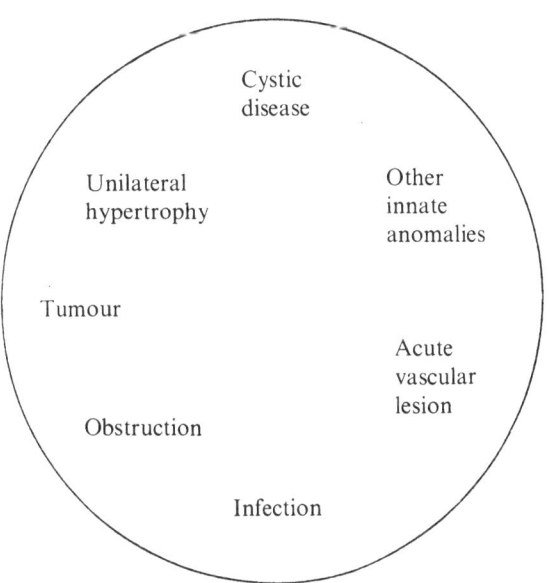

1. *Cystic disease*
   Multicystic kidney
   Multilocular cyst (sometimes termed
       lymphangiomatous cyst)
   Cystic dysplasia
   Simple cyst

2. *Other innate anomalies*
   Duplication
   Fused crossed ectopia

3. *Acute vascularisation*
   Renal venous thrombosis
   Infarction

4. *Infection*
   Acute pyelonephritis
   Pyonephrosis (may be with perinephric abscess)
   Xanthogranulomatous pyelonephritis
   Tuberculoma
   Echinoccosis

5. *Obstruction*
   Acute
   Protracted
   Acute on chronic (See Chapter 3 for causes)

6. *Tumour*
   Wilms' tumour
   Benign mesoblastic nephroma
   Sarcoma
   Renal carcinoma in late childhood

7. *Unilateral hypertrophy*
   A feature of atrophy or growth failure in the
       contralateral kidney – causes include:
       Aplasia
       Hypoplasia
       Severe dysplasia
       Nephrectomy (total or partial)
   Parenchymal damage as in:
       Pyelonephritic scarring and reflux nephrop-
       athy
       Tuberculosis
       Obstructive atrophy
       Postunilateral renal venous thrombosis
       Trauma
       Radiation

13.3 Small Kidneys

Causes of dimunitive kidneys may be considered as
follows. More than one cause may be present in any

particular infant or child; for example obstruction
with infection may give rise to small kidneys with
features of obstructive atrophy and pyelonephritic
scarring.

Small Kidneys

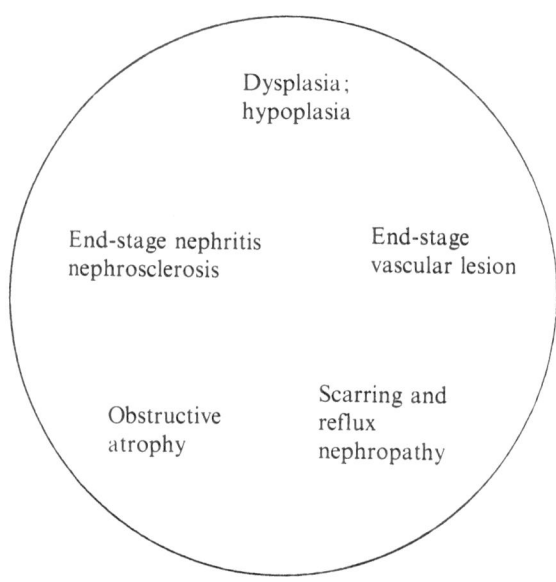

1. *Dysplasia, hypoplasia*
   Bilateral hypoplasia (maybe segmental)
   Bilateral cystic dysplasia
   Urethral valves (and other congenital obstruction)
   Syndromes: e.g. prune belly syndrome, Laurence–Moon–Biedl syndrome, Jeune's syndrome (asphyxiating thoracic dystrophy: synonym thoraco-pelvic-phalangeal syndrome)

2. *End-stage vascular lesion*
   Bilateral renal venous thrombosis
   Arterial; emboli/occlusive diseases (Chapter 12)
   Cortical necrosis
   Medullary necrosis

3. *Scarring and reflux nephropathy*
   Kidney may show localised or generalised
       changes with growth failure
   Reflux is not always demonstrable at time of
       discovery of renal lesions
   Reflux may be associated with other lesions such
       as urethral valves, urethral polyps, ectopic
       ureterocoele, neuropathic bladder

4. *Obstructive atrophy*
   Any cause of obstruction especially protracted
       obstruction may lead to atrophy
   Causes listed in Chapter 3

5. *End-stage nephritis; nephrosclerosis*
   Chronic nephritis, may be preceded by definable acute stage or due to a variety of causes, including radiation nephritis and nephritis as one feature of generalised disease (e. g. Henoch–Schönlein disease)
   Nephrosclerosis, generally described in conjunction with changes in the kidney due to hypertension

When *one* kidney is small and the contralateral kidney is of essentially normal structure then it undergoes compensatory hypertrophy. Accordingly, the causes for a kidney being small are found on page 194, which lists causes of compensatory hypertrophy in a kidney which is in consequence enlarged.

13.4 Renal Malposition

When the kidney is not normally located a meaningful interpretation of this finding may depend on closely relating observations concerning the kidney with all information which is available from other sources. This is evident in the analysis which follows.

Renal Malposition

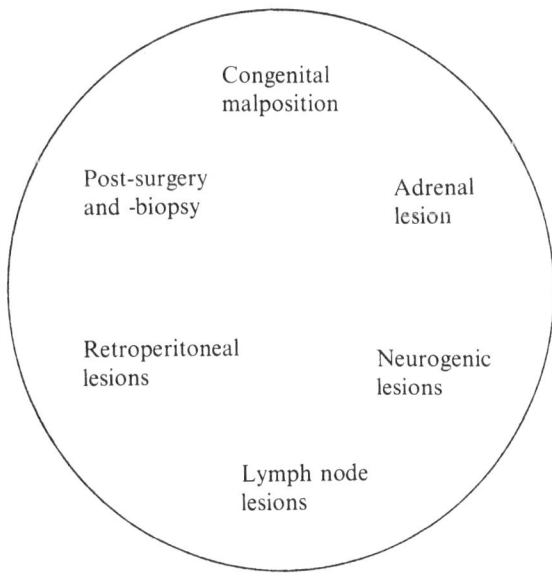

1. *Congenital malposition*
   In thorax (with diaphragmatic defect)
   In pelvis
   Intermediate degrees of malascent
   Rotation – usually pelvis lies anteriorly

Horseshoe kidney
Fused crossed ectopia
Congenital spinal defects

2. *Adrenal lesion*
   Haemorrhage
   Abscess
   Neoplasm – benign or malignant and may be endocrinologically active

3. *Neurogenic lesions*
   Neuroblastoma
   Ganglioneuroma
   Neurfibromatosis

4. *Lymph node lesions*
   Lymphoma
   Ovarian/testicular malignancy
   Chronic granulomatous disease
   Extramedullary haematopoeisis

5. *Other retroperitoneal lesions*
   Perinephric abscess and psoas abscess
   Haemorrhage after trauma and biopsy
   Retroperitoneal sarcoma

6. *Post-surgery and -biopsy*
   Bleeding after surgery or biopsy or urine leakage may displace the kidney; the renal malposition may persist long after the acute incident; calcification may follow such haemorrhage

13.5 Renal Calcification

The topics of nephrocalcinosis and nephrolithiasis have been discussed in Chapter 5. No apology is offered for not including the following causes in that discussion; these causes are renal infarcts, trauma, phleboliths in renal arterio-venous malformations, sarcoidosis, milk–alkali syndrome, hyperthyroidism, steroid treatment and penicillamine treatment. In the paediatric age range these entities when associated with renal calcification amount to quirks of rare disorders and sometimes their unsatisfactory management or unmanageable status.

13.6 Dilated Ureters

Ureteric dilatation may be unilateral or bilateral. It may affect single or duplex systems. The causes are almost infinite in number and variety. Here is a selection.

Dilated Ureters

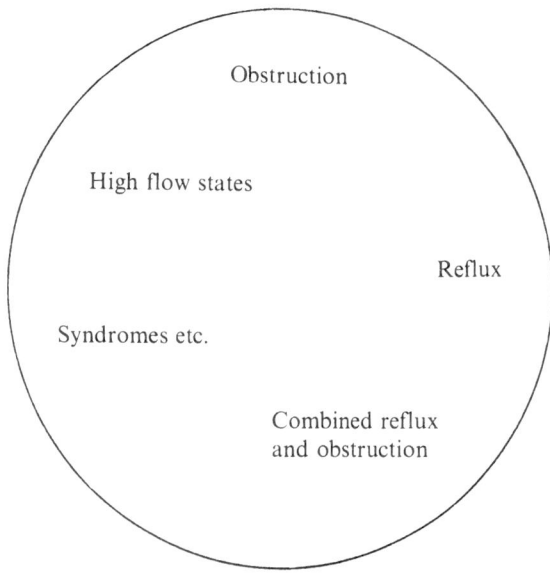

1. *Obstruction*
   Causes of obstruction are given in Chapter 3: ureteric dilatation is a sequel to those lesions lying below the pelvi-ureteric junction.
   Extrinsic mass lesions are an important source of ureteric dilatation; they include pelvic mass lesions including neurofibromatosis and severe rectal dilatation due to faecal retention.

2. *Reflux*
   Severe reflux is associated with ureteric dilatation, which varies and usually increases when the child micturates;
   Ureteric dilatation may follow or persist after reimplantation (see Chapter 4).

3. *Combined reflux and obstruction*
   Lower urinary tract obstruction from any cause may be associated with reflux.
   Ureteric dilatation is then usually considerable and kidney function poor.

4. *Syndromes, etc.*, a miscellany
   Prune belly syndrome
   Pseudo-prune-belly syndrome
   Adynamic syndrome
   Ehlers-Danlos syndrome
   Hypoprolinaemia

5. *High flow states*
   Diabetes insipidus
   Nephrogenic diabetes insipidus
   Chronic renal failure

Although ureteric dilatation often denotes obstruction distally this is not always the case.

13.7 Ureteric Displacement

Virtually all lesions which cause renal malposition are also associated with ureteric displacement. However, there are in addition other types of ureteric displacement and sometimes the displacement is pathognomonic for the lesion, notably in retrocaval ureter, ectopic ureterocoele and retroperitoneal fibrosis. In spina bifida, with a lesion in the lumbar region associated with severe kyphosis, the middle third of the ureters may approach the midline. The total dysplasia of the absent abdominal muscles syndrome is characterised by dilated ureters which meander across the retroperitoneum. Severe lower tract obstruction causes ureteric dilatation and tortuosity. Large pelvic mass lesions may displace the lower third of the ureters and in exstrophy the lowermost part of each ureter enters the bladder at its inferior aspect. Rarely, neurogenic lesions, such as ganglioneuroma or neurofibromatosis, may displace the ureter without affecting either renal position or vesical configuration.

13.8 Large Bladder

Enlargement of the bladder may be a clinical finding, or a finding at IVU, cystography or echography. The bladder may seem to be large at all times or after micturition its capacity may not appear large. Nevertheless, bladder enlargement is an entity. And so the causes for this phenomenon need to be identified.

1. *Habit*
   Variations in habit produce bladder enlargement: however, this is always a feature of the child and never of the infant.

2. *Obstruction*
   Bladder enlargement is associated with those organic lesions which affect the urethra; these are listed in Chapter 3.

3. *Severe vesico-ureteric reflux*
   Reflux is discussed in Chapter 4; bladder enlargement due to reflux only occurs when the reflux is severe when the upper tract is dilated.

Bladder Enlargement

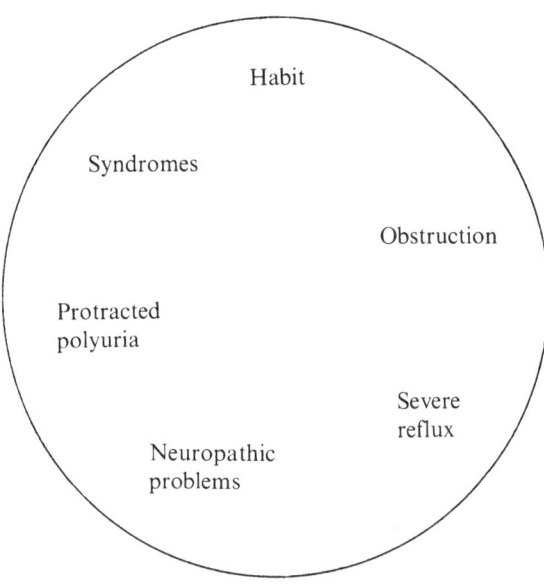

4. *Neuropathic problems*
   The cause may be an obvious spinal lesion or surgery (often with sepsis) in the pelvis for ano-rectal anomaly or Hirschsprung's disease – in other neuropathic bladder problems the bladder usually is not large.

5. *Protracted polyuria*
   Often this gives ureteric dilatation also; causes include:
   Diabetes insipidus from any cause
   Nephrogenic diabetes insipidus
   Chronic renal failure

6. *Syndromes*
   The underlying diagnosis, as with the prune belly syndrome or the adynamic syndrome is usually obvious on other grounds.

13.9 Small Bladder

The bladder may be small when affected by an inflammatory process – these include acute cystitis, chronic cystitis in the form of tuberculous or bilharzial lesions and opportunistic infections such as may occur in patients with chronic granulomatous disease or malignancies undergoing therapy. Direct infiltrations such as those which may occur in leukaemia or in neurofibromatosis reduce bladder capacity. The neuropathic bladder (whatever the cause) is often small. Large pelvic and abdominal masses may reduce bladder capacity, but in such circumstances there is almost always bladder displacement as well.

13.10 Bladder Displacement

Mass lesions in the vicinity of the bladder frequently displace it and impress its contours. The capacity of the bladder may be reduced if its drainage remains unimpeded. Very often mass lesions affect the base of the bladder and the proximal part of the urethra; when this happens obstruction often ensues and the bladder capacity increases as drainage is impaired. Causes of bladder displacement may be grouped in this way:

Bladder Displacement

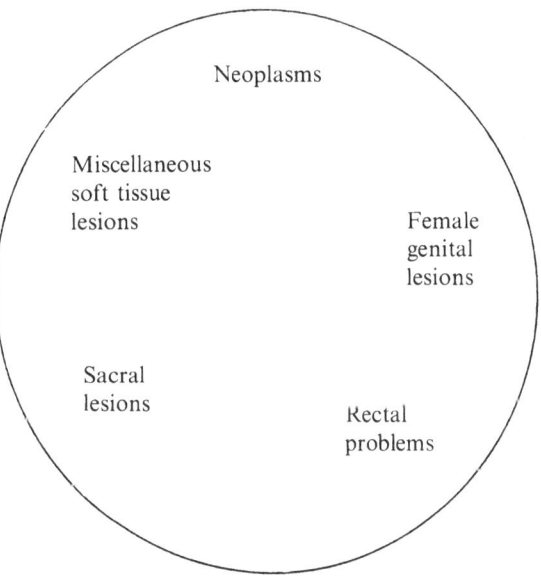

1. *Neoplasms*
   Rhabdomyosarcoma (solid or polypoid)
   Teratomas and dermoids (sacrococcygeal or genital)
   Pelvic bone and other malignancies (e. g. Ewing's sarcoma)

2. *Female Genital Lesions*
   Canalization failures leading to hydrometrocolpos, haematometrocolpos, etc.
   Ovarian mass lesions; benign cysts and malignancies are listed in Chapter 10 and the effect on the bladder is usually of peripheral importance.

3. *Rectal problems*
   Principally, faecal retention due to altered habit or anorectal surgery

4. *Sacral lesions*
   Presacral meningocoele, abscess or neoplasm

5. *Miscellaneous soft tissue lesions*
   Trauma and haemorrhage, maybe with a pelvic bone fracture
   Variety of soft tissue lesions; neurofibromatosis haemangioma, lipomas, fibromatous lesions, sarcoma
   Inflammatory lesions; pelvic abscess from any cause, appendix abscess, cellulitis

Syndromes with Renal Malformations

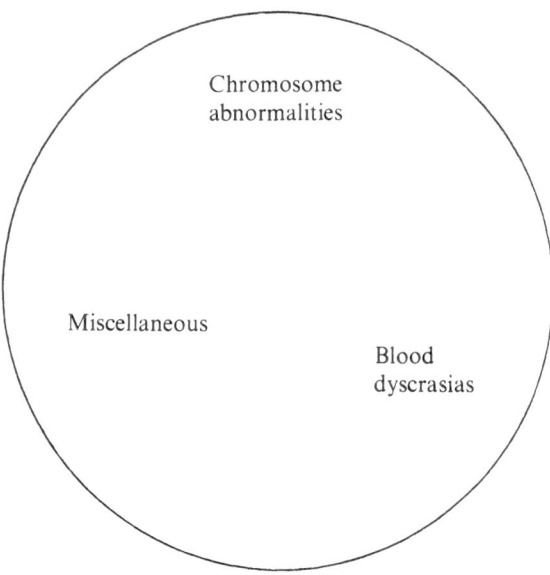

13.11 Space Occupying Lesions in Bladder

Simple direct observation will show whether the particular lesion is solely intravesical or whether it has an attachment or relationship to the wall of the bladder. Sometimes, the lesion occupies the bladder base and the vesico-urethral junction; when this happens the bladder may be obstructed. Bladder lesions which are generally and demonstrably freely within the lumen are foreign bodies, blood clot and calculus. A calculus may impact in the vesico-urethral junction producing vesical obstruction.
Of the lesions producing obstruction to bladder emptying, but which have an association with the vesical wall, there are ectopic ureterocoele and polypoid rhabdomyosarcoma; differentiation between these two is not difficult. More difficult may be the distinction between malignant polypoid rhabdomyosarcoma, mural polyps and intravesical myomas and haemangiomas; endoscopy and biopsy can be decisive. Conditions like cystitis cystica, neurofibromatosis and vesical paraganglioneuromas have their own specific additional connotations.

1. *Chromosome abnormalities*
   Turner's syndrome XO
   Trisomy 18
   18q syndrome
   13q syndrome
   21q syndrome

2. *Blood dyscrasias*
   Fanconi pancytopaenia syndrome
   Radial aplasia–thrombocytopaenia syndrome

3. *Miscellaneous group with unrelated multisystem involvement*
   Meckel–Gruber syndrome
   Oro-facial-digital syndrome
   Zellweger syndrome
   Ehlers–Danlos syndrome
   Rubenstein–Taybi syndrome
   Russell–Silver syndrome
   Thanatophoric dwarfism
   Klippel–Feil syndrome
   Noonan's syndrome

13.12 Syndromes with Associated Renal Malformations

A miscellany of syndromes may be associated with congenital abnormalities of the kidneys. The malformations cover a wide range; such as aplasia, duplication, horseshoe kidney or renal ectopia; and usually are not specific for a given syndrome.

13.13 Syndromes Associated with Renal Cysts

Cystic disease of the kidneys may occur as a specific renal finding in a wide range of syndromes. In some, the renal changes are important in the clinical management of the patient, and determine the eventual outcome, as in Jeune's syndrome. In others renal cysts are incidental findings and the involvement of other systems, and the pattern of involvement of other systems, determines diagnosis and prognosis.

Syndromes with Renal Cysts

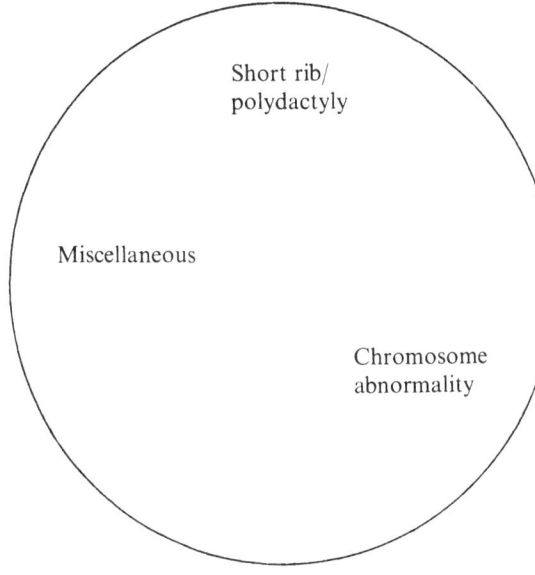

1. *Syndromes with short ribs and polydactyly*
   Jeune's asphyxiating thoracic dystrophy
   Majewski syndrome
   Saldino–Noonan syndrome
   Meckel's syndrome

2. *Chromosome abnormalities*
   Triploidy syndrome

3. *Miscellaneous group*
   Cerebro-hepato-renal syndrome
   Congenital hemihypertrophy syndrome
   Beckwith–Wiedemann syndrome
   Laurence–Moon–Biedl syndrome
   Tuberous sclerosis
   Von Hippel–Lindau syndrome
   Familial juvenile nephronophthisis syndrome
   Polycythaemia with tumours and cysts
   Potter's syndrome

13.14 Syndromes Associated with Nephropathy

These syndromes form a large miscellaneous collection which do not conform to subgrouping. In some syndromes the renal changes predominate and renal failure may be the outcome. In others the nephropathy is mild and does not determine the prognosis.

Fabry's syndrome
Löwe syndrome
Nail–patella syndrome
Zellweger syndrome
Johanson-Blizzard syndrome
Laurence–Moon–Biedl. syndrome
Alport's syndrome
Jeune's asphyxiating thoracic dystrophy
Bartter's syndrome
Fanconi–De Toni syndrome
Goodpasture syndrome
Idiopathic hypercalcaemia syndrome
   (synonym Williams' syndrome)
Familial juvenile nephronophthisis
Henoch–Schönlein purpura
Von Gierke's purpura
Osteolysis with nephropathy
Wegener's granulomatosis

13.15 Congenital Renal Anomalies Associated with Other System Involvement

There is a greater than random tendency for congenital renal abnormalities to be associated with congenital abnormalities of other systems. The malformations are probably related to some event occurring at a critical stage of intrauterine development of the involved systems, and this event is probably before the seventh week of foetal life.

Renal Anomalies may be Associated with

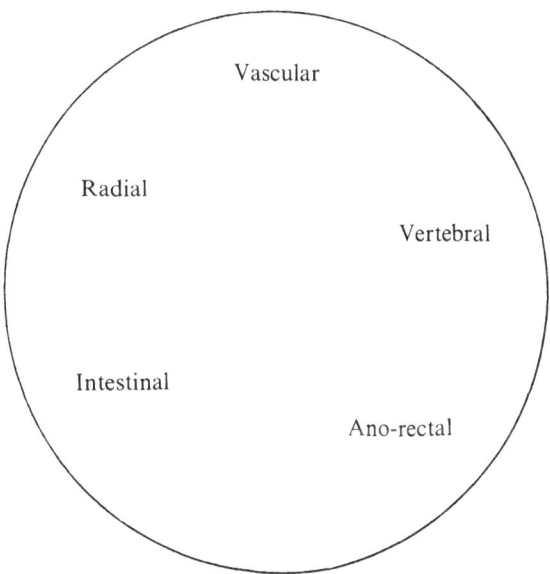

1. *Vascular anomalies*
   Congenital heart disease commonly V. S. D.
   Single umbilical artery

2. *Vertebral anomalies*
   May occur at any level in the spine
   In the dorsal region may be associated with rib changes
   There may be increased segmentation, e. g. 13 pairs of ribs or six lumbar vertebrae

3. *Ano-rectal anomalies*
   Vary from a simple covered anus to a high rectal atresia with a recto-vesical fistula

4. *Other intestinal anomalies*
   Oesophageal atresia with or without a tracheo-oesophageal fistula
   Duodenal stenosis or atresia

5. *Radial anomalies*
   Unilateral or bilateral radial hypoplasia or aplasia
   Preaxial polydactyly; commonly a bifid terminal phalanx of the thumb
   The lower limbs may also have preaxial involvement

13.16 Hemihypertrophy

Hemihypertrophy is a clinical finding which may be associated with a wide range of abnormalities. The importance of recognising hemihypertrophy as a presenting feature is that it may be associated with a number of malignant tumours.

1. *Tumours*
   Renal – Wilms'
   Adrenal – neuroblastoma
      Adrenal cortical tumours
   Hepatic – hepatoblastoma

2. *Vascular anomalies leading to overgrowth*
   Klippel–Trenaunay syndrome
   Neurofibromatosis
   Macrodystrophia lipomatosa

3. *Renal*
   Medullary sponge kidney
   Beckwith–Wiedemann syndrome

4. *Miscellaneous*
   Ehlers–Danlos syndrome
   Pyloric stenosis

Hemihypertrophy

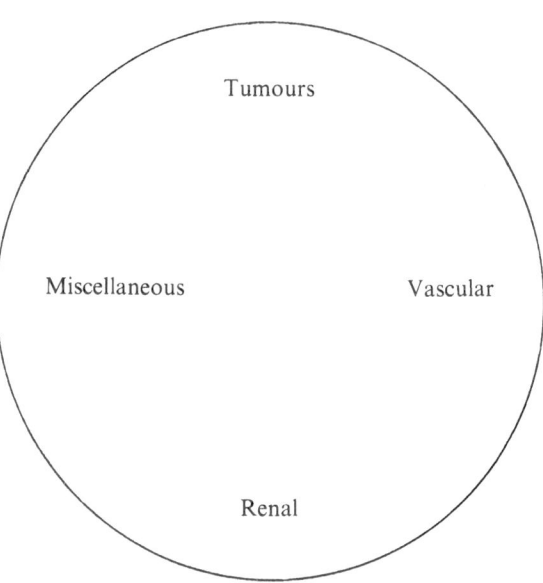

13.17 Conclusion

In clinical evaluation and investigation the objective is to establish a reasonable measure of confidence. The information which accrues provides the basis for deduction as to cause. The pathways of deduction are very often not along straight lines, with a linear branching pattern, no matter how much one might ideally wish them to be so. In reaching a position of confidence about diagnosis and cause, elements of judgment are essential. Stated simply, what is needed is the fastet route to common sense.

There is no point and it is not kind to subject infants and children to the flak of the various batteries of the investigatory armamentarium, once reasonable confidence is there. Confidence is related to the next phase of clinical management and so a rational approach is to ascertain from the clinical team if any additional information is required before management progresses. When contemplating and choosing any additional investigations, think of what they entail and the likely diagnostic yield. For example, with these standards in mind, lymphangiography is very time consuming, unpleasant for the child and the contrast medium has the unhappy habit of by-passing and so not demonstrating a possible lesion at the site of concern. At the other end of the scale ultrasound studies are non-invasive, well tolerated and frequently decisive. Based on the information available about the individual child's problem clinical management is instituted in the anticipation this will have a favourable outcome for the child. Thus, the process leading to management is essentially one of induction.

The clinical problems of the individual child or infant very often have long-term consequences. Irrespective of whether patients are managed medically or surgically it is very often essential to plan follow-up investigations. A base-line of information is needed against which subsequent progress can be evaluated and the objective of this is to secure the best potential for future well-being. When formulating programmes for follow-up it is wise to think incisively. For example, in children with urinary infections who are over about 5 years of age, once the kidneys have been shown to have a normal structure and there is no major lesion affecting the lower urinary tract, follow-up studies may be strictly limited; repeat echography can show continuing and normal renal development. Essential information should always be secured safely and with an economy of style. Information about a child's problem establishes a position of knowledge which leads, by a process of induction, to clinical action. The techniques used to obtain information vary and so the information is of various types; this means that, when looking at information and the method by which it is obtained, preferences are considered and choices are made. But investigating and imaging are an evolving process. In sequence and with the use of each technique, additional information becomes available. In this way the circle of necessary knowledge is circumscribed and so there is drawn the full circle.

14 Subject Index

Urology in Childhood

By D.I. Williams, T.M. Barratt, H.B. Eckstein,
S.M. Kohlinsky, G.H. Newns, P.E. Polany,
J.D. Singer
1974. 218 figures. XXIII, 458 pages
(Handbuch der Urologie/Encyclopedia of
Urology, Band 15, Supplement)
ISBN 3-540-06406-0

G.B. Bradač, R. Oberson
Angiography in Cerebro-Arterial Occlusive Diseases

Including Computer Tomography and Radio-
nuclide Methods
1979. 144 figures in 341 separate illustrations.
IX, 228 pages
ISBN 3-540-08898-9
Distribution rights for Japan:
Igaku Shoin Ltd., Tokyo

B.J. Cremin, P. Beighton
Bone Dysplasias of Infancy

A Radiological Atlas
Foreword from R.O. Murray
1978. 55 figures in 124 separate illustrations.
4 tables. XIII, 109 pages
ISBN 3-540-08816-4

S.N. Hassani
Real Time Ophthalmic Ultrasonography

In collaboration with R.L. Bard
1978. 423 figures. XXI, 214 pages
ISBN 3-540-90318-6

Diagnostic Radiology

Supplement
Radionuclides in Urology – Urological Ultrasono-
graphy – Percutaneous Puncture Nephrostomy
By L. Andersson, I. Fernström, G.R. Leopold,
J.U. Schlegel, L.B. Talner
Editor: L. Andersson
1977. 88 figures. X, 199 pages
(Handbuch der Urologie/Encyclopedia of
Urology, Band 5, Teil 1)
ISBN 3-540-07896-7

F.P. Probst
The Prosencephalies

Morphology, Neuroradiological Appearances and
Differential Diagnosis.
In cooperation with A. Brun,
I. Pascual-Castroviejo
1979. 93 figures, 3 tables. IX, 145 pages
ISBN 3-540-09318-4

Clinical Computer Tomography

Head and Trunk
Editor: A. Baert, L. Jeanmart, A. Wackenheim
1978. 414 figures, 2 tables. VIII, 261 pages
ISBN 3-540-08458-4
Distribution rights for Japan:
Igaku Shoin Ltd., Tokyo

Computerized Axial Tomography

An Anatomic Atlas of Serial Sections of the Human
Body. Anatomy – Radiology – Scanner
By J. Gambarelli, G. Guérinel, L. Chevrot,
M. Mattèi
With the technical collaboration of R. Galliano,
S. Nazarian. Drawings by J.P. Jacomy. Photo-
graphies by D. Amy, M. Soler
1977. 550 figures, some in color. VI, 286 pages
ISBN 3-540-07961-0

The Diagnostic Limitations of Computerised Axial Tomography

Editor: J. Bories
1978. 175 figures, 52 tables. IX, 220 pages
ISBN 3-540-08593-9
Distribution rights for Japan:
Nankodo Co. Ltd., Tokyo

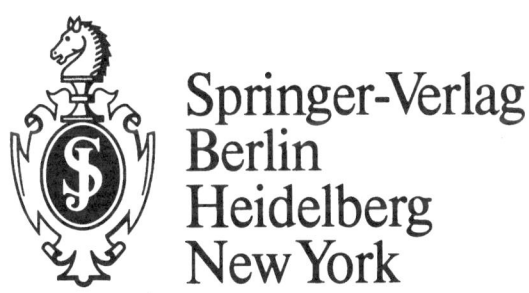

Springer-Verlag
Berlin
Heidelberg
New York

Pediatric Radiology

Roentgenology, Nuclear Medicine, Ultrasonics, Computed Tomography

ISSN 0301-0449   Title No. 247

Editorial Board: W. E. Berdon, A. R. Chrispin, B. J. Cremin, G. Currarino, P. Deffrenne, A. Doberti, A. Domenech, J. S. Dunbar, K.-D. Ebel, O. A. Eklöf, C. Fauré, Z. Fruchter, A. Giedion, C. A. Gooding, J. L. Gwinn, G. B. C. Harris, G. Iannaccone, H. J. Kaufmann, K. Knapp, K. Kozlowski, M. A. Lassrich, C. Manzano, W. Porstmann, A. Rubin, J. Sauvegrain, F. N. Silverman, E. B. Singleton, J. Sutcliffe, E. Willich.

As a result of the rapid advances made in recent decades, pediatric radiology has become a significant, independent, and clinically important speciality. In order to fulfill the increasing need of child-health specialtists for keeping fully abreast with all major developments in this new field, **Pediatric Radiology,** the only journal devoted exclusively to the various aspects of pediatric radiology was founded in 1973.

It publishes the following types of material:

1. Original papers report progress and results from all areas of pediatric radiology and its related fields.
2. Review articles and annotations reflect the present state of knowledge in special areas or summarize limited themes in which discussion has led to clearly defined conclusions.
3. Short Reports are either case reports or short statements of facts and analysis, or preliminary communications
4. Technology, methodology, new apparatus, and auxiliary equipment together with modifications of standard techniques are discussed.
5. **Pediatric Radiology** presents a continuing statement of the world literatrue in pediatric radiology and related fields.

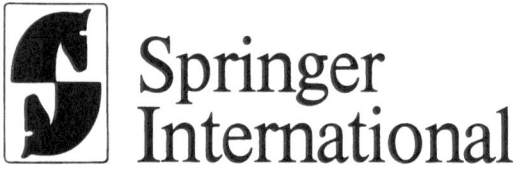 Springer International

Urologic Radiology

A Journal of Diagnostic Imaging

Title No. 290

Editors in Chief: J. Becker, New York, NY, USA; M. A. Bosniak, New York, NY, USA; H. Saxton, London, Great Britain

Editors: M. D. Blaufox, A. Davidson, M. Elkin, R. Friedenberg, R. R. Hattery, R. Kendall, A. F. Lalli, R. L. Lebowitz, J. Lowenstein, B. L. McClennan, R. C. Pfister, H. M. Pollak, R. C. Sanders, L. Talner, J. R. Thornbury, K. Waterhouse, D. M. Witten

Urological Radiology is a publication dedicated to the study of the urinary tract by the use of radiography, including angiography, ultrasound, nuclear medicine, computed tomography, invasive techniques and associated modalities.

The editorial board of the journal is composed of physicians of international reputation of the United States and Europe, with specialities in radiology, urology, nephrology and pathology.

The publication of original papers, technical notes and case reports as well as invited review articles make up the content of this journal. **Urologic Radiology** emphasizes a clinically oriented approach, but pertinent investigative works with clinical application are invited as well.

The journal publishes manuscripts on the latest developments in uroradiology and will also, on occasion, review controversial subjects in depth. Case reports are selected for publication, not only for their rarity, but more importantly for their educational value.

A constant monitoring of the newly developing diagnostic modalities in uroradiology is considered to be an important part of the scope of **Urologic Radiology.** It will define and evaluate the role of these techniques in patient diagnosis and management.

To complish these goals the journal promply reviews submitted manuscripts to assure rapid publication.